Clinical Application of Hemodialysis and Its Adverse Effects

Clinical Application of Hemodialysis and Its Adverse Effects

Editors

Shuzo Kobayashi
Takayasu Ohtake

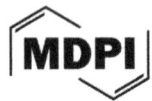

Basel • Beijing • Wuhan • Barcelona • Belgrade • Novi Sad • Cluj • Manchester

Editors
Shuzo Kobayashi
Shonan Kamakura General
Hospital
Kamakura
Japan

Takayasu Ohtake
Shonan Kamakura General
Hospital
Kamakura
Japan

Editorial Office
MDPI
St. Alban-Anlage 66
4052 Basel, Switzerland

This is a reprint of articles from the Special Issue published online in the open access journal *Journal of Clinical Medicine* (ISSN 2077-0383) (available at: https://www.mdpi.com/journal/jcm/special_issues/Hemodialysis_Adverse_Effects).

For citation purposes, cite each article independently as indicated on the article page online and as indicated below:

Lastname, A.A.; Lastname, B.B. Article Title. *Journal Name* **Year**, *Volume Number*, Page Range.

ISBN 978-3-7258-0929-5 (Hbk)
ISBN 978-3-7258-0930-1 (PDF)
doi.org/10.3390/books978-3-7258-0930-1

Cover image courtesy of Shuzo Kobayashi

© 2024 by the authors. Articles in this book are Open Access and distributed under the Creative Commons Attribution (CC BY) license. The book as a whole is distributed by MDPI under the terms and conditions of the Creative Commons Attribution-NonCommercial-NoDerivs (CC BY-NC-ND) license.

Contents

About the Editors vii

Preface ix

Shuzo Kobayashi and Takayasu Ohtake
The Characteristics of Dialysis Membranes: Benefits of the AN69 Membrane in Hemodialysis Patients
Reprinted from: *J. Clin. Med.* **2023**, *12*, 1123, doi:10.3390/jcm12031123 1

Didier Sánchez-Ospina, Sebastián Mas-Fontao, Carolina Gracia-Iguacel, Alejandro Avello, Marina González de Rivera, Maddalen Mujika-Marticorena and Emilio Gonzalez-Parra
Displacing the Burden: A Review of Protein-Bound Uremic Toxin Clearance Strategies in Chronic Kidney Disease
Reprinted from: *J. Clin. Med.* **2024**, *13*, 1428, doi:10.3390/jcm13051428 18

Ricardo Peralta, Luís Sousa and António Filipe Cristovão
Cannulation Technique of Vascular Access in Hemodialysis and the Impact on the Arteriovenous Fistula Survival: Systematic Review and Meta-Analysis
Reprinted from: *J. Clin. Med.* **2023**, *12*, 5946, doi:10.3390/jcm12185946 34

Junko Ishida and Akihiko Kato
Recent Advances in the Nutritional Screening, Assessment, and Treatment of Japanese Patients on Hemodialysis
Reprinted from: *J. Clin. Med.* **2023**, *12*, 2113, doi:10.3390/jcm12062113 46

Hirotaka Fukasawa, Ryuichi Furuya, Mai Kaneko, Daisuke Nakagami, Yuri Ishino, Shuhei Kitamoto, et al.
Clinical Significance of Trace Element Zinc in Patients with Chronic Kidney Disease
Reprinted from: *J. Clin. Med.* **2023**, *12*, 1667, doi:10.3390/jcm12041667 64

Daisuke Katagiri and Kan Kikuchi
The Impact and Treatment of COVID-19 in Hemodialysis Patients
Reprinted from: *J. Clin. Med.* **2023**, *12*, 838, doi:10.3390/jcm12030838 72

Shuzo Kobayashi, Yasuhiro Mochida, Kunihiro Ishioka, Machiko Oka, Kyoko Maesato, et al.
Malnutrition and Insulin Resistance May Interact with Metabolic Syndrome in Prevalent Hemodialysis Patients
Reprinted from: *J. Clin. Med.* **2023**, *12*, 2239, doi:10.3390/jcm12062239 79

Yoshitaka Kumada, Norikazu Kawai, Narihiro Ishida, Yasuhito Nakamura, Hiroshi Takahashi, Satoru Ohshima, et al.
Combined Prognostic Value of Preprocedural Protein–Energy Wasting and Inflammation Status for Amputation and/or Mortality after Lower-Extremity Revascularization in Hemodialysis Patients with Peripheral Arterial Disease
Reprinted from: *J. Clin. Med.* **2024**, *13*, 126, doi:10.3390/jcm13010126 90

Masao Iwagami, Yuka Kanemura, Naru Morita, Toshitaka Yajima, Masafumi Fukagawa and Shuzo Kobayashi
Association of Hyperkalemia and Hypokalemia with Patient Characteristics and Clinical Outcomes in Japanese Hemodialysis (HD) Patients
Reprinted from: *J. Clin. Med.* **2023**, *12*, 2115, doi:10.3390/jcm12062115 101

Koji Hashimoto, Makoto Harada, Yosuke Yamada, Taro Kanno, Yutaka Kanno and Yuji Kamijo
Impact of Vascular Access Flow Suppression Surgery on Cervical Artery Circulation: A Retrospective Observational Study
Reprinted from: *J. Clin. Med.* **2024**, *13*, 641, doi:10.3390/jcm13030641 . . . . **116**

Piotr Olczyk, Patryk Jerzak, Krzysztof Letachowicz, Tomasz Gołębiowski, Magdalena Krajewska and Mariusz Kusztal
The Influence of Healthy Habits on Cognitive Functions in a Group of Hemodialysis Patients
Reprinted from: *J. Clin. Med.* **2023**, *12*, 2042, doi:10.3390/jcm12052042 . . . . **126**

Agnieszka Zakrzewska, Jan Biedunkiewicz, Michał Komorniczak, Magdalena Jankowska, Katarzyna Jasiulewicz, Natalia Płonka, et al.
Intradialytic Tolerance and Recovery Time in Different High-Efficiency Hemodialysis Modalities
Reprinted from: *J. Clin. Med.* **2024**, *13*, 326, doi:10.3390/jcm13020326 . . . . **137**

Suthiya Anumas, Sithichai Kunawathanakul, Pichaya Tantiyavarong, Pajaree Krisanapan and Pattharawin Pattharanitima
Predictors for Unsuccessful Reductions in Hemodialysis Frequency during the Pandemic
Reprinted from: *J. Clin. Med.* **2023**, *12*, 2550, doi:10.3390/jcm12072550 . . . . **150**

Špela Bogataj, Jernej Pajek, Blaž Slonjšak and Vanja Peršič
Prevalence of Impaired Physical Mobility in Dialysis Patients: A Single-Centre Cross-Sectional Study
Reprinted from: *J. Clin. Med.* **2023**, *12*, 6634, doi:10.3390/jcm12206634 . . . . **160**

About the Editors

Shuzo Kobayashi

I am currently working as the CEO of Shonan Kamakura General Hospital in Kamakura, Japan (669 beds), and am also the executive managing director of the board members in Tokushukai General Incorporated Association (the 12th biggest medical group in the world based on annual revenue). I am very active as a councilor for several scientific and medical professional societies: the Japanese Society of Nephrology, Japanese Society of Internal Medicine, and the Japanese Society for Dialysis Therapy. In addition, I am the President of the Japanese Society of Foot Care Medicine. I obtained my MD degree in 1980 and postgraduate training that led to a PhD degree in 1986 from Hamamatsu University School of Medicine in Hamamatsu, Japan. I then worked as a visiting assistant professor at the Department of Pathology, University of Texas. Following this, I worked as the Chairman of Internal Medicine, the Chief of the Kidney & Dialysis Center, and the Deputy Executive Director of the Shonan Kamakura General Hospital. I am the author of more than 300 research papers and I continue to be active in clinical research as an expert in nephrology, vascular medicine, and regenerative medicine.

I have been appointed as an outstanding reviewer of the committee of PMDA (Pharmaceuticals and Medical Devices Agency). Additionally, I have been appointed as the Director of the Shonan Research Institute of Innovative Medicine (sRIIM), which belongs to our hospital.

Takayasu Ohtake

I am the Vice President and Director of Regenerative Medicine at Shonan Kamakura General Hospital. My specialties include nephrology, regenerative medicine, and atherosclerosis including cardiovascular diseases, peripheral artery disease, and vascular calcification. I am actively working to develop a new effective regenerative cell therapy against severe acute kidney injury and progressive chronic kidney disease.

Preface

The incidence of end-stage renal disease (ESRD) reached 3.7 million in 2016, and it has been increasing by 5~6% every year. Along with an increase in older patients with ESRD, several important pathophysiologies, including accelerating systemic atherosclerosis, vascular calcification, malnutrition, inflammation, frailty, cognitive disturbance, and so on, have recently been discovered in hemodialysis (HD) patients. These disease states complexly impact unfavorable events and prognosis in HD patients. The excessive removal of essential substances in the body, or, on the contrary, the insufficient removal of harmful substances by HD treatment, might be linked to pathophysiology in HD patients. On the other hand, dialysis treatment has made significant progress. Several dialysis membranes and modalities may be selected when considering patient status.

Based on the abovementioned background, we introduce a Special Issue titled "Clinical Application of Hemodialysis and Its Adverse Effects" in the Journal of Clinical Medicine. As Guest Editors, we are pleased that fourteen clinically important articles have been published in our Special Issue from June 2022 to January 2024. We are profoundly grateful to all authors and collaborators. We also extend our thanks to Barret Zhang for his kind support as an Assistant Editor.

Shuzo Kobayashi and Takayasu Ohtake
Editors

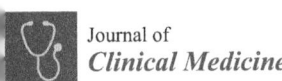

Review

The Characteristics of Dialysis Membranes: Benefits of the AN69 Membrane in Hemodialysis Patients

Shuzo Kobayashi * and Takayasu Ohtake

Kidney Disease and Transplant Center, Shonan Kamakura General Hospital, 1370-1 Okamoto, Kamakura-City 247-8533, Kanagawa, Japan
* Correspondence: shuzo@shonankamakura.or.jp

Abstract: Patients undergoing hemodialysis (HD) experience serious cardiovascular complications, through malnutrition, inflammation, and atherosclerosis. Amputation for peripheral arterial disease (PAD) is more prevalent in patients undergoing HD than in the general population. In addition, revascularization procedures in dialysis patients are often associated with subsequent amputation and high mortality rates. To improve the prognosis of dialysis patients, malnutrition and inflammation must be properly treated, which necessitates a better understanding of the characteristics of dialysis membranes. Herein, the characteristics of several dialysis membranes were studied, with a special reference to the AN69 membrane, noting several similarities to low-density lipoprotein (LDL)-apheresis, which is also applicable for the treatment of PAD. Both systems (LDL-apheresis and AN69) have anti-inflammatory and anti-thrombogenic effects because they use a negatively charged surface for extracorporeal adsorptive filtration from the blood/plasma, and contact phase activation. The concomitant use of both these therapeutic systems may have additive therapeutic benefits in HD patients. Here, we reviewed the characteristics of dialysis membranes and benefits of the AN69 membrane in dialysis patients.

Keywords: hemodialysis; dialysis membrane; AN69; PAD; LDL-apheresis

Citation: Kobayashi, S.; Ohtake, T. The Characteristics of Dialysis Membranes: Benefits of the AN69 Membrane in Hemodialysis Patients. *J. Clin. Med.* **2023**, *12*, 1123. https://doi.org/10.3390/jcm12031123

Academic Editors: Juan F. Navarro-González and Giacomo Garibotto

Received: 12 December 2022
Revised: 11 January 2023
Accepted: 18 January 2023
Published: 31 January 2023

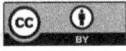

Copyright: © 2023 by the authors. Licensee MDPI, Basel, Switzerland. This article is an open access article distributed under the terms and conditions of the Creative Commons Attribution (CC BY) license (https:// creativecommons.org/licenses/by/ 4.0/).

1. Burden of Chronic Hemodialysis (HD) in Japan: Epidemiological and Economic Perspectives

Japan is estimated to have the highest number of dialysis patients, and this number continues to increase every year [1]. Estimates from the Japanese Society for Dialysis Therapy indicate that currently, one out of 385.1 Japanese citizens are dialysis patients. The number of chronic dialysis patients per million in 2016 had increased to 2596.7 from 2557.0 in 2015, and at the end of 2016, 76,836 patients were undergoing hemodiafiltration (HDF) and 635 patients were treated by home hemodialysis (HD) therapy, indicating an increase of 63 patients from 2015 [2]. At the end of 2017, the number of chronic dialysis patients had reached 334,505, an increase of 4896 patients from 2016 [2]. However, the number of peritoneal dialysis (PD) patients has gradually decreased since 2014, the number of PD patients in 2015 and 2016 being 9322 and 9021, respectively. Again, 20.3% of the PD patients were on combination therapy with either HD or HDF therapy [1]. Japan is also plagued by an increase in the proportion of elderly patients (70 years and above) who remain on dialysis [3]. The financial burden of renal diseases is particularly high, with the average medical cost being 14.5 times higher in individuals with renal disease than in those without renal disease/dialysis. In Japan, the estimated medical costs incurred for treating renal diseases were approximately 1.546 trillion yen in 2016, accounting for 3.8% of the total healthcare expenditure that year [4]. In Japan, in-center dialysis, home dialysis, and transplantation are the available options for the treatment of end-stage renal disease (ESRD); however, the use of transplantation and home dialysis is generally very low [4].

2. Risk Factors and Complications Associated with Chronic HD

In Japan, HD is considered as a mainstream renal replacement therapy and used in 95% of patients suffering from chronic kidney disease (CKD) [5]. The most common reasons for dialysis use in Japanese patients include diabetic nephropathy (38.8%), chronic glomerulonephritis (28.8%), and nephrosclerosis (9.9%) [2]. Diabetes mellitus is a well-known risk factor for CKD. Recent estimates indicate that the cumulative survival of chronic HD patients with poor glycemic control is significantly lower than that of patients with fair or good glycemic control [6].

Cardiovascular disease (CVD) is the main cause of mortality in dialysis patients [7]. The increased cardiovascular risk in CKD patients may be attributed to hypertension that may occur due to the activation of the renin–angiotensin–aldosterone system, vascular calcification associated with abnormal metabolism of calcium and phosphorus, and the specific dyslipidemia of CKD, chronic inflammation, malnutrition, oxidative stress, and uremic factors [7,8].

Observational studies in Japanese dialysis patients have demonstrated a close relationship between dyslipidemia (hyper-low-density lipoprotein (LDL) cholesterolemia, hypo-high-density lipoprotein (HDL) cholesterolemia, hypertriglyceridemia, and/or hyper-non-HDL-cholesterolemia), the severity of atherosclerosis, and the risk of myocardial infarction. 'The Japanese Society for Dialysis Therapy Guidelines for Management of Cardiovascular Diseases in Patients on Chronic Hemodialysis' suggest that dyslipidemia is an independent risk factor for CVD, as it is closely associated with atherosclerosis, CVD, and myocardial infarction [9].

Hypertension in HD patients plays an important role in the development of CVD. Because of the variability of blood pressure within a week, weekly averaged blood pressure (WAB) is a useful prognostic marker for evaluating hypertension in HD patients [10].

Peripheral arterial disease (PAD), defined as obstructive atherosclerosis of the lower extremities, is associated with an increased risk of cardiovascular events, and an increased mortality rate in HD patients [11]. Moreover, PAD is characterized by a high morbidity rate in dialysis patients related to vascular calcification and a high mortality rate related to lower limb amputation. Vascular calcification is induced by PAD, and is difficult to treat [12,13]. Vascular calcification reportedly increases with a decline of glomerular filtration ratio (GFR) [14]. Both the prevalence and severity of PAD in HD patients are closely associated with arterial calcification in the lower limbs [15]. Arterial abnormalities may be caused by rheological abnormalities [16]. Compared to those in healthy individuals, leukocyte aggregates are increased in HD patients. Increased platelet/leukocyte aggregates are associated with atherosclerosis in these patients [16].

Moreover, patients undergoing dialysis often complain of uncomfortable symptoms such as pruritus, irritability, depression, insomnia, and intradialytic hypotension. The common pathogenesis of these dialysis-related complications could be explained by the uremic retention of solutes and bio-incompatibility of dialysis therapy, which may in turn lead to microinflammation [17]. With respect to these complications, malnutrition, inflammation, and atherosclerosis are the most important aspects to consider, as they cause the highest morbidity and mortality among dialysis patients [18]. In subsequent sections, we will discuss in detail the various dialysis-related complications and their clinical impact on patients undergoing chronic HD.

3. Malnutrition, Inflammation, and Atherosclerosis in HD: The Heart of the Matter

Malnutrition–inflammation–atherosclerosis (MIA) syndrome, CKD-related mineral and bone disorder (CKD-MBD), and cardio-renal-anemia (CRA) syndrome interact with each other in the setting of renal disease. MIA syndrome is a complex of microinflammation, malnutrition, and atherosclerosis, which mutually interact and form a vicious cycle leading to advanced atherosclerosis in dialysis patients [19]. CRA syndrome is a vicious complex of cardiovascular disease, renal failure, and anemia, which also form a vicious circle, with each one capable of causing or worsening of other components [20]. CKD-MBD includes abnormal mineral metabolism, deranged bone turnover and mineralization, and widespread distribution of ectopic calcification in soft tissues, including vascular calcification (medial calcification). Fibroblast growth factor-23 (FGF23) and its co-receptor, Klotho, are thought to have a central role in atherosclerosis and CKD-MBD [21]. Inflammation plays a central role in all the three conditions (Figure 1) [22].

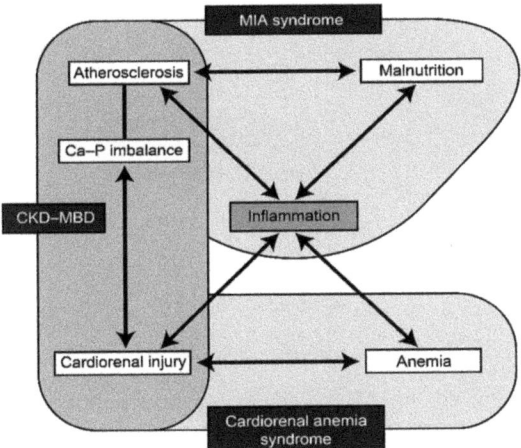

Figure 1. Interaction between malnutrition, inflammation, and atherosclerosis in chronic kidney disease [22]. MIA: malnutrition–inflammation–atherosclerosis; Ca: Calcium; P: Phosphorus; CKD-MBD: chronic kidney diseases-related mineral and bone disorder.

4. Malnutrition and HD: Critical Connection

Malnutrition is common in HD patients and is a powerful predictor of morbidity and mortality. In chronic HD patients, low concentrations of serum albumin, blood urea nitrogen (BUN), serum creatinine, and low relative body weight are significantly associated with an increased risk of mortality. Malnutrition has been reported in 23–76% of HD patients and is dependent on factors such as the quality of dialysis therapy, case mix, comorbid conditions, and age [23]. Anorexia, hormonal and metabolic derangements, decreased nutrient intake, and catabolic factors are associated with the dialysis procedure selected. Additionally, the structure of the dialysis membrane plays an important role in dialysis-related malnutrition [24].

The elderly population undergoing dialysis has distinct characteristic features: malnutrition, protein-energy wasting (PEW), frailty, and sarcopenia [25]. A study conducted by Yasui et al. indicated that 15% of Japanese patients on HD have PEW. These findings further suggest that reduced muscle mass, lack of exercise, chronic inflammation, unintentional low dietary energy intake, and insulin resistance are the major contributing factors for PEW [26]. The optimum protein and calorie intake does not effectively help combat malnutrition in chronic HD patients. This is because multifactorial derangements cause malnutrition in chronic HD patients rather than poor nutritional intake alone [27].

5. Inflammation and HD

Numerous complications of chronic dialysis are attributed to inflammation, via monocyte release of interleukin (IL)-1, the master cytokine of inflammation. The development of inflammation in CKD begins well before the need for chronic dialysis. Elevated levels of inflammatory biomarkers such as IL-6 and C-reactive protein (CRP) suggest that CKD and chronic dialysis can both be regarded as low-grade inflammatory processes [28]. Multiple factors contribute to the chronic inflammatory activation in patients undergoing dialysis. The contributing factors for higher levels of circulating cytokines include decreased cytokine clearance and increased production of the cytokines, uremic milieu, epigenetic influences, infectious and thrombotic events, dialysis procedure, dysbiosis, adipose tissue metabolism, and comorbid conditions (Figure 2) [28]. Procedure-related factors that cause inflammation in dialysis patients include the use of nonsterile dialysate or non-biocompatible membranes and back leakage of dialysate across membranes [29].

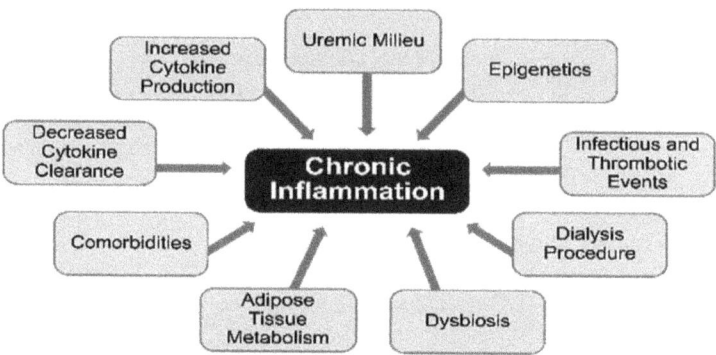

Figure 2. Inflammation in dialysis patients [28].

Increased levels of inflammatory markers are associated with adverse clinical outcomes, including all-cause mortality, cardiovascular events, kidney disease progression, PEW, diminished motor function, and cognitive impairment. Other adverse consequences of elevated inflammatory markers include CKD-MBD, anemia, and insulin resistance [28].

6. Atherosclerosis in HD: PAD-Associated Heightened Risk of Cardiovascular Events

The risk of atherosclerosis is high in patients undergoing HD, which can lead to the development of PAD [30,31]. PAD is defined as obstructive atherosclerosis of the lower extremities and is associated with an increased risk of cardiovascular events and an increased mortality rate in HD patients [11]. A recent study in Japan reported a high prevalence rate of PAD in HD patients [30,31]. Several factors that are unique to dialysis patients may predispose them to the development of PAD, including manifestations of kidney disease, such as hyperparathyroidism, chronic inflammation, and hyperphosphatemia [11]. Because of its progressive nature, screening and diagnosis of PAD in dialysis patients are of utmost importance. Furthermore, neglecting PAD could lead to an increased risk of cardiovascular events and even amputation [11]. The ankle–brachial blood pressure index (ABI) is used as the standard tool to detect PAD. However, due to the presence of vascular calcification, ABI yields false-negative results. Therefore, skin perfusion pressure (SPP) is a more useful tool for detecting PAD in HD patients, with 84.9% accuracy [32].

Among non-dialysis patients with PAD, 1% to 3% with claudication underwent amputation within five years. Amputation for PAD is more prevalent in patients with ESRD than in the general population. In addition, revascularization procedures among dialysis patients are often associated with subsequent amputation and high mortality at the end of one year [11].

A high incidence of major amputation or death is a major clinical problem in HD patients. In chronic HD patients, critical limb ischemia (CLI) from isolated infra-popliteal artery disease is frequently observed and is usually treated with endovascular therapy (EVT) and lower extremity bypass surgery [33]. In a study by Nakano et al., the amputation-free survival (AFS) rates after EVT and bypass surgery were 66% and 61%, respectively, at 1 year [34]. However, an important limitation is that the angiographic restenosis rate is extremely high in patients with CLI after EVT or bypass surgery [35]. The study revealed that within a year after EVT, 70% of the patients with PAD underwent revascularization.

7. Physicochemical Structures and Key Features of Different Dialysis Membranes

Different Types of Dialysis Membranes and Their Features

To reduce cardiovascular events, of importance to note is choosing an appropriate dialysis membrane. Dialysis membrane materials can be classified into three groups: unsubstituted cellulose, substituted (modified) cellulose, and synthetic [36–38]. Initially, unsubstituted cellulose membranes of large thickness and small pore size were used for HD. These membranes are inefficient for small solute removal and have side effects such as elevated levels of complement activation. Regenerated cellulose membranes were later developed via chemical modification to improve their biocompatibility by replacing their hydroxyl groups with acetate groups, such as cellulose acetate (CA), cellulose diacetate (CDA), or cellulose triacetate (CTA). Other membranes developed from regenerated cellulose have relatively better performance, including diethylaminoethyl (DEAE)-substituted cellulose and multilayer vitamin E-coated cellulose [39]. Subsequently, several types of synthetic membranes have been developed from different materials, such as polysulfone (PSu) [40], polyamide, polymethyl methacrylate, and polyacrylonitrile (PAN). Atherosclerosis, commonly observed in HD patients, is associated with an increase in leukocyte/platelet aggregates. Arterial abnormalities also result from rheological anomalies in the blood. In this context, vitamin E-coated hemodialyzers improve atherosclerotic changes in HD patients through positive effects on rheology in addition to antioxidant effects. It also helps to reduce the required erythropoietin (EPO) dose during HD [39].

The different types of dialysis membranes and their key features are listed in Table 1.

Table 1. Different types of dialysis membranes and their key features.

Biomaterial of Dialysis Membrane	Common Name	Key Features	
		Chemical Properties	Clinical Significance
Cellulose	Cuprophan (CU)	• Composed of regenerated cellulose, consisting of linear chains of glucose rings with free surface hydroxyl groups • Highly hydrophilic and uniform porosity	• Low cost • Good diffusive transport properties for small solutes
DEAE-substituted cellulose	Hemophan	• Regenerated cellulose membrane with positively charged DEAE substance substituting 1% hydroxyl moieties	• Higher suppression of complement activation • Adsorbs heparin, causing blood coagulation
Cellulose diacetate and triacetate	CA, CTA	• Modified cellulose membranes developed by substituting free hydroxyl groups on cellulose membrane surface with CA, or diacetate (80% substitution), or CTA (90% substitution) • More hydrophobic than regenerated cellulose membranes	• Lower complement activation vs. unsubstituted cellulose
Multilayer vitamin-E coated cellulose	Excebrane	• Developed by covalent binding of synthetic block polymers (oleyl alcohol and vitamin-E moieties) to hydroxyl groups on cellulose • Decreased activation of mononuclear cells and lower levels of proinflammatory cytokine, IL-6	• Has antioxidant effects and reduces thrombosis • Decreased activation of mononuclear cells and lower levels of proinflammatory cytokine, IL-6
Polysulfone	F-series Optiflux series	• Synthetic polymeric membrane made from petroleum • Hydrophobic in nature and mostly included with pore-forming hydrophilic agents	• Relatively low diffusion rates for small solutes (to overcome this disadvantage, polyvinylpyrrolidone is added during the manufacturing process.)
Polyamide	Polyflux series	• Derived from synthetic polymer, polyamide • Strongly asymmetric membrane structure	• Due to hydrophobic sites, allows endotoxin retention • Owing to minimal interaction with blood components, provides improved biocompatibility

Table 1. Cont.

Biomaterial of Dialysis Membrane	Common Name	Key Features	
		Chemical Properties	Clinical Significance
Polyacrylonitrile and methacrylate	PAN	• Synthetic membrane • Hydrophobic	• Adsorbs proteins and cells on their surface
Poly(methyl methacrylate)	PMMA	• Synthetic membrane • Hydrophobic	• Adsorbs proteins and cells on their surface
Polyethersulfone	PES	• Synthetic membrane • Hydrophobic	• Adsorbs proteins and cells on their surface
Polycarbonate	Polycarbonate	• Synthetic membrane • Hydrophobic	• Causes activation of proteins and cells

(From [36–40], CU: Cuprophan; CA: Cellulose acetate or diacetate; CTA: Cellulose triacetate; DEAE: Diethylaminoethyl; PAN: Polyacrylonitrile; PMMA: Poly (methyl methacrylate); PES: Polyethersulfone.

8. Impact of Dialysis Membranes on Clinical Outcomes

Reports indicate that the clinical outcomes of chronic HD patients are influenced by the type of dialyzer membrane used. This is particularly dependent on the solute mass transport efficiency and bio(in)compatibility of the dialyzer membrane [41,42].

The solute mass transport is mostly represented by the flux characteristics of the membrane and is expressed as the ultrafiltration (UF) coefficient in mL/mmHg/h. This represents the water permeability of the membrane [41,42].

Various reactions may be triggered by the contact of blood with the artificial surface of an inadequately biocompatible dialysis system. These interactions include leukocyte, complement, and thrombocyte activation, coagulation, and production of cytokines, free-oxygen radicals, β2-microglobulin, bradykinin, and other events. Reactions caused by inadequate biocompatibility may injure the patient. Hence, biocompatibility is considered one of the leading areas of concern in dialysis treatment. Dialysis membranes that cause minimal activation of plasma proteins or cellular cascades can be considered biocompatible.

9. Unique Biocompatibility and Selective Adsorptive Properties of the AN69 Membrane

Introduction and History of the AN69 Membrane

The development of a synthetic membrane for use in dialysis was initiated in 1969 by a company named Rhône-Poulenc, following a request from the French government. This led to the development of the AN69 membrane. A copolymer of sodium methallyl sulfonate and acrylonitrile was used to manufacture an AN69 membrane. The unique feature of the AN69 membrane is that it is hydrophilic in nature compared with other synthetic membranes. This is because of the presence of sulfonate groups that create a hydrogel structure by attracting water, thereby providing hydraulic permeability with highly diffusive properties [43]. The AN69 membrane was first produced as a flat sheet; however, since 1980, it has been developed as a hollow fiber. The AN69 membrane has evolved continuously since its development in the early 1970s to meet the challenges and requirements of dialysis therapy. Its continuous advancement in thickness and internal diameter has led to improved performance. In the 1980s, the dialyzer manufacturing process was modified to allow sterilization by γ-radiation, instead of ethylene oxide [43]. The use of the AN69 membrane has been found to be associated with improved efficiency, reduced treatment duration, reduced risk of peripheral neuropathy, and improved clinical outcomes and quality of life. This paved the way for the initiation of volume-controlled, high-flux dialysis [43].

10. Key Features of the AN69 Membrane

Adsorptive Features

The microstructure and chemical composition of the AN69 membrane facilitate the bulk absorption of low-molecular-weight proteins, such as basic proteins and inflammatory mediators. The adsorptive property of the AN69 membrane, specifically for basic medium-sized proteins, distinguishes it from other adsorptive membranes and synthetic high-flux dialysis membranes [43]. A study demonstrated that low-molecular-weight acidic proteins can be eliminated by filtration on negatively charged membranes (such as AN69) or uncharged membranes. Conversely, basic low-molecular-weight proteins can be removed by specific ionic interactions on the AN69 membrane [44]. The superior biocompatibility of the AN69 membrane is due to its unique adsorptive capacity for anaphylatoxin and inflammatory complement factors [43].

The hallmark features of the AN69 membrane are its high permeability to fluids, including a broad range of uremic retention products, and its excellent biocompatibility, measured using either novel or conventional indicators [43].

11. Effect on Inflammatory Response

During HD, exposure of the blood to foreign surfaces activates various defense mechanisms, including coagulation, fibrinolysis, and complement activation, via an alternative pathway. In turn, complement activation leads to impairment of the host defense, as a result of increased consumption of complement proteins [45]. It has been observed that the intensity of complement activation varies with the type of membrane used: for example, with cellulose (CU), a much more marked activation is observed when compared to synthetic PAN membrane [46].

Several studies have demonstrated that the AN69 membrane has a lower ability to activate the complement system because of its adsorptive properties when compared to other membranes, such as CA dialyzers and CU membranes [46–49].

Adverse effects of dialysis, such as fever, hypotension, and acute-phase inflammatory reactions, are linked to the production of activated monocytes and macrophages. These were IL-1, tumor necrosis factor (TNF)-α, and IL-6. Compared to the other membranes such as CU, the AN69 membrane neither induces cytokine production nor causes the activation of mononuclear cells [50,51]. Moreover, no changes in neutrophil and monocyte counts occur during HD with the AN69 membrane, unlike with the CU membrane [52].

Since high-flux dialysis membranes, such as the AN69 membrane, are highly permeable, concerns regarding their potential to permit the passage of cytokine-inducing residues across these membranes, either through back-diffusion or back-filtration, have been raised. However, in vitro studies have shown that the AN69 membrane is not permeable to specific types of bacterial endotoxins compared with the permeability of other membranes [53,54].

Recent advances in the manufacturing technique of dialysis membranes enabled the development of a new hemofilter with an AN69 surface-treated membrane (Oxiris) [55]. It provides high absorbance of endotoxin (negatively charged) and cytokines and excellent anti-thrombogenicity because of its positively charged surface [56,57]. Case series and studies have reported the hemofilter's validity in reducing cytokine concentrations in COVID-19 patients [58–60].

12. Effect on Oxidative Stress and Carbonyl Stress

In addition to increased inflammation, HD is often associated with oxidative stress due to the activation of white blood cells, which triggers the generation of reactive oxygen species (ROS) and the loss of antioxidants during dialysis. Oxidative stress increases the risk of morbidity and mortality in this patient population and could be measured as advanced oxidation protein products in the plasma of uremic patients [61,62].

Evidence indicates that the AN69 membrane provides more protection from oxidative stress in HD patients than other membranes such as CDA [63]. Carbonyl stress is also implicated in long-term complications, such as atherosclerosis or dialysis-related amyloidosis, in ESRD patients [64,65]. Increased levels of advanced glycation end products (AGEs), which contribute to uremic toxicity, result from the accumulation of carbonyl AGE precursors in uremic plasma [66]. The effect of the AN69 membrane on carbonyl stress marker levels was similar to those of other membranes in a single HD session. However, in patients who were switched from PSu to the AN69 membrane, the carbonyl stress marker levels reduced to the control level [66].

13. Hemocompatibility

A high fibrinogen concentration is associated with increased cardiovascular risk and accelerated atherosclerosis. The AN69 membrane has good hemocompatibility, as it induces a lower thrombotic response, and fibrinogen and erythrocyte sedimentation rates are higher in non-biocompatible membranes [66].

14. Negative Charge

During the 1990s, the incidence of hypersensitivity reactions in HD patients, especially in those using electronegatively charged PAN membranes (AN69), increased significantly. This was due to the widespread use of antihypertensive drugs, such as angiotensin-I-converting enzyme inhibitors (ACEi) [67]. These inhibitors prevented the normal breakdown of bradykinin, the chief mediator of hypersensitivity reactions that occur during HD [68,69]. Similar reactions have also been reported with the use of PSu and other synthetic membranes during dialysis. The Evaluation of the Losartan in Hemodialysis (ELHE) study, which assessed the efficacy of an alternative antihypertensive drug, losartan, for HD patients, indicated a lower prevalence of anaphylactoid reactions compared to the use of ACEi when used in combination with the AN69 membrane [70]. To neutralize the electronegativity of the AN69 membrane and lower the generation of kinins, a membrane was developed with a coating of polyethyleneimine, called the AN69-ST (ST for surface treated) membrane [43]. They demonstrated lower adsorption of high-molecular–weight kininogen and contact-phase activation than the regular AN69 membrane [71].

15. Functional Similarities of AN69 with LDL-Apheresis

LDL-Apheresis is the process of removing LDLs from the plasma and was originally used for familial hyperlipidemia patients. Recommendations for initiation of LDL-apheresis in patients affected by hypercholesterolemia are controvercial, as no study demonstrated definitively improved survival with LDL-apheresis. International guidelines and systematic review recommend to consider LDL-apheresis in homozygotes or those with analogous phenotypes if the patient has already been treated with diet and pharmacotherapy and LDL cholesterol levels still remain higher than cut-off values based on age and cardiovascular state [72,73].

There are several methods to remove LDL cholesterol from the blood. These include heparin-induced extracorpoeral LDL cholesterol precipitation, immunoadsorption, double filtration plasma pheresis of lipoproteins, and liposorber system. Through selective adsorption, liposorber system LDL-apheresis removes LDL from plasma using negatively charged dextran beads [74]. In addition to the lipid-lowering function, several other beneficial effects of LDL-apheresis have been reported, including anti-inflammatory, anti-atherogenic, and anti-thrombotic effects [74,75]. Owing to its pleotropic benefits, LDL-apheresis is effective against PAD in HD patients, through the reduction of LDL, coagulation factors, and ROS production [76]. In this context, it is important to note that LDL-apheresis has several functional similarities with the AN69 membrane. Both of these systems use a negatively charged surface for extracorporeal adsorptive filtration from the blood/plasma, and contact phase activation has been associated with both these systems [77]. Similar to AN69, LDL-apheresis therapy leads to a reduced generation of cytokines and CRP and improved macrophage function, thereby eliciting its anti-inflammatory role. Similar to the protective role of AN69 in oxidative stress, LDL-apheresis lowers the ROS generation by leukocytes. As observed in the case of AN69, LDL-apheresis also improves hemorheology by increasing blood viscosity and lowering coagulant and fibrinogen levels [74].

In addition to the beneficial effects of AN69, it is associated with fewer complications in HD patients, even those with PAD, as compared to those associated with other common membranes [78]. LDL-apheresis has also been successfully used in HD patients with complications such as PAD, owing to its pleiotropic benefits other than lipid-lowering effects [74,78]. Therefore, the concomitant use of both these therapeutic systems in specific patients, such as those with PAD, may provide additive therapeutic benefits in such HD patients.

16. Clinical Evidence of AN69 Membrane Use in Chronic HD Patients

The AN69 membrane is one such membrane that has favorable effects on dialysis because of its well-balanced removal of low-molecular–weight proteins and small solutes [10]. In this section, we will discuss the clinical evidence highlighting the benefits of AN69 membrane use in patients undergoing HD. Table 2 lists the different clinical studies evaluating the different effects of the AN69 membrane in the chronic HD setting.

Table 2. Membrane in chronic hemodialysis patients.

Author and Year	Study Type	Study Details	Dialysis Membranes Involved
Furuta et al., 2011 [78]	A crossover study to compare HD efficiency and effects on nutritional, hemodynamic, and inflammatory conditions of polysulfone and AN69 membranes in elderly (aged 75 years or older) HD patients.	Twenty-eight elderly maintenance HD patients were treated with polysulfone for 3 months, followed by AN69 for the next 3 months, then switched back to polysulfone for 3 months.	Polysulfone and AN69
Nakada et al., 2014 [79]	Crossover trial to study the efficacy of long-term use of PAN hemodialyzer in elderly dialysis patients with mild PAD.	Six chronic HD patients were switched from polysulfone to AN69 membrane and observed for 72 weeks.	AN69 and polysulfone membrane
Yokomatsu et al., 2014 [80]	Comparative study to assess amino acid loss into dialysate during HD with 3 different membranes.	Nine maintenance HD patients were studied, who received HD for more than 3 months. Dialysate samples were evaluated for measurement of amino acid loss.	Nonhydrophilic PEPA (FLX-15GW, Nikkiso), hydrophilic PEPA (FDX-150GW, Nikkiso), PAN/AN69 membrane (H12-4000, Gambro)
Kuragano et al., 2013 [81]	Single-center study; measured changes in serum hepcidin levels during HD with different membranes.	Comprised ex vivo and in vivo studies. In the ex vivo study, a mini-dialyzer made of either polysulfone or AN69 was used to circulate blood from healthy volunteers, followed by measurement of serum hepcidin levels. In the in vivo study, 10 healthy individuals and 28 maintenance HD patients were included. After treatment with the polysulfone membrane, AN69 was used in the following weeks and serum hepcidin levels were measured.	APS-SA® (hollow fiber, composed of polysulfone membrane), and H12-3400® (flat-sheet, AN69)
Latrou 2002 [82]	Comparative study to evaluate the effects of HD membranes on production of PAF.	The study was conducted among 10 HD patients who were first treated with the CU membrane and then the AN69 membrane in the following week. Along with changes in the PAF levels at different time points, platelet and leukocyte counts and the extent of complement activation were studied.	CU and AN69 membranes
Chandran 1993 [83]	A ten-year analysis to study patient survival on PAN/AN69 HD.	This was a retrospective single-center study conducted to analyze the 10-year survival of 352 HD patients on PAN/AN69 membrane.	PAN/AN69 membrane

(From [78–83], MIA: malnutrition, inflammation, and atherosclerosis; HD: hemodialysis; AN69-ST: AN69 surface-treated; ESRD: end-stage renal disease; PAN: polyacrylonitrile; PAD: peripheral arterial disease; PEPA: polyester–polymer alloy; PAF: platelet-activating factor; CU: cuprophan.

17. Effect on Solute Removal, Hemodynamic Parameters, and Nutritional Status

A crossover study conducted by Furuta et al. [78] among 28 elderly maintenance HD (MHD) patients aged 75 years or older compared AN69 with PSu membrane with respect to solute removal during HD, hemodynamic condition, and nutritional status after three months of treatment. In the last session of the first PSu period and the AN69 period, pre-and post-serum levels of IL-6 were measured and calculated for reduction ratio. At the start of the study and the last session of each membrane period, pre-HD serum total protein, albumin, total cholesterol, triglyceride levels were measured to compare the nutritional status among each treatment period. The study findings indicated that the reduction ratio for the inflammatory cytokine IL-6 was significantly higher for AN69 compared to PSu membrane ($p < 0.05$). This could be attributed to the negative charge present on the AN69 membrane surface that facilitates adsorption of various inflammatory cytokines such as IL-10, IL-6, and IL-18. The study findings also indicated that after three months of AN69 use, serum albumin, total protein, and cholesterol levels increased significantly and returned to baseline after switching back to PSu (Figure 3). Furthermore, the frequency of saline use to treat hypotension episodes decreased significantly during HD with AN69. The study revealed that, in elderly MHD patients, AN69 use led to improvements in both chronic inflammatory conditions and malnutrition. Therefore, for elderly HD patients, AN69 may be the preferred membrane for dialysis.

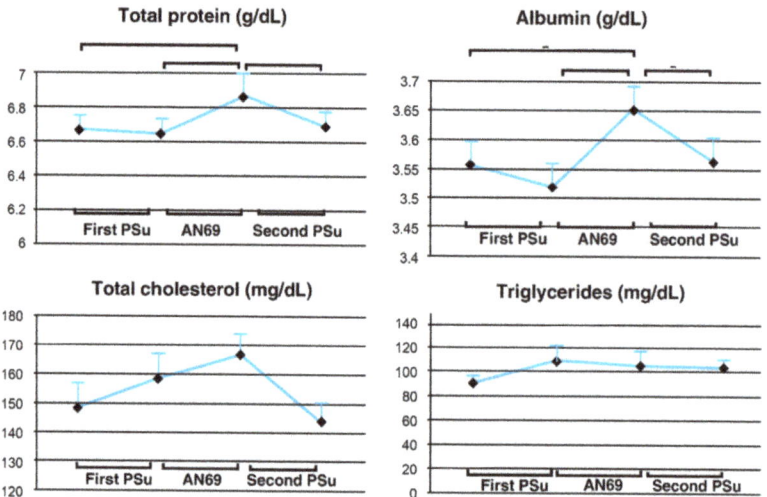

Figure 3. Changes in the nutritional indices during the PSu and AN69 periods [78]. PSu: polysulfone, AN69: acrylonitrile 69.

18. Effects on Solute Removal and Nutritional Status of Older HD Patients with Mild PAD

18.1. Crossover Trial

A crossover trial [79] comparing the solute removal properties of AN69 and PSu membranes was conducted among six elderly patients with mild PAD (mean age: 70.8 ± 9.0 years) with stable hemodynamics and no detectable anemia; the patients were administered four-hour HD thrice a week; dialyzers were switched every two weeks, and parameters such as reduction rate, clearance, clear space, and amount of low-molecular-weight protein, β2-microglobulin, and low-molecular-weight solutes including creatinine, urea nitrogen, and inorganic phosphorus were evaluated. The reduction rate and removal amount of amino acids and albumin were also determined. Although AN69 was less efficient than PSu in the removal of β2-microglobulin and creatinine, the overall dialysis efficiency for the removal of low-molecular-weight solutes was similar for both membranes. Albumin leakage and amino acid removal were significantly lower in the case of AN69 than in PSu. The study concluded that, owing to the negative charge and pore size, albumin removal by AN69 was significantly lower than that of the other membranes, and that the use of AN69 may ameliorate the deterioration of symptoms in HD patients.

18.2. Long-Term Benefits

A study included eight elderly patients (mean age: 72.1 ± 10.6 years) who were switched from PSu membrane to AN69 and observed for 72 weeks to determine the long-term effects of AN69 use. Analyses for nutritional benefits and long-term effects included measurements of albumin levels and various parameters from blood, such as β2-microglobulin, CRP, low-density lipoprotein (LDL), fibrinogen, nitrogen oxide, hemoglobin, ferritin, and renal anemia. Both serum albumin and the geriatric nutritional risk index (GNRI) were maintained at stable levels. The GNRI level was maintained above 92, which is the target level for HD patients. All the parameters studied to assess the nutritional status, such as normalized protein catabolic rate, dry weight, and creatinine generation rate, remained stable throughout long-term use of the AN69 membrane. CRP and LDL levels are associated with the development of atherosclerosis. Although the patients had atherosclerosis, AN69 did not significantly alter the levels of CRP and LDL. No significant changes occurred in β2-microglobulin levels. The hemoglobin levels remained favorable and stable. Overall, in elderly HD patients with mild PAD, AN69 demonstrated good biocompatibility and HD efficiency [79].

19. Effect on Amino-Acid Loss into Dialysate during HD

Another study [80] conducted in Japan among nine maintenance HD patients evaluated the amino acid losses using three types of membranes: hydrophilic and nonhydrophilic polyester–polymer alloy membranes and the AN69 membrane. In the same order, patients received treatments with all three membranes at one-month intervals, without membrane reuse. Standard HD was administered three times a week for 3 to 4 h. Significant differences in the losses of tryptophan, cystine, phenylalanine, and ornithine were observed between the HD membranes (Table 3). The total amino acid loss was 72.1 ± 22.5 mg/L for the AN69 membrane, and 83.3 ± 16.1 mg/L and 85.7 ± 27.2 mg/L for nonhydrophilic and hydrophilic polyester–polymer alloy membranes, respectively [80].

Table 3. Clinical Evidence on Benefits of AN69 in Inflammation, Malnutrition, and Peripheral Arterial Disease Associated with Hemodialysis.

Amino Acids	Hydrophilic PEPA	Non-Hydrophilic PEPA	AN69	*p*-Value
Ornithine	2.0 ± 0.6	2.0 ± 0.4	1.4 ± 0.4	0.008 *
Phenylalanine	2.4 ± 0.9	2.3 ± 0.5	1.8 ± 0.8	0.005 **
Tryptophan	0.6 ± 0.2	0.7 ± 0.2	0.4 ± 0.2	0.002 **
Cystine	2.8 ± 1.4	3.2 ± 0.7	2.0 ± 0.7	0.004 **

PEPA: Polyester–polymer alloy; * $p \leq 0.05$; ** $p \leq 0.005$.

Therefore, compared to polyester–polymer alloy membranes, AN69 leads to lower amino acid loss, thereby implying a better nutritional state with its use in maintenance HD (MHD) patients.

20. Other Benefits of the AN69 Membrane in HD Patients

20.1. Effect on Serum Hepcidin Levels

CKD patients have a dysregulated iron metabolism, leading to anemia of chronic disease (ACD). Liver hormone hepcidin controls iron homeostasis. Hepcidin is a negative regulator of intestinal iron absorption and iron release from macrophages. Hepcidin induces degradation of the iron exporter ferroportin to reduce iron entry into plasma from dietary sources and body stores. Iron deficiency and erythropoietic drive suppress hepcidin production to provide adequate iron for erythropoiesis [84]. Hepcidin excess, as a consequence of inflammation, decreased renal clearance, and reduced erythropoietin production, is suspected to cause the dysregulation of iron metabolism, resulting in ACD.

20.1.1. Ex Vivo Study

An ex vivo study [81] was performed using 50 mL of whole blood collected from healthy volunteers circulated for 2 h in a microcircuit with mini-dialyzers (acrylonitrile-co-methallyl sulfonate [AN69] or PSu without ultrafiltration). The levels of hepcidin-25 were measured in the blood samples at 0, 60, and 120 min. The study demonstrated that although serum hepcidin 25 levels increased after the ex vivo session with PS, they significantly decreased with AN69 after one and two hours (mean change ratio: $-68 \pm 39\%$).

20.1.2. In Vivo Study

An in vivo study included the collection of blood samples with 28 MHD patients at the start and end of HD sessions with the PS or AN69 membrane. The serum levels of hepcidin 20, 22, and 25 were measured using liquid chromatography tandem mass spectrometry. The serum levels of urea nitrogen and β2-microglobulin were also measured. The study findings indicated that the reduction of β2-microglobulin was significantly higher for PSu ($62.4 \pm 6.5\%$) than for the AN69 membrane ($29.2 \pm 8.2\%$). However, the reduction ratios of hepcidin 20, 22, and 25 did not significantly differ between the PS and AN69 membranes [81].

The study thus demonstrated that the AN69 membrane had the potential to remove hepcidin because of its high adsorptive capacity, whereas PSu removed serum hepcidin because of its high solute-removing potential. In consideration of the high adsorptive capacity of the AN69 membrane for hepcidin, HD patients treated with AN69 membrane might need less quality of intravenous iron administration.

21. Production of Platelet-Activating Factor (PAF)

PAF is produced by different cells, such as macrophages, monocytes, platelets, neutrophils, and endothelial cells, via activation from immune or nonimmune stimuli. Apart from other biological functions, PAF mediates allergic responses. Interaction between blood cells and HD membranes stimulates PAF production. Therefore, the blood concentration of PAF is regarded as one of the important indices of membrane biocompatibility.

The production of PAF during HD with a CU membrane has been established; however, with the AN-69 PAN membrane, this has not been clearly linked. To assess this, a study [84] was conducted among 10 HD patients, who were subjected to HD with CU and AN-69 membranes for two consecutive weeks (first week with CU and second week with AN-69). The blood PAF levels and leukocyte and platelet counts were measured during the third HD session of each week and at different time points (0, 2, 5, 15, 30, 60, 180, and 240 min), while the circulating levels of the C3a-desArg and SC5b-9 were measured at 0, 5, 15, 60, and 240 min. The study results showed that circulating PAF levels were detectable at all time points during HD with AN-69 (PAF_{AN-69}) and CU (PAF_{CU}) membranes [83].

The study findings showed that at all time intervals $PAF_{AN-69} < PAF_{CU}$, statistically significant differences (s) existed only at 15, 30, 60, 180, and 240 min between the two membranes. The highest PAF_{AN-69} and PAF_{CU} levels occurred at 5 and 15 min, respectively, during dialysis. Similar observations were made for the reduction in circulating leukocytes and C3a-desArg levels. The maximum reduction in platelet count was observed after two minutes of dialysis initiation for both membranes. The study concluded that although AN69 led to the production of PAF, circulating PAF levels were lower at all time intervals during HD with the AN 69 membrane when compared with the CU membrane. This study confirmed that PAF production with both the membranes probably contributed to thrombocytopenia and leukopenia.

22. Effect on Patient Survival

A retrospective single-center study assessed the survival characteristics over a 10-year period of 340 HD patients who were hemodialyzed exclusively on PAN (polyacrylonitrile) or AN69 membranes and compared it with national data collected by the US Renal Data System (USRDS). The USRDS, established in 1989, is the largest national ESRD and CKD surveillance system in the United States. USRDS covers Medicare and non-Medicare ESRD patients, and Medicare CKD patients. USRDS is a stand-alone database on the diagnosis and demographic characteristics of ESRD patients, along with biochemical data, dialysis information, hospitalization, and deaths. The characteristics of 340 HD patients using PAN or AN69 membranes were: age of 55.89 ± 0.9 years (mean ± SE) and HD duration of 922.99 ± 47.58 days. The diagnostic categories were diabetic nephropathy (30%), glomerulonephritis (23.5%), hypertensive nephrosclerosis (18.5%), and others (28%). Corresponding information about age, mean duration of HD, and cause of renal failure in USRDS database were not provided in the manuscript [83]. The number of expected deaths in 340 patients according to the USRDS database was 190, whereas the number of the observed actual deaths in patients on PAN/AN69 membranes was only 120, a high significant difference at a p value of <0.0001 (Table 4) [83]. A comparison with the national data collected by the USRDS revealed that AN69 improved survival in HD membranes, possibly due to its better removal of 'intermediate molecules' and low-molecular-weight uremic toxins by AN69 [83].

Table 4. Survival of hemodialysis patients treated with PAN/AN69 membrane [83].

No. of Patients on PAN/AN69 in Authors' HD Center	Age (Mean ± SE)	HD Duration (Days)	Expected Mortality from USRDS Database	Observed Mortality	p-Value
340	55.89 ± 0.9	922.99 ± 47.58	189.89	120	<0.001

PAN: Polyacrylonitrile; SE: Standard error.

23. Conclusions

As Japan has a relatively large number of dialysis patients, evaluating of the performance of dialysis membranes, in terms of biocompatibility, long-term benefits, and lowered dialysis-associated complications, is of paramount importance. The constantly increasing number of elderly patients on long-term dialysis in Japan is another issue of concern and therefore requires careful consideration of the appropriate dialysis membranes.

The AN69 membrane has several advantages over other dialysis membranes. The key features of the AN69 membrane is its high permeability and selective absorptive property. The AN69 membrane improves nutritional status, lowers inflammation in patients undergoing dialysis, and leads to lower amino acid loss, implying a better nutritional state with its use in MHD patients. The AN69 membrane demonstrates good biocompatibility and HD efficiency in the setting of atherosclerosis and PAD in dialysis patients. Moreover, the safety profile of the AN69 membrane broadens its applicability and highlights its importance as the membrane of choice in chronic HD patients.

Author Contributions: Conceptualization and writing, S.K.; Supervision and editing, T.O. All authors have read and agreed to the published version of the manuscript.

Funding: This research received no external funding.

Institutional Review Board Statement: There is no need for permission from IRB in this review article.

Informed Consent Statement: There is no need for informed consent in this review article.

Data Availability Statement: There is no data to provide for reasonable request in this review article.

Conflicts of Interest: Author receives lecture and advisory fee from Kaneka Co., Ltd. (Tokyo, Japan).

References

1. Masakane, I.; Taniguchi, M.; Nakai, S.; Tsuchida, K.; Wada, A.; Ogata, S.; Hasegawa, T.; Hamano, T.; Hanafusa, N.; Hoshino, J.; et al. Annual Dialysis Data Report 2016, JSDT Renal Data Registry. *Ren. Replace. Ther.* **2018**, *4*, 45. [CrossRef]
2. Nitta, K.; Masakane, I.; Hanafusa, N.; Taniguchi, M.; Hasegawa, T.; Nakai, S.; Goto, S.; Wada, A.; Hamano, T.; Hoshino, J.; et al. Annual dialysis data report 2017, JSDT Renal Data Registry. *Ren. Replace. Ther.* **2019**, *5*, 53. [CrossRef]
3. Hanafusa, N.; Nitta, K.; Tsuchiya, K. The characteristics of the older dialysis population-heterogeneity and another type of altered risk factor patterns. *Ren. Replace. Ther.* **2017**, *3*, 29. [CrossRef]
4. Nawata, K.; Kimura, M. Evaluation of medical costs of kidney diseases and risk factors in Japan. *Health* **2017**, *9*, 1734–1749. [CrossRef]
5. Watanabe, Y.; Yamagata, K.; Nishi, S.; Hirakata, H.; Hanafusa, N.; Saito, C.; Hattori, M.; Itami, N.; Komatsu, Y.; Kawaguchi, Y.; et al. Japanese society for dialysis therapy clinical guideline for "Hemodialysis initiation for maintenance hemodialysis". *Ther. Apher. Dial.* **2015**, *19* (Suppl. S1), 93–107. [CrossRef]
6. Oomichi, T.; Emoto, M.; Tabata, T.; Morioka, T.; Tsujimoto, Y.; Tahara, H.; Shoji, T.; Nishizawa, Y. Impact of glycemic control on survival of diabetic patients on chronic regular hemodialysis: A 7-year observational study. *Diabetes Care* **2006**, *29*, 1496–1500. [CrossRef]
7. Cozzolino, M.; Mangano, M.; Stucchi, A.; Ciceri, P.; Conte, F.; Galassi, A. Cardiovascular disease in dialysis patients. *Nephrol. Dial. Transpl.* **2018**, *33* (Suppl. S3), iii28–iii34. [CrossRef]
8. Nishida, M.; Ando, M.; Iwamoto, Y.; Tsuchiya, K.; Nitta, K. New insight into atherosclerosis in hemodialysis patients: Overexpression of scavenger receptor and macrophage colony-stimulating factor genes. *Nephron. Extra* **2016**, *6*, 22–30. [CrossRef]
9. Hirakata, H.; Nitta, K.; Inaba, M.; Shoji, T.; Fujii, H.; Kobayashi, S.; Tabei, K.; Joki, N.; Hase, H.; Nishimura, M.; et al. Therapy. Japanese Society for Dialysis Therapy guidelines for management of cardiovascular diseases in patients on chronic hemodialysis. *Ther. Apher. Dial.* **2012**, *16*, 387–435. [CrossRef]
10. Moriya, H.; Oka, M.; Maesato, K.; Mano, T.; Ikee, R.; Ohtake, T.; Kobayashi, S. Weekly averaged blood pressure is more important than a single-point blood pressure measurement in the risk stratification of dialysis patients. *Clin. J. Am. Soc. Nephrol.* **2008**, *3*, 416–422. [CrossRef]
11. DeLoach, S.S.; Mohler, E.R., III. Peripheral arterial disease: A guide for nephrologists. *Clin. J. Am. Soc. Nephrol.* **2007**, *2*, 839–846. [CrossRef] [PubMed]
12. Kobayashi, S. Cardiovascular events in hemodialysis patients: Challenging against vascular calcification. *Ann. Vasc. Dis.* **2017**, *10*, 1–7. [CrossRef] [PubMed]
13. Kobayashi, S. Cardiovascular events in Chronic Kidney Disease (CKD)–An importance of vascular calcification and microcirculatory impairment. *Ren. Replace. Ther.* **2016**, *2*, 55. [CrossRef]
14. Kobayashi, S.; Oka, M.; Maesato, K.; Ikee, R.; Mano, T.; Moriya, H.; Ohtake, T. Coronary artery calcification, ADMA, and insulin resistance in CKD patients. *Clin. J. Am. Soc. Nephrol.* **2008**, *3*, 1289–1295. [CrossRef] [PubMed]
15. Ohtake, T.; Oka, M.; Ikee, R.; Mochida, Y.; Ishioka, K.; Moriya, H.; Hidaka, S.; Kobayashi, S. Impact of lower limbs' arterial calcification on the prevalence and severity of PAD in patients on hemodialysis. *J. Vasc. Surg.* **2011**, *53*, 676–683. [CrossRef]
16. Kobayashi, S.; Miyamoto, M.; Kurumatani, H.; Oka, M.; Maesato, K.; Mano, T.; Ikee, R.; Moriya, H.; Ohtake, T. Increased leukocyte aggregates are associated with atherosclerosis in patients with hemodialysis. *Hemodial. Int.* **2009**, *13*, 286–292. [CrossRef]
17. Masakane, I. How to prescribe hemodialysis or hemodiafiltration in order to ameliorate dialysis-related symptoms and complications. *Contrib. Nephrol.* **2011**, *168*, 53–63.
18. Tonbul, H.Z.; Demir, M.; Altintepe, L.; Güney, I.; Yeter, E.; Türk, S.; Yeksan, M.; Yildiz, A. Malnutrition-inflammation-atherosclerosis (MIA) syndrome components in hemodialysis and peritoneal dialysis patients. *Ren. Fail.* **2006**, *28*, 287–294. [CrossRef]
19. Stenvinkel, P. Inflammatory and atherosclerotic interactions in the depleted uremic patient. *Blood Purif.* **2001**, *19*, 53–61. [CrossRef]
20. Silverberg, D.S.; Wexler, D.; Blum, M.; Schwartz, D.; Wollman, Y.; Iaina, A. Erythropoietin should be part of congestive heart failure management. *Kidney Int.* **2003**, *64*, S40–S47. [CrossRef]
21. Cianciolo, G.; Galassi, A.; Capelli, I.; Schillaci, R.; La Manna, G.; Cozzolino, M. Klotho-FGF23, cardiovascular disease, and vascular calcification: Black or white? *Current Vasc. Pharmacol.* **2018**, *16*, 143–156. [CrossRef] [PubMed]
22. Tsuruya, K.; Eriguchi, M. Cardiorenal syndrome in chronic kidney disease. *Curr. Opin. Nephrol. Hypertens.* **2015**, *24*, 154–162. [CrossRef] [PubMed]
23. Qureshi, A.R.; Alvestrand, A.; Danielsson, A.; Divino-Filho, J.C.; Gutierrez, A.; Lindholm, B.; Bergstrom, J. Factors predicting malnutrition in hemodialysis patients: A cross-sectional study. *Kidney Int.* **1998**, *53*, 773–782. [CrossRef] [PubMed]
24. Parker, T.F., III; Wingard, R.L.; Husni, L.; Ikizler, T.A.; Parker, R.A.; Hakim, R.M. Effect of the membrane biocompatibility on nutritional parameters in chronic hemodialysis patients. *Kidney Int.* **1996**, *49*, 551–556. [CrossRef] [PubMed]
25. Hanafusa, N.; Tsuchiya, K.; Nitta, K. Malnutrition-wasting conditions in older dialysis patients: An individualized approach. *Contrib. Nephrol.* **2019**, *198*, 12–20. [PubMed]
26. Yasui, S.; Shirai, Y.; Tanimura, M.; Matsuura, S.; Saito, Y.; Miyata, K.; Ishikawa, E.; Miki, C.; Hamada, Y. Prevalence of protein-energy wasting (PEW) and evaluation of diagnostic criteria in Japanese maintenance hemodialysis patients. *Asia Pac. J. Clin. Nutr.* **2016**, *25*, 292–299. [CrossRef]
27. Lorember, F.M. Malnutrition in Chronic Kidney Disease. *Front. Pediatr.* **2018**, *6*, 161. [CrossRef]

28. Nowak, K.L.; Chonchol, M. Does inflammation affect outcomes in dialysis patients? *Semin. Dial.* **2018**, *31*, 388–397. [CrossRef]
29. Kaysen, G.A. Inflammation: Cause of vascular disease and malnutrition in dialysis patients. *Semin. Nephrol.* **2004**, *24*, 431–436. [CrossRef]
30. Ishioka, K.; Ohtake, T.; Moriya, H.; Mochida, Y.; Oka, M.; Maesato, K.; Hidaka, S.; Kobayashi, S. High prevalence of peripheral arterial disease (PAD) in incident hemodialysis patients: Screening by ankle-brachial index (ABI) and skin perfusion pressure (SPP) Measurement. *Ren. Replace. Ther.* **2018**, *4*, 27. [CrossRef]
31. Harada, M.; Matsuzawa, R.; Aoyama, N.; Uemura, K.; Horiguchi, Y.; Yoneyama, J.; Hoshi, K.; Yoneki, K.; Watanabe, T.; Shimoda, T.; et al. Asymptomatic peripheral artery disease and mortality in patients on hemodialysis. *Ren. Replace. Ther.* **2018**, *4*, 17. [CrossRef]
32. Okamoto, K.; Oka, M.; Maesato, K.; Ikee, R.; Mano, T.; Moriya, H.; Ohtake, T.; Kobayashi, S. Peripheral arterial occlusive disease is more prevalent in patients with hemodialysis: Comparison with the findings of multidetector-row computed tomography. *Am. J. Kidney Dis.* **2006**, *48*, 269–276. [CrossRef]
33. Kumada, Y.; Nogaki, H.; Ishii, H.; Aoyama, T.; Kamoi, D.; Takahashi, H.; Murohara, T. Clinical outcome after infrapopliteal bypass surgery in chronic hemodialysis patients with critical limb ischemia. *J. Vasc. Surg.* **2015**, *61*, 400–404. [CrossRef] [PubMed]
34. Nakano, M.; Hirano, K.; Yamauchi, Y.; Iida, O.; Soga, Y.; Kawasaki, D.; Yamaoka, T.; Suemasu, N.; Suzuki, K. Three-year clinical outcome after infrapopliteal angioplasty for critical limb ischemia in hemodialysis patients with minor or major tissue loss. *Catheter. Cardiovasc. Interv.* **2015**, *86*, 289–298. [CrossRef] [PubMed]
35. Iida, O.; Soga, Y.; Kawasaki, D.; Hirano, K.; Yamaoka, T.; Suzuki, K.; Miyashita, Y.; Yokoi, H.; Takahara, M.; Uematsu, M. Angiographic restenosis and its clinical impact after infrapopliteal angioplasty. *Eur. J. Vasc. Endovasc. Surg.* **2012**, *44*, 425–431. [CrossRef] [PubMed]
36. Grooteman, M.P.C.; Nubé, M.J. Impact of the type of dialyser on the clinical outcome in chronic haemodialysis patients: Does it really matter? *Nephrol. Dial. Transplant.* **2004**, *19*, 2965–2970. [CrossRef] [PubMed]
37. Yamashita, A.C.; Sakurai, K. *Dialysis Membranes—Physicochemical Structures and Features, Updates in Hemodialysis*; IntechOpen: London, UK, 2015. [CrossRef]
38. Liangos, O.; Jaber, B.L. Dialyzer Structure and Membrane Biocompatibility. *Stud. Comput. Intell.* **2013**, *404*, 427–480.
39. Kobayashi, S.; Moriya, H.; Aso, K.; Ohtake, T. Vitamin E-bonded hemodialyzer improves atherosclerosis associated with a rheological improvement of circulating red blood cells. *Kidney Int.* **2003**, *63*, 1881–1887. [CrossRef]
40. Ronco, C.; Crepaldi, C.; Brendolan, A.; Bragantini, L.; D'Intini, V.; Inguaggiato, P.; Bonello, M.; Krause, B.; Deppisch, R.; Goehl, H.; et al. Evolution of synthetic membranes for blood purification: The case of the Polyflux family. *Nephrol. Dial. Transplant.* **2003**, *18* (Suppl. S7), vii10–vii20. [CrossRef]
41. Hoenich, N.A. Update on the biocompatibility of hemodialysis membranes. *Hong Kong J. Nephrol.* **2004**, *6*, 74–78. [CrossRef]
42. Opatrný, K., Jr. Clinical importance of biocompatibility and its effect on haemodialysis treatment. *Nephrol. Dial. Transplant.* **2003**, *18* (Suppl. S5), v41–v44. [CrossRef]
43. Thomas, M.; Moriyama, K.; Ledebo, I. AN69: Evolution of the world's first high permeability membrane. *Contrib. Nephrol.* **2011**, *173*, 119–129.
44. Moachon, N.; Boullange, C.; Fraud, S.; Vial, E.; Thomas, M.; Quash, G. Influence of the charge of low molecular weight proteins on their efficacy of filtration and/or adsorption on dialysis membranes with different intrinsic properties. *Biomaterials* **2002**, *23*, 651–658. [CrossRef]
45. Poppelaars, F.; Faria, B.; Gaya da Costa, M.; Franssen, C.F.M.; van Son, W.J.; Berger, S.P.; Daha, M.R.; Seelen, M.A. The Complement System in Dialysis: A Forgotten Story? *Front. Immunol.* **2018**, *25*, 71. [CrossRef]
46. Chenoweth, D.E. Complement activation during hemodialysis: Clinical observations, proposed mechanisms, and theoretical implications. *Artif. Organs.* **1984**, *8*, 281–290. [CrossRef] [PubMed]
47. Pascual, M.; Schifferli, J.A. Adsorption of complement factor D by polyacrylonitrile dialysis membranes. *Kidney Int.* **1993**, *43*, 903–911. [CrossRef] [PubMed]
48. Kandus, A.; Ponikvar, R.; Drinovec, J.; Kladnik, S.; Ivanovich, P. Anaphylatoxins C3a and C5a adsorption on acrylonitrile membrane of hollow-fiber and plate dialyzer–an in vivo study. *Int. J. Artif. Organs.* **1990**, *13*, 176–180. [CrossRef] [PubMed]
49. Cheung, A.K.; Chenoweth, D.E.; Otsuka, D.; Henderson, L.W. Compartmental distribution of complement activation products in artificial kidneys. *Kidney Int.* **1986**, *30*, 74–80. [CrossRef]
50. Herbelin, A.; Nguyen, A.T.; Urena, P.; Descamps-Latscha, B. Induction of cytokines by dialysis membranes in normal whole blood: A new in vitro assay for evaluating membrane biocompatibility. *Blood Purif.* **1992**, *10*, 40–52. [CrossRef]
51. Carracedo, J.; Ramírez, R.; Martin-Malo, A.; Rodríguez, M.; Aljama, P. Nonbiocompatible hemodialysis membranes induce apoptosis in mononuclear cells: The role of G-proteins. *J. Am. Soc. Nephrol.* **1998**, *9*, 46–53. [CrossRef]
52. Stuard, S.; Carreno, M.P.; Poignet, J.L.; Albertazzi, A.; Haeffner-Cavaillon, N. A major role for CD62P/CD15s interaction in leukocyte margination during hemodialysis. *Kidney Int.* **1995**, *48*, 93–102. [CrossRef]
53. Evans, R.C.; Holmes, C.J. In vitro study of the transfer of cytokine-inducing substances across selected high-flux hemodialysis membranes. *Blood Purif.* **1991**, *9*, 92–101. [CrossRef] [PubMed]
54. Laude-Sharp, M.; Caroff, M.; Simard, L.; Pusineri, C.; Kazatchkine, M.D.; Haeffner-Cavaillon, N. Induction of IL-1 during hemodialysis: Transmembrane passage of intact endotoxins (LPS). *Kidney Int.* **1990**, *38*, 1089–1094. [CrossRef] [PubMed]

55. Hattori, N.; Oda, S. Cytokine-adsorbing hemofilter: Old but new modality for septic acute kidney injury. *Ren. Replace. Ther.* **2016**, *2*, 41. [CrossRef]
56. Yamada, H.; Ohtsuru, S. Blood purification could tackle COVID-19? *J. Intensive Care* **2021**, *9*, 74. [CrossRef] [PubMed]
57. Schwindenhammer, V.; Girardot, T.; Chaulier, K.; Grégoire, A.; Monard, C.; Huriaux, L.; Illinger, J.; Leray, V.; Uberti, T.; Crozon-Clauzel, J.; et al. oXiris use in septic shock: Experience of two French centres. *Blood Purif.* **2019**, *47* (Suppl. S3), 29–35. [CrossRef] [PubMed]
58. Zhang, H.; Zhu, G.; Yan, L.; Lu, Y.; Fang, Q.; Shao, F. The adsorbing filter Oxiris in severe coronavirus disease 2019 patients: A case series. *Artif. Organs.* **2020**, *44*, 1296–1302. [CrossRef]
59. Peerapornratana, S.; Sirivongrangson, P.; Tungsanga, S.; Tiankanon, K.; Kulvichit, W.; Putcharoen, O.; Kellum, J.A.; Srisawat, N. Endotoxin adsorbent therapy in severe COVID-19 pneumonia. *Blood Purif.* **2022**, *51*, 47–54. [CrossRef]
60. Villa, G.; Romagnoli, S.; De Rosa, S.; Greco, M.; Resta, M.; Montin, D.P.; Prato, F.; Patera, F.; Ferrari, F.; Rotongo, G.; et al. Blood purification therapy with a hemofilter featured enhanced adsorptive properties for cytokine removal in patients presenting COVID-19: A pilot study. *Crit. Care* **2020**, *24*, 605. [CrossRef]
61. Liakopoulos, V.; Roumeliotis, S.; Zarogiannis, S.; Eleftheriadis, T.; Mertens, P.R. Oxidative stress in hemodialysis: Causative mechanisms, clinical implications, and possible therapeutic interventions. *Semin. Dial.* **2019**, *32*, 58–71. [CrossRef]
62. Witko-Sarsat, V.; Friedlander, M.; Capeillère-Blandin, C.; Nguyen-Khoa, T.; Nguyen, A.T.; Zingraff, J.; Jungers, P.; Descamps-Latscha, B. Advanced oxidation protein products as a novel marker of oxidative stress in uremia. *Kidney Int.* **1996**, *49*, 1304–1313. [CrossRef] [PubMed]
63. Biasioli, S.; Schiavon, R.; Petrosino, L.; Cavallini, L.; Cavalcanti, G.; De Fanti, E. Dialysis kinetics of homocysteine and reactive oxygen species. *ASAIO J.* **1998**, *44*, M423-32. [CrossRef] [PubMed]
64. Jadoul, M.; Ueda, Y.; Yasuda, Y.; Saito, A.; Robert, A.; Ishida, N.; Kurokawa, K.; Van Ypersele De Strihou, C.; Miyata, T. Influence of hemodialysis membrane type on pentosidine plasma level, a marker of "carbonyl stress". *Kidney Int.* **1999**, *55*, 2487–2492. [CrossRef] [PubMed]
65. Hörl, W.H. Hemodialysis membranes: Interleukins, biocompatibility, and middle molecules. *J. Am. Soc. Nephrol.* **2002**, *13* (Suppl. S1), S62–S71. [PubMed]
66. Brouillard, M.; Reade, R.; Boulanger, E.; Cardon, G.; Dracon, M.; Dequiedt, P.; Pagniez, D. Erythrocyte sedimentation rate, an underestimated tool in chronic renal failure. *Nephrol. Dial. Transplant.* **1996**, *11*, 2244–2247. [CrossRef] [PubMed]
67. Désormeaux, A.; Moreau, M.E.; Lepage, Y.; Chanard, J.; Adam, A. The effect of electronegativity and angiotensin-converting enzyme inhibition on the kinin-forming capacity of polyacrylonitrile dialysis membranes. *Biomaterials* **2008**, *29*, 1139–1146. [CrossRef]
68. Verresen, L.; Fink, E.; Lemke, H.D.; Vanrenterghem, Y. Bradykinin is a mediator of anaphylactoid reactions during hemodialysis with AN69 membranes. *Kidney Int.* **1994**, *45*, 1497–1503. [CrossRef]
69. Coppo, R.; Amore, A.; Cirina, P.; Scelfo, B.; Giacchino, F.; Comune, L.; Atti, M.; Renaux, J.L. Bradykinin and nitric oxide generation by dialysis membranes can be blunted by alkaline rinsing solutions. *Kidney Int.* **2000**, *58*, 881–888. [CrossRef]
70. Saracho, R.; Martin-Malo, A.; Martinez, I.; Aljama, P.; Montenegro, J. Evaluation of the Losartan in Hemodialysis (ELHE) study. *Kidney Int. Suppl.* **1998**, *68*, S125–S129. [CrossRef]
71. Thomas, M.; Valette, P.; Mausset, A.L.; Déjardin, P. High molecular weight kininogen adsorption on hemodialysis membranes: Influence of pH and relationship with contact phase activation of blood plasma. influence of pre-treatment with poly(ethyleneimine). *Int. J. Artif. Organs.* **2000**, *23*, 20–26. [CrossRef]
72. Authors/Task Force Members; ESC committee for practice guidelines (CPG); ESC national cardiac societies: 2019 ESC/EAS guidelines for the management of dyslipidaemias: Lipid modification to reduce cardiovascular risk. *Atherosclerosis* **2019**, *290*, 140–205. [CrossRef] [PubMed]
73. Wang, A.; Richhariya, A.; Gandra, S.R.; Calimlim, B.; Kim, L.; Quek, R.G.W.; Nordyke, R.J.; Toth, P.P. Systematic review of low-density lipoprotein cholesterol apheresis for the treatment of familial hypercholesterolemia. *J. Am. Heart Assoc.* **2016**, *5*, e003294. [CrossRef] [PubMed]
74. Kobayashi, S. Applications of LDL-apheresis in nephrology. *Clin. Exp. Nephrol.* **2008**, *12*, 9–15. [CrossRef] [PubMed]
75. Varga, V.E.; Lőrincz, H.; Zsíros, N.; Fülöp, P.; Seres, I.; Paragh, G.; Balla, J.; Harangi, M. Impact of selective LDL apheresis on serum chemerin levels in patients with hypercholesterolemia. *Lipids. Health Dis.* **2016**, *15*, 182. [CrossRef] [PubMed]
76. Hara, T.; Kiyomoto, H.; Hitomi, H.; Moriwaki, K.; Ihara, G.; Kaifu, K.; Fujita, H.; Higashiyama, C.; Nishiyama, A.; Kohno, M. Low-density lipoprotein apheresis for haemodialysis patients with peripheral arterial disease reduces reactive oxygen species production via suppression of NADPH oxidase gene expression in leucocytes. *Nephrol. Dial. Transplant.* **2009**, *24*, 3818–3825. [CrossRef] [PubMed]
77. Krieter, D.H.; Steinke, J.; Kerkhoff, M.; Fink, E.; Lemke, H.D.; Zingler, C.; Müller, G.A.; Schuff-Werner, P. Contact activation in low-density lipoprotein apheresis systems. *Artif. Organs.* **2005**, *29*, 47–52. [CrossRef]
78. Furuta, M.; Kuragano, T.; Kida, A.; Kitamura, R.; Nanami, M.; Otaki, Y.; Nonoguchi, H.; Matsumoto, A.; Nakanishi, T. A crossover study of the acrylonitrile-co-methallyl sulfonate and polysulfone membranes for elderly hemodialysis patients: The effect on hemodynamic, nutritional, and inflammatory conditions. *ASAIO J.* **2011**, *57*, 293–299. [CrossRef]
79. Nakada, H.; Kashiwagi, T.; Iino, Y.; Katayama, Y. Therapeutic effects of the long-term use of PAN membrane dialyzer in hemodialysis patients: Efficacy in old dialysis patients with mild PAD. *J. Nippon. Med. Sch.* **2014**, *81*, 221–235. [CrossRef]

80. Yokomatsu, A.; Fujikawa, T.; Toya, Y.; Shino-Kakimoto, M.; Itoh, Y.; Mitsuhashi, H.; Tamura, K.; Hirawa, N.; Yasuda, G.; Umemura, S. Loss of amino acids into dialysate during hemodialysis using hydrophilic and nonhydrophilic polyester-polymer alloy and polyacrylonitrile membrane dialyzers. *Ther. Apher. Dial.* **2014**, *18*, 340–346. [CrossRef]
81. Kuragano, T.; Furuta, M.; Shimonaka, Y.; Kida, A.; Yahiro, M.; Otaki, Y.; Hasuike, Y.; Matsumoto, A.; Nakanishi, T. The removal of serum hepcidin by different dialysis membranes. *Int. J. Artif. Organs.* **2013**, *36*, 633–639. [CrossRef]
82. Iatrou, C.; Afentakis, N.; Nomikos, T.; Dinas, C.; Stavropoulos-Giokas, C.; Antonopoulou, S. Is platelet-activating factor produced during hemodialysis with AN-69 polyacrylonitrile membrane? *Nephron* **2002**, *91*, 86–93.
83. Chandran, P.K.; Liggett, R.; Kirkpatrick, B. Patient survival on PAN/AN69 membrane hemodialysis: A ten-year analysis. *J. Am. Soc. Nephrol.* **1993**, *4*, 1199–1204. [CrossRef] [PubMed]
84. Babitt, J.L.; Eisenga, M.F.; Haase, V.H.; Kshirsagar, A.V.; Levin, A.; Locatelli, F.; Małyszko, J.; Swinkels, D.W.; Tarng, D.-C.; Cheung, M.; et al. Controversies in optimal anemia management: Conclusions from a Kidney Disease: Improving Global Outcomes (KDIGO) conference. *Kidney Int.* **2021**, *99*, 1280–1295. [CrossRef] [PubMed]

Disclaimer/Publisher's Note: The statements, opinions and data contained in all publications are solely those of the individual author(s) and contributor(s) and not of MDPI and/or the editor(s). MDPI and/or the editor(s) disclaim responsibility for any injury to people or property resulting from any ideas, methods, instructions or products referred to in the content.

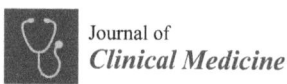
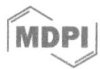

Review

Displacing the Burden: A Review of Protein-Bound Uremic Toxin Clearance Strategies in Chronic Kidney Disease

Didier Sánchez-Ospina [1,†], Sebastián Mas-Fontao [2,3,4,†], Carolina Gracia-Iguacel [5], Alejandro Avello [5], Marina González de Rivera [5], Maddalen Mujika-Marticorena [1] and Emilio Gonzalez-Parra [2,5,*]

1. Servicio Análisis Clínicos, Hospital Universitario de Burgos, 09006 Burgos, Spain; sliverco41@gmail.com (D.S.-O.); mmujika@saludcastillayleon.es (M.M.-M.)
2. IIS-Fundación Jiménez Díaz, 28040 Madrid, Spain; smas@fjd.es
3. Centro de Investigación Biomédica en Red de Diabetes y Enfermedades Metabólicas Asociadas (CIBERDEM), 28029 Madrid, Spain
4. Faculty of Medicine and Biomedicine, Universidad Alfonso X el Sabio (UAX), 28037 Madrid, Spain
5. Department of Nephrology and Hypertension, IIS-Fundación Jiménez Díaz, Univerdad Autonoma de madrid, 28049 Madrid, Spain; cgraciai@quironsalud.es (C.G.-I.); alejandro.avello@quironsalud.es (A.A.); marina.grivera@fjd.es (M.G.d.R.)
* Correspondence: egonzalezspa@senefro.org
† These authors contributed equally to this work.

Abstract: Uremic toxins (UTs), particularly protein-bound uremic toxins (PBUTs), accumulate in chronic kidney disease (CKD) patients, causing significant health complications like uremic syndrome, cardiovascular disease, and immune dysfunction. The binding of PBUTs to plasma proteins such as albumin presents a formidable challenge for clearance, as conventional dialysis is often insufficient. With advancements in the classification and understanding of UTs, spearheaded by the European Uremic Toxins (EUTox) working group, over 120 molecules have been identified, prompting the development of alternative therapeutic strategies. Innovations such as online hemodiafiltration aim to enhance the removal process, while novel adsorptive therapies offer a means to address the high affinity of PBUTs to plasma proteins. Furthermore, the exploration of molecular displacers, designed to increase the free fraction of PBUTs, represents a cutting-edge approach to facilitate their dialytic clearance. Despite these advancements, the clinical application of displacers requires more research to confirm their efficacy and safety. The pursuit of such innovative treatments is crucial for improving the management of uremic toxicity and the overall prognosis of CKD patients, emphasizing the need for ongoing research and clinical trials.

Keywords: chronic kidney disease; uremic toxins; protein-bound uremic toxins; adsorptive therapies; molecular displacers

1. Introduction

Chronic kidney disease (CKD), a global health challenge, impacts an estimated 10–15% of the world's population [1]. In 2017, around 843.6 million individuals were affected, as recent studies on the global CKD prevalence indicate [2]. This rise is partly attributed to the increased incidence of diabetes, hypertension, obesity, and aging populations [3], alongside improved access to renal replacement therapies in economically developing nations [4].

CKD stages are independently linked to heightened cardiovascular event risks, decreased quality-adjusted life years, and high morbidity and mortality rates. From 1990 to 2017, the CKD-related global mortality surged by 41.5%, ranking it as the 12th leading death cause worldwide [5]. By 2040, it is projected to become the 5th leading cause of global mortality [6].

One CKD consequence is the gradual decline of glomerular filtration, leading to metabolic waste product accumulation in the bloodstream, known as uremic toxins (UTs).

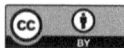

These toxins are associated with the uremic syndrome, presenting symptoms like nausea, vomiting, asthenia, anorexia, and pruritus due to their detrimental pathophysiological effects [7].

2. Definition and Classification of Uremic Toxins

Definition of Uremic Toxins: Uremic toxins (UTs), pivotal to the pathology of chronic kidney disease (CKD), are metabolic by-products typically excreted by healthy kidneys. In CKD, however, diminished glomerular filtration, particularly at rates below 60 mL/min/ 1.73 m^2, results in their accrual in the bloodstream. UTs emerge from diverse origins, including the degradation of endogenous and bacterial proteins and the consumption of certain foods [8]. The complex pathophysiological mechanisms they trigger include inflammation, oxidative stress, cellular trans-differentiation, mitochondrial dysfunction, intestinal barrier impairment, and gut microbiota alterations [9,10].

In 1999, the European Uremic Toxins (EUTox) working group, spearheaded by Vanholder and colleagues, established a classical definition and classification of UTs. This definition, recently scrutinized for its breadth and precision, laid out five criteria for classifying an organic solute as a uremic toxin:

(a) Chemical Identification and Analysis: The compound must be chemically identifiable, with quantitative analysis feasible in biological fluids.
(b) Elevated Levels in Uremia: The total and plasma levels should be higher in uremic subjects than in non-uremic individuals.
(c) Clinical Relevance: Elevated concentrations should correlate with specific uremic dysfunctions and/or symptoms that decrease or disappear when the concentration is reduced.
(d) Biological Activity: There must be evidence of biological activity, consistent with clinical changes observed in uremic syndrome, demonstrated in in vivo, ex vivo, or in vitro studies.
(e) Concentration Consistency: Concentrations in these studies should reflect those found in bodily fluids or tissues of uremic patients.

In 2003, EUTox introduced a UT classification based on the physicochemical properties influencing their clearance during conventional hemodialysis [11]:

- Small Hydrophilic Toxins (<500 Da): These include compounds like urea (60 Da) and uric acid. Conventional hemodialysis effectively removes them using diffusion as the primary transport mechanism [12].
- Medium-Sized Toxins (≥500 Da): Examples are β2 microglobulin (11.8 kDa) and parathyroid hormone (9.5 kDa). While convective transport can remove some of these toxins, their size hinders efficient elimination [13].
- Protein-Bound Toxins (PBUTs): This category encompasses molecules with low molecular weight, such as indoxyl sulfate and p-cresyl sulfate, which exhibit more than 80% plasma protein binding. Despite their inherently low molecular weight, clearance is negatively affected due to the lower concentration of unbound toxin at the dialysate side surface of the membrane.

The expanding knowledge of UTs, with over 120 molecules identified to date [14], coupled with advancements in hemodialysis techniques, has necessitated a re-evaluation of the definition and classification of uremic retention solutes [15]. The prior classification's limitations, such as the inaccuracy in capturing the variable protein binding of uremic solutes and its application solely to conventional hemodialysis, are now being addressed. This re-examination considers factors like solute compartmentalization within the body and alternative strategies for uremia reduction, such as preserving residual renal function and employing adsorption and convection techniques. Some of the most relevant PBUTs for dialysis adequacy are shown in Table 1.

Table 1. Albumin-binding percentages of common protein-bound uremic toxins (PBUTs) (adapted from Shi et al. [16]).

Uremic Toxin	Albumin Binding %
Indoxyl Sulfate (IS)	90–95%
p-Cresyl Sulfate (pCS)	90–95%
Hippuric Acid (HA)	>40%
Indole-3-Acetic (IAA)	>30%
3-Carboxy-4-Methyl-5-Propyl-2-Furanpropionate (CMPF)	>40%

3. Protein-Bound Toxins: Main Types and Molecular Weight

Characteristics of Protein-Bound Uremic Toxins (PBUTs): Protein-bound uremic toxins (PBUTs) are a distinct class of toxins characterized by their strong affinity to plasma proteins, particularly albumin. This binding complicates their elimination via conventional dialysis techniques. The European Group for the study of Uremic Toxins (EUTox) recognized 25 PBUTs in 2003 [11], further categorizing them based on their originating compounds into groups like phenols, indoles, hippurates, polyamines, advanced glycation end products (AGEs), and peptides or small and medium-sized proteins, including leptin and retinol-binding protein. The binding affinity of these toxins for albumin varies, with indoxyl sulfate (IS), 3-carboxy-4-methyl-5-propyl-2-furanpropanoic acid (CMPF), p-cresyl sulfate, hippuric acid, and indoleacetic acid exhibiting the highest affinity.

Formation and Elimination: The genesis of PBUTs primarily occurs in the intestine, where dietary proteins undergo metabolism by the intestinal microbiota, producing precursors that later form toxins. This intestinal origin underscores the increasing importance of studying the gut microbiome in preventing renal disease [17]. The plasma levels of PBUTs consist of the free fraction and the protein-bound fraction, with the toxicity largely attributed to the free fraction. This aspect becomes particularly significant in malnourished patients with hypoalbuminemia, as they exhibit a higher concentration of the free fraction, leading to more severe uremic symptoms.

Molecular Weight and Protein-Binding Considerations: PBUTs typically have a molecular weight under 500 Da. However, their protein binding confers them with an effectively larger molecular size. Notably, the peptide group among PBUTs, including leptin and retinol-binding protein, exhibits significantly higher molecular weights of 16,000 Da and 21,200 Da, respectively.

Being the most abundant plasma protein, albumin plays a crucial role in binding various compounds, including uremic toxins and drugs, due to its two binding sites for toxins: one high-affinity site and one low-affinity site and specificities [18]. It has multiple binding sites that can interact with uremic toxins, including at least two drug-binding sites [19]. The most studied binding sites, known as site I and site II, have been identified for their ability to bind a variety of drugs and metabolites [20]. Additionally, modeling suggests that albumin contains two binding sites for toxins, a single high-affinity site and a second low-affinity site [21] (Figure 1).

Affinity and Specificity: Interactions between albumin and toxins can be hydrophobic, electrostatic, or through hydrogen bonding. Studies have also shown that albumin has specific binding sites for anionic, neutral, and cationic ligands, indicating its versatility in binding different types of compounds [22]. The nature and strength of these interactions depend on the chemical structure of the toxin and the physiological conditions, such as the pH and the presence of other ligands. Several factors can influence albumin's ability to bind uremic toxins:

(a) Post-Translational Modifications: Glycation, oxidation, and other changes in albumin can alter its structure and, therefore, its binding capacity. In patients with chronic kidney disease, these modifications are more common and can affect albumin's transport function [20].

(b) Competition with Other Molecules: The presence of drugs and other metabolites in plasma may compete with uremic toxins for binding sites on albumin, affecting its ability to neutralize these toxins [23,24].
(c) Changes in pH and Electrolytes: Variations in the blood pH and electrolyte levels, common in patients with renal insufficiency, can modify albumin's structure and its affinity for uremic toxins. Albumin's spatial structures are sensitive to changes in the acid–base balance, common in patients with renal insufficiency, and their tertiary structures change considerably with pH variations [25,26].

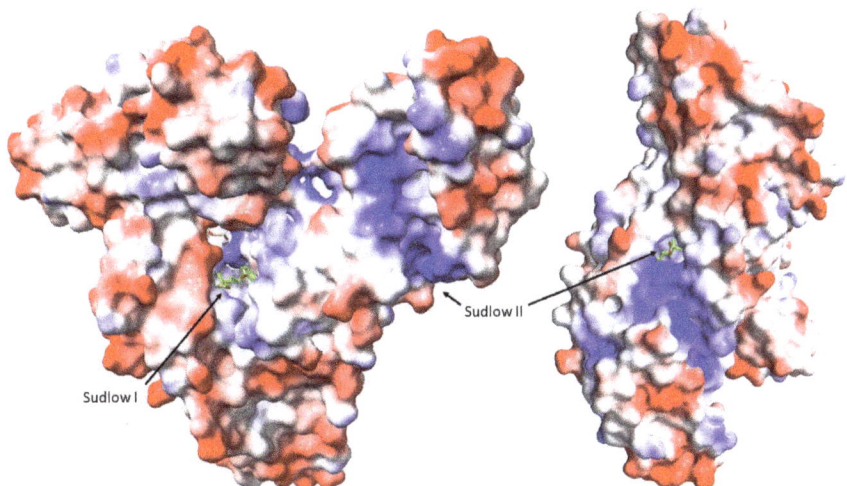

Figure 1. Location of Sudlow sites I and II (black arrows) on a human albumin molecule complexed with Gemfibrozil (PDB ID: 7QFE) [27], depicted using Coulombic electrostatic potential (ESP) color coding (coloring gradient that spans from red, indicating negative potential to blue, signifying positive potential) in ChimeraX.

4. Effects of Protein-Bound Uremic Toxins

Protein-bound uremic toxins (PBUTs) are not merely waste products; their accumulation in chronic kidney disease (CKD) can lead to a range of systemic effects. These toxins, particularly notorious for their harmful influence on various tissues, significantly impact the cardiovascular system. Studies have elucidated the multifaceted roles of PBUTs in instigating renal fibrosis, vascular calcification, anemia, peripheral arterial disease, adynamic bone disease, insulin resistance, malnutrition, and immune system deficiency [7,28].

- Endothelial Dysfunction: Endothelial dysfunction caused by PBUTs is closely related to the development of cardiovascular diseases in patients with chronic kidney disease. PBUTs can cause structural damage, inflammation, and a decrease in endothelium-dependent vasodilation [29,30]. Furthermore, endothelial dysfunction is associated with the progression of chronic kidney disease and albuminuria [31]. Patients undergoing dialysis for chronic kidney disease exhibit a markedly diminished endothelial response to stimuli when compared to a control group of healthy individuals. This reduced response is evident across various assessment parameters, including both shear stress and biochemical agents, indicative of compromised endothelial function [32]. PBUTs can decrease nitric oxide production in endothelial cells by inhibiting endothelial nitric oxide synthase (eNOS) activity and expression [33]. PBUTs, like indoxyl sulfate, act as prooxidant and proinflammatory agents, which are associated with changes in the hemostatic system, increased oxidative stress, and monocyte activation. Additionally, this leads to a prothrombotic state through the activation of prothrombotic factors such as tissue factor and factor Xa [34], and the formation of endothelial microparticles.

High levels of indoxyl sulfate (IS) and p-cresol sulfate (PCS) in the serum have been used to predict cardiovascular events and are also implicated in vascular disease, including arteriosclerosis, endothelial inflammation, oxidative stress, and vascular calcification [35].

Most cardiovascular complications associated with chronic kidney disease are secondary to the activation of prooxidative/inflammatory pathways through human AhR activation. PBUTs have been recognized as endogenous agonists of AhR [36]. The aryl hydrocarbon receptor (AhR) is a transcription factor found in the cell's cytoplasm in its inactive form. It has been demonstrated that AhR is more stimulated in stage 3 chronic kidney disease patients, directly associated with higher IS levels and inversely proportional to epidermal growth factor receptor (EGFR) levels [37].

- Prooxidant and Proinflammatory Actions: Indoxyl sulfate acts as both a prooxidant and proinflammatory agent, linked with changes in the hemostatic system, increased oxidative stress, and monocyte activation. This leads to a prothrombotic state through the activation of prothrombotic factors such as tissue factor and factor Xa [34], and the formation of endothelial microparticles.
- Cardiorenal Syndrome: The accumulation of PBUTs, particularly IS, in cardiomyocytes is linked to increased production of inflammatory cytokines such as IL1, IL6, and TNF-α [38]. These toxins have been associated with pro-arrhythmogenic effects and atrial fibrillation [35]. Studies have also noted structural and functional changes in cardiomyocytes, including reduced spontaneous contraction and irregularity, following exposure to toxins like p-cresol sulfate (PCS) [39].
- Immune System Dysfunction: Patients with chronic kidney disease present immune system dysfunction due to various causes, such as the dialysis process, vitamin D deficiency, and a sustained systemic inflammatory state due to elevated PBUT, which can alter the innate immune response [40]. Among the main PBUTs related to immune system activation are IS, PCS, and p-cresyl glucuronide, among the most well-known [41,42].

IS acts as a prooxidant and proinflammatory agent, triggering immune responses and stimulating chronic kidney disease progression. Increased plasma IS has been associated with changes in the coagulation cascade, increased oxidative stress, and monocyte activation [43]. This molecule shows a positive correlation with neopterin, a molecule generated by macrophages and monocytes after being stimulated by IFN-gamma produced by activated T cells. As a result, a high production of reactive oxygen species (ROS) and an increase in the expression of cell adhesion molecules (CAM) can be observed, promoting monocyte–endothelial cell interaction, leading to vascular inflammation and endothelial dysfunction. PBUTs affect both the innate and adaptive immune systems through multiple mechanisms, resulting in the development of systemic pathologies in humans, highlighting the importance of studying them, and advancements in this field would greatly improve the clinical management of these patients.

Kidney

Accumulation of indoxyl sulfate (IS) can lead to the deterioration of the remaining renal nephrons, primarily within proximal tubular cells, thereby stimulating glomerulosclerosis, renal fibrosis, and the progression of chronic kidney disease (CKD). This process contributes to an increased expression of pro-collagen alpha 1, transforming growth factor beta 1 (TGF-β1), and tissue inhibitor of metalloproteinase 1 (TIMP-1) genes, resulting in further nephron loss and thereby accelerating CKD progression [44]

There is evidence that elevated levels of p-cresyl sulfate (PCS) in the kidneys lead to increased expression of proinflammatory cytokines and genes in renal tubular cells, along with activation of the renin–angiotensin–aldosterone system (RAAS) and epithelial–mesenchymal transition, culminating in fibrosis and nephrosclerosis [45]. Moreover, elevated PCS levels are associated with reduced Klotho expression through methylation of the Klotho gene, contributing to renal cell senescence [46].

5. PBUT Clearance Strategies

Conventional dialysis remains the primary treatment modality for patients with end-stage chronic kidney disease (CKD). Nevertheless, the effective removal of protein-bound uremic toxins (PBUTs) presents a significant challenge in these patients, attributed to their high affinity for protein binding. This limitation is not adequately addressed by current conventional methods. There is a scarcity of long-term evidence, as most efforts to enhance the clearance of these toxins remain experimental. Furthermore, regarding the techniques currently employed, such as prolonged and frequent dialysis, there are no comprehensive studies that evaluate the long-term outcomes of PBUT removal in comparison to other techniques [47].

5.1. Conventional Dialysis Efficacy on Protein-Bound Uremic Toxins (PBUTs)

Conventional dialysis methods, including hemodialysis and peritoneal dialysis, have not been proven effective in significantly reducing the levels of PBUTs [48,49]. When focusing on protein-bound toxins, it becomes evident that they play a critical role in patients undergoing dialysis due to the inability of the dialysis membrane to filter them effectively. Various studies have focused on this issue, adopting different approaches [50]. Although advancements in membrane technology and purification techniques have shown varying degrees of success in decreasing the free fraction of certain toxins, the clinical significance of these reductions remains under active investigation. Some membranes, especially those with high sieving coefficients, have been promising in enhancing toxin purification. However, their overall efficacy varies depending on the toxin type and clinical scenario, see Table 2 [51].

Table 2. Efficacy of different clearance strategies for protein-bound uremic toxins (PBUTs), comparing dialysis techniques, the role of residual renal function, online hemodiafiltration, expanded hemodialysis, and adsorptive therapies. IS, indoxyl sulfate; p-CS, p-cresyl sulfate; HA, hippuric acid; IAA, indole acetic acid.

Clearance Strategy	Tested PBUT	Clearance Efficiency	Clinical Effects and Conclusions	Ref.
		Dialysis Techniques		
Convectional HD	pCS and IS	Less than 50%	Alternative strategies promise to be more efficient	[48]
	pCS, IS and CMPF	29%, 32% and 0%, respectively		[49]
	pCS, IS and inorganic phosphate	No significant clearance	Need to focus on different approaches	[50]
Prolonged Convectional HD	pCS, IS, IAA, CMPF and HA	IAA, IS and pCS at the borderline of significance		[47]
	pCS	Significantly less than other soluble molecules	Convection can provide superior protein-bound solute removal compared with high-flux HD	[52]
Residual Renal Function	IS, pCS, IAA, HA, p-cresyl glucuronide, kynurenine, kynurenic acid	Only IS decreased by 8.0%	RRF is an important determinant of PBUT plasma concentrations in HD patients	[53]
	pCS and IS	1.7% and 2%, respectively	The implementation of theOWHD plus LPD strategy may be useful for lowering PBUTs	[54]
	IS, pCS, HA and phenylacetylglutamine	Significantly less than the rates of urea and creatinine	An increase in treatment frequency would be required to significantly reduce the plasma levels of PBUTs	[55]
Online HDF	pCS and IS	Free IS and free and total pCS remained unaltered	Current HDF techniques have only limited impact on IS and pCS plasma levels in the short and also long term	[56]

Table 2. Cont.

Clearance Strategy	Tested PBUT	Clearance Efficiency	Clinical Effects and Conclusions	Ref.
Expanded HD	IS and pCS	No statistically significant clearance	The clearance did not differ between the HF-HD, post-OL-HDF, and MCO-HD	[57]
	pCS and IS	No statistically significant clearance		[58]
Adsorptive Therapies				
Oral absorbents (AST-120)	IS	Dose dependent decreased levels	To determine whether this effect can attenuate the progression of CKD	[59]
	pCS, IS and phenyl sulfate	Reduction of IS (total 45.7%; free 70.4%) pCS (total 31.1%: free, 63.5%) and phenyl sulfate (free 50.6%)	AST-120 has additive effects on the continuous reduction of some PBUTs in anuric patients in HD	[60]
Activated charcoal	pCS and IS	Increase in the clearance of protein-bound solutes without altering the clearance of unbound solutes	Increasing the dialysate flow without the addition of sorbent, had a similar effect	[61]
Hexadecyl-immobilized cellulose bead (HICB)	IS, pCS, IAA and phenyl sulfate	34% decrease in free form, no change in total	Need to develop more effective materials to adsorb PBUTs selectively	[62]
Ordered nanoporous adsorbent material (CMK-3 type)	IS and HA	Significant reduction in the free form but not the total form	The IS removal is slightly lower than the corresponding one for HA	[63]
Divinylbenzene-polyvinylpyrrolidone (DVB-PVP)	IS and pCS	In vitro 54% IS and 56% PCS, In vivo efficient only for IS plasma levels	Symbiotic treatment with DVB-PVP HD decreased IS and pCS; this study provides the first line of evidence on the synergistic action of gut microbiota modulation and an absorption-based approach	[64]

It appears that no membrane or technique, regardless of its high sieving coefficient, has been able to adequately purify these toxins. They may demonstrate a reduction in the free fraction, but this represents a very modest clinical impact, as the free fraction constitutes a minimal portion of the total toxin amount. However, the use of albumin in dialysate, by promoting binding with a high flow, demonstrates that standard dialysis membranes are not the limiting factor due to the low molecular weights of PBUTs but rather its protein binding [51].

In recent years, the clearance profiles of state-of-the-art hemodialysis membranes have seen significant improvements. Several characteristics must be considered in the evaluation of new membranes. These include new permeability rates, the hydrophilic or hydrophobic nature of the membranes, adsorption capacity, and electrical potential [65]. Additionally, the onset of molecular weight retention, molecular weight limit, and mass transfer area coefficient must be measured [66].

Conventional dialysis poorly clears them because only the free solute portion contributes to the concentration gradient that drives their diffusion from plasma to dialysate. The extent to which protein binding limits the removal of PBUTs depends on multiple factors, including the dialyzer size, dialysate flow, and the strength of the protein binding itself. Despite the rapid dissociation of PBUTs from albumin, studies by T. Meyer demonstrate that significantly increasing the dialysate flow with standard dialyzers can approximately quadruple the PBUT removal [51].

5.2. Conventional Dialysis: Importance of Dialysis Time

One of the most crucial factors in the efficacy of uremic toxin elimination is the dialysis time. The duration of the dialysis session is a critical determinant to ensure adequate clearance. Generally, longer dialysis sessions allow for more effective removal of PBUTs [67]. The reason is that the small-sized free fraction is cleared, balancing with the albumin-bound fraction released from anchoring to maintain the free fraction ratio. The longer the hemodialysis (HD) session, the progressively more free fraction is cleared. The clearance is the same per minute but is more constant and frequent [47]. Dissociation of the protein-bound form requires time; a conventional dialysis session is too short to prevent the new equilibrium of PBUTs strongly bound to albumin [68]. But to drive this transfer, what is needed is merely more clearance of the free fraction of the PBUTs within the dialyzer (as with more frequent dialysis with the same blood, more time on dialysis, or increasing the dialysate flow). PBUTs' clearance increases when the free form is removed in long conventional dialysis, while it does not change with extended convective dialysis [52]. Association/dissociation of PBUTs and albumin happens during the time of blood passing through a hollow fiber dialyzer, when a strong chemical gradient is promoted by a rapid dialysate flow.

Prolonging the HD time through extended nocturnal HD removes a larger amount of PBUTs. Cornelis et al. observed higher PCS and IS clearance in long nocturnal dialysis, although the plasma concentrations did not change when the HD duration increased from 4 to 8 h [69]. Much of the problem is also in the slow diffusive transfer of PBUTs and mid-large dialysate toxins from cells to interstitium to blood. Long dialysis also provides time for this transfer [70].

5.3. Importance of Residual Renal Function

Residual renal function is important in reducing PBUTs [53,54]. The native kidney eliminates PBUTs mainly as free forms, while the total forms of IS and pCS are eliminated only 2% and 1.7%, respectively. Dialysis clears the total forms similarly to the native kidney, while it clears only 20–30% of free forms compared to the native kidney [55].

5.4. Online Hemodiafiltration: Role of Convection

Convection increases the elimination of uremic toxins during dialysis, especially medium- or large-sized ones [71]. However, PBUTs' clearance with convective techniques has not shown conclusive data on their efficacy. One study demonstrated a lower pCS concentration and higher elimination in predilutional 60 L online hemodiafiltration compared to postdilutional 20 L. In addition to free PBUTs, small-sized toxins, including urea and creatinine, are better eliminated in predilutional HDF than postdilutional [52]. However, another study showed a greater reduction in both free and protein-bound PBUTs in postdilutional online HDF [56].

5.5. Expanded HD

Medium cutoff (MCO) dialyzers, also known as expanded dialysis, cannot increase PBUT elimination [57,58].

5.6. Adsorptive Therapies

Adsorptive therapies represent an innovative strategy for addressing uremic toxin removal in CKD patients. Despite their effectiveness, technical complications such as cost, biocompatibility and material saturation limit their use (Table 2).

These therapies rely on the ability of certain adsorbent materials to selectively capture PBUTs from the bloodstream, not only the free fraction but also the protein-bound fraction, due to their high affinity for these molecules [72].

The mechanism of action involves the interaction between PBUTs and adsorbent materials. When the patient's blood or dialysate flows through an adsorptive therapy device, uremic toxins bind to the adsorbent surface due to chemical and physical forces. Once bound, they do not detach, causing material saturation depending on the surface. Activated carbon's high adsorption capacity and other adsorbent materials have led to a significant reduction in toxin concentrations in CKD patients [73–76].

Among the adsorbent materials used is activated charcoal, which significantly improves toxin clearance when used simultaneously with conventional HD [61] or with hemo-perfusion [62]. Activated carbon has a high specific surface area and exceptional adsorptive properties [77].

Besides charcoal, many molecules, primarily celluloses or polymers, have been used. Hexadecyl chains immobilized in cellulose pores have been used simultaneously with conventional HD, resulting in a 34% decrease in the free form of IS, while the total IS barely changed [62].

CMK-3 is a silica- and carbon-based nanoporous sorbent [78]. The CMK-3 sorbent presents two different types of pores, micropores and mesopores [63], showing a high adsorption level on the free fraction of PBUTs. In another study [64] with two different resins, one with a sorbent based on divinylbenzene attached to a highly biocompatible polymer and cellulose with hexadecyl chains, showed a significant reduction in the free form rather than the total PBUTs. The difficulty in reducing the total PBUTs could be due to the constant disturbance of the balance between the free and protein-bound forms [68]. Initially, the unbound fraction undergoes elimination, resulting in a disruption of equilibrium between the bound fraction and the extravascular compartments. The dissociation does not occur until the concentration of the unbound fraction decreases, a process that unfolds gradually due to its dialysis over the course of the session. Despite the rapid dissociation capacity of albumin [79], the equilibrium is eventually restored as the bound fraction is gradually released. However, the passage of toxins from the tissue compartment to the blood is very slow and constitutes the most limiting factor. The degree of binding is related to the concentration of PBUTs around the albumin. As the unbound concentration decreases, especially below the dissociation constant level, the PBUTs have to leave the albumin. If a sorbent treatment removes free PBUTs but not the total, it is because the albumin has bound PBUTs in its course around the body. This mechanism may elucidate the augmentation in the binding percentage observed in certain studies, along with the potential modulation of equilibrium by variables such as the pH [68].

Efforts have also been directed toward enhancing this adsorption process through the application of prior plasma separation. While this method has shown promise, it is characterized by its labor-intensive and costly nature [75,76]. T. Meyer has observed that using a conventional high-permeability dialyzer and standard dialysis system provided total solute clearances of about 18 mL/min for p-cresol sulfate, and 19 mL/min for indoxyl sulfate, when dialyzing blood with these tightly bound solutes [51]. The dialyzers with a carbon-block recirculating system had clearances of about 45 mL/min for p-cresol sulfate and 61 mL/min for indoxyl sulfate when operating alone, without removing small toxins such as urea. When operated in series, the clearances of the carbon-regenerated dialysis system and regular dialysis system had clearances for PBUTs that were additive. These clearances were with standard high-permeability dialyzers, and the only change was the increase in dialysate flow rate to 1000 mL/min that is made possible by regeneration of the dialysate by an activated carbon block. So, 80% binding or even 90% is not so high that significant clearances are made impossible with standard dialysis membranes. A high dialysate flow rate maintains the gradient for removal by diminishing the dialysate concentration right at the membrane surface. Suspended charcoal particles in the dialysate can do the same thing as a very high dialysate flow rate [51]

Challenges and Future Directions of Adsorptive Therapies

Despite the promising benefits of adsorptive therapies, there are challenges that must be addressed. These include optimizing adsorbent materials, therapy duration, and managing potential side effects. Furthermore, more research is needed to fully understand the impact of these therapies on the quality of life of CKD patients [73].

6. Protein-Bound Uremic Toxin Displacers

The concept of displacing protein-bound uremic toxins (PBUTs) from their binding sites on plasma proteins, particularly albumin, offers a novel therapeutic approach in the management of chronic kidney disease (CKD). This strategy aims to increase the free fraction of these toxins, thereby facilitating their removal through dialysis.

6.1. The Role of Displacers

Displacers work by competing with PBUTs for binding sites on plasma proteins. This competition results in an increased concentration of the free, unbound fraction of the toxins, which is more amenable to dialysis clearance. Albumin, the principal transporter protein in blood plasma, has specific subdomains that bind to toxins through non-covalent bonds. The competition for these binding sites by displacers is a critical mechanism for enhancing toxin removal [80]. Figure 2 show the mechanism of displacers' action on PBUTs.

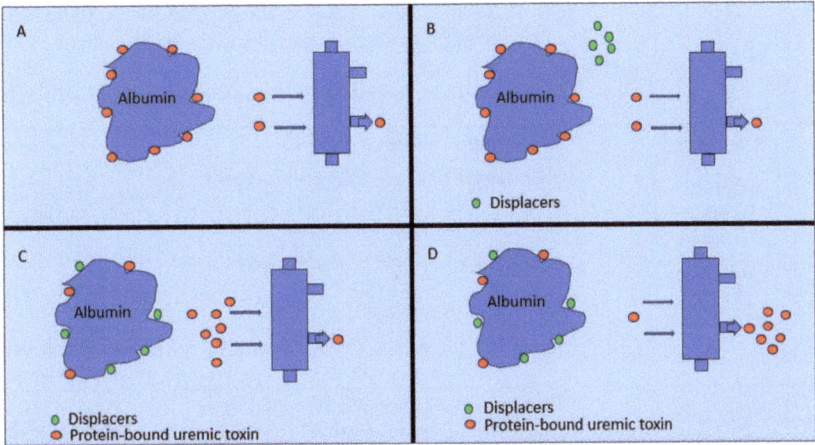

Figure 2. Mechanism of displacer action on albumin-bound uremic toxins. (**A**) Albumin (blue) with bound uremic toxins (red); (**B**) displacers (green) introduced; (**C**) displacers bind to albumin, releasing toxins; and (**D**) free uremic toxins increase post-displacement and are eliminated through hemodialysis.

6.2. The Affinity for Albumin of Uremic Toxins (UTs)

Some uremic toxins, as mentioned, exhibit a notable affinity for proteins. These toxins predominantly bind to the Sudlow sites I and II on albumin [7,81]. This characteristic plays a crucial role in their pharmacokinetics and the difficulty of their removal through conventional dialysis procedures. Other uremic toxins, such as hippuric acid (HA), indole-3-acetic acid (IAA), and 3-carboxy-4-methyl-5-propyl-2-furanpropionate (CMPF), also show affinity to albumin, albeit to a lesser extent, as depicted in Table 1.

The affinity for albumin of the various studied molecules allows for an in vitro analysis of the competition occurring at protein binding sites when these compounds are administered as shown in Table 3. This competition leads to a decrease in protein binding sites and consequently an increase in the concentration of free UTs susceptible to dialysis [82].

6.3. Major Described Displacers

- Ibuprofen: A nonsteroidal anti-inflammatory drug (NSAID) with high protein-binding capacity, ibuprofen effectively displaces PBUTs such as p-cresyl sulfate (pCS) and indoxyl sulfate (IS) from albumin. However, its long-term use poses risks like gastrointestinal and renal complications [83]. Cellulose membranes embedded with ibuprofen have been developed, which exhibit a 1.2-fold increase in the removal of protein-bound uremic toxins (PBUTs). This performance is slightly lower than that achieved with ibuprofen perfusion, yet it comes without the associated potential risks [84].

- Furosemide: This diuretic shows a high affinity for albumin and can increase the free fraction of certain UTs like hippuric acid. Combined with ibuprofen, it enhances the displacement of toxins like IS [80].
- Tryptophan: Being the precursor of IS through intestinal microbiota metabolism, tryptophan shares structural similarities with some uremic toxins. It can bind to the Sudlow site II on albumin. A concentration of 1 mM of tryptophan increases the free fraction of IS and p-CS by a factor of 2, demonstrating its ability to compete with these toxins for albumin-binding sites [85].
- Non-Esterified Fatty Acids (NEFA): NEFAs have shown a high capacity to increase the free fraction of UTs such as IS and pCS [86]. However, high concentrations of these molecules are required to achieve this effect, which may predispose patients to adverse effects, and in the case of NEFA, there is a high risk of hemolysis at the concentrations necessary for the displacing effect on UTs.

Table 3. Effects of various displacers on the removal of PBUTs in dialysis therapies.

Displacer	Effect on PBUT Removal	Considerations	References
Ibuprofen (1 mM)	Free fraction of IS and pCS increased by a factor 3 No impact on HA removal	Handling high doses can be a risk for HD patients	[80]
Furosemide (1 mM)	Free fraction of IS and pCS increased by a factor of 1.3 HA by a factor of 1.5	Side effects such as ototoxicity	[80]
Ibuprofen + Furosemide	Increased the removal of IS by a factor of 3 and IAA by a factor of 2	Enhanced PBUT displacement but increased the risk of side effects	[80]
Tryptophan (1 mM)	Free fraction of IS and pCS increased by a factor of 2.0 No impact on HA removal	Could increase uremic syndrome	[80,85]
Non-esterified fatty acids (NEFAs)	High capacity to increase free fraction of IS and pCS	High doses required Risk of hemolysis	[86]
Salvianolic acids	In vitro, increased the dialysis efficiency of IS and pCS by 99.13% and 142.00%, and in vivo (rats), by 135.61% and 272.13%	Need to test these results in patients	[87]

- Salvianolic Acids: Salvianolic acids, including lithospermic acid (LA), salvianolic acid A (SaA), tanshinol (DSS), caffeic acid (CA), salvianolic acid B (SaB), protocatechuic aldehyde (PA), and rosmarinic acid (RA), are molecules with high affinity for albumin receptors, significantly increasing the free concentration of UTs. This effect depends on their plasma concentration [87].

6.4. Efficacy and Safety

While experimental studies have shown promising results with displacers, their clinical efficacy and safety are not fully established. Comprehensive clinical trials are required to validate their effectiveness in reducing UT levels over time [88].

The potential side effects and clinical limitations of long-term use of some displacers, such as ibuprofen and furosemide, necessitate careful consideration of their application.

6.5. Future Directions for Displacer Use

Some challenges in implementing these molecules as standard treatment include the following:

Risk of Side Effects: Certain displacers, such as ibuprofen or furosemide, have clinical limitations in chronic use, potentially causing unwanted side effects such as hypertension or decreased residual diuresis in the case of ibuprofen or furosemide-induced ototoxicity [89].

An additional concern is that displacement compounds may result in elevated intracellular concentrations of PBUTs, which are demonstrably more toxic than their bound counterparts.

Dosage and Administration: The complexity of treatment regimens in patients with chronic kidney disease is influenced by the types of molecules and doses studied so far. Ideally, displacers with minimal side effects and, if possible, even health benefits, such as fatty acids and tryptophan, should be chosen [82].

Need for More Research: More research is required to fully understand the dynamics of toxin binding and displacement under different physiological and pathological conditions, as well as to identify the most effective and safe displacers for clinical practice [82].

Cost-Effectiveness Considerations: The introduction of new therapies in clinical practice should also consider cost-effectiveness aspects, especially in the context of chronic kidney disease, where costs are already high.

7. Conclusions

The management of chronic kidney disease (CKD) and its complications, particularly relating to the accumulation of protein-bound uremic toxins (PBUTs), presents a complex and evolving challenge. This comprehensive review has explored the multifaceted aspects of PBUTs, from their definition, classification, and systemic effects, to the emerging strategies for their clearance and potential future treatments.

It is clear that PBUTs play a significant role in the pathology of CKD, contributing to a range of systemic effects, particularly on cardiovascular health and immune function. The binding of these toxins to plasma proteins, notably albumin, underscores the complexities involved in their clearance.

Conventional dialysis techniques, such as hemodialysis and peritoneal dialysis, have limited efficacy in removing PBUTs due to their high protein-binding nature. The length of dialysis sessions and the maintenance of residual renal function are crucial factors in enhancing toxin clearance. The exploration of online hemodiafiltration and the use of medium cutoff (MCO) dialyzers represent significant strides in improving dialysis efficacy. However, the effectiveness of these methods specifically for PBUTs needs further investigation and clinical validation.

Adsorptive therapies and the use of displacers offer promising avenues for more effective removal of PBUTs. Adsorptive therapies, particularly with activated carbon and other novel materials, show potential in enhancing toxin clearance. Displacers, such as ibuprofen, furosemide, and tryptophan, aim to increase the free fraction of PBUTs, thereby facilitating their removal. Yet, their clinical efficacy, safety, and long-term application require careful evaluation and further research. Critical areas for further exploration include the development and refinement of dialysis techniques and cleansing concepts tailored to the treatment of uremic patients, the investigation of a standard dialyzer with standard sorbent (activated charcoal) in dialysis with a high dialysate flow, novel adsorptive materials, and the clinical implementation of toxin displacers. Each of these areas presents its own set of challenges and opportunities, particularly in terms of efficacy, safety, and cost-effectiveness.

In conclusion, while significant progress has been made in understanding and managing PBUTs in CKD, ongoing research and innovation are critical. Future studies should focus on optimizing current treatment modalities, exploring new therapeutic strategies, and understanding the long-term implications of these treatments on patient outcomes and quality of life. The ultimate goal remains enhancing the standard of care for CKD patients, reducing the burden of uremic toxicity and improving overall health outcomes. At present, offering specific recommendations is challenging due to the complexities associated with PBUT elimination. The insights presented in this review are based on studies aimed at reducing PBUTs in clinical practice. Until more effective strategies are implemented, the most rational approach to eliminating these toxins in patients involves maintaining residual renal function. This necessitates proper and hypotension-free dialysis. Among various techniques, daily dialysis has been shown to achieve superior clearance. Time continues to be a critical factor in the effective removal of these molecules.

Author Contributions: Conceptualization, E.G.-P. and D.S.-O.; writing—original draft preparation, D.S.-O., S.M.-F., C.G.-I., A.A., M.G.d.R., M.M.-M. and E.G.-P.; writing—review and editing, S.M.-F. and E.G.-P.; visualization S.M.-F.; supervision, E.G.-P.; funding acquisition, E.G.-P. and S.M.-F. All authors have read and agreed to the published version of the manuscript.

Funding: This research received no external funding. The research groups of S.M.-F. and E.G.-P. are funded by the Ministerio de Economia, Industria y competitividad: FIS/Fondos FEDER (PI20/00487; PI21/01430). The funders had no role in study design, data collection and analysis, decision to publish, or preparation of the manuscript.

Data Availability Statement: Not applicable.

Conflicts of Interest: The authors declare no conflicts of interest.

References

1. Hill, N.R.; Fatoba, S.T.; Oke, J.L.; Hirst, J.A.; O'Callaghan, C.A.; Lasserson, D.S.; Hobbs, F.D.R. Global Prevalence of Chronic Kidney Disease—A Systematic Review and Meta-Analysis. *PLoS ONE* **2016**, *11*, e0158765. [CrossRef] [PubMed]
2. Jager, K.J.; Kovesdy, C.; Langham, R.; Rosenberg, M.; Jha, V.; Zoccali, C. A Single Number for Advocacy and Communication-Worldwide More than 850 Million Individuals Have Kidney Diseases. *Kidney Int.* **2019**, *96*, 1048–1050. [CrossRef] [PubMed]
3. Kovesdy, C.P. Epidemiology of Chronic Kidney Disease: An Update 2022. *Kidney Int. Suppl.* **2022**, *12*, 7–11. [CrossRef] [PubMed]
4. Thurlow, J.S.; Joshi, M.; Yan, G.; Norris, K.C.; Agodoa, L.Y.; Yuan, C.M.; Nee, R. Global Epidemiology of End-Stage Kidney Disease and Disparities in Kidney Replacement Therapy. *Am. J. Nephrol.* **2021**, *52*, 98–107. [CrossRef] [PubMed]
5. Cockwell, P.; Fisher, L.-A. The Global Burden of Chronic Kidney Disease. *Lancet* **2020**, *395*, 662–664. [CrossRef] [PubMed]
6. Foreman, K.J.; Marquez, N.; Dolgert, A.; Fukutaki, K.; Fullman, N.; McGaughey, M.; Pletcher, M.A.; Smith, A.E.; Tang, K.; Yuan, C.-W.; et al. Forecasting Life Expectancy, Years of Life Lost, and All-Cause and Cause-Specific Mortality for 250 Causes of Death: Reference and Alternative Scenarios for 2016-40 for 195 Countries and Territories. *Lancet* **2018**, *392*, 2052–2090. [CrossRef] [PubMed]
7. Duranton, F.; Cohen, G.; De Smet, R.; Rodriguez, M.; Jankowski, J.; Vanholder, R.; Argiles, A. European Uremic Toxin Work Group Normal and Pathologic Concentrations of Uremic Toxins. *J. Am. Soc. Nephrol.* **2012**, *23*, 1258–1270. [CrossRef] [PubMed]
8. Fernandez-Prado, R.; Esteras, R.; Perez-Gomez, M.V.; Gracia-Iguacel, C.; Gonzalez-Parra, E.; Sanz, A.B.; Ortiz, A.; Sanchez-Niño, M.D. Nutrients Turned into Toxins: Microbiota Modulation of Nutrient Properties in Chronic Kidney Disease. *Nutrients* **2017**, *9*, 489. [CrossRef]
9. Koppe, L.; Fouque, D.; Soulage, C.O. The Role of Gut Microbiota and Diet on Uremic Retention Solutes Production in the Context of Chronic Kidney Disease. *Toxins* **2018**, *10*, 155. [CrossRef]
10. Popkov, V.A.; Silachev, D.N.; Zalevsky, A.O.; Zorov, D.B.; Plotnikov, E.Y. Mitochondria as a Source and a Target for Uremic Toxins. *Int. J. Mol. Sci.* **2019**, *20*, 3094. [CrossRef]
11. Vanholder, R.; De Smet, R.; Glorieux, G.; Argilés, A.; Baurmeister, U.; Brunet, P.; Clark, W.; Cohen, G.; De Deyn, P.P.; Deppisch, R.; et al. Review on Uremic Toxins: Classification, Concentration, and Interindividual Variability. *Kidney Int.* **2003**, *63*, 1934–1943. [CrossRef] [PubMed]
12. Neirynck, N.; Vanholder, R.; Schepers, E.; Eloot, S.; Pletinck, A.; Glorieux, G. An Update on Uremic Toxins. *Int. Urol. Nephrol.* **2013**, *45*, 139–150. [CrossRef]
13. Clark, W.R.; Dehghani, N.L.; Narsimhan, V.; Ronco, C. Uremic Toxins and Their Relation to Dialysis Efficacy. *Blood Purif.* **2019**, *48*, 299–314. [CrossRef]
14. List of Uremic Solutes—Uremic Solutes Database. Available online: https://database.uremic-toxins.org/soluteList.php (accessed on 4 December 2023).
15. Rosner, M.H.; Reis, T.; Husain-Syed, F.; Vanholder, R.; Hutchison, C.; Stenvinkel, P.; Blankestijn, P.J.; Cozzolino, M.; Juillard, L.; Kashani, K.; et al. Classification of Uremic Toxins and Their Role in Kidney Failure. *Clin. J. Am. Soc. Nephrol.* **2021**, *16*, 1918–1928. [CrossRef] [PubMed]
16. Shi, Y.; Tian, H.; Wang, Y.; Shen, Y.; Zhu, Q.; Ding, F. Effect of Ionic Strength, pH and Chemical Displacers on the Percentage Protein Binding of Protein-Bound Uremic Toxins. *Blood Purif.* **2019**, *47*, 351–360. [CrossRef]
17. Hobby, G.P.; Karaduta, O.; Dusio, G.F.; Singh, M.; Zybailov, B.L.; Arthur, J.M. Chronic Kidney Disease and the Gut Microbiome. *Am. J. Physiol. Renal Physiol.* **2019**, *316*, F1211–F1217. [CrossRef]
18. Kragh-Hansen, U.; Chuang, V.T.G.; Otagiri, M. Practical Aspects of the Ligand-Binding and Enzymatic Properties of Human Serum Albumin. *Biol. Pharm. Bull.* **2002**, *25*, 695–704. [CrossRef] [PubMed]
19. Awasthi, S.; Murugan, N.A.; Saraswathi, N.T. Advanced Glycation End Products Modulate Structure and Drug Binding Properties of Albumin. *Mol. Pharm.* **2015**, *12*, 3312–3322. [CrossRef]

20. Viaene, L.; Annaert, P.; de Loor, H.; Poesen, R.; Evenepoel, P.; Meijers, B. Albumin Is the Main Plasma Binding Protein for Indoxyl Sulfate and P-Cresyl Sulfate. *Biopharm. Drug Dispos.* **2013**, *34*, 165–175. [CrossRef]
21. Sudlow, G.; Birkett, D.J.; Wade, D.N. The Characterization of Two Specific Drug Binding Sites on Human Serum Albumin. *Mol. Pharmacol.* **1975**, *11*, 824–832.
22. Meijers, B.K.I.; De Loor, H.; Bammens, B.; Verbeke, K.; Vanrenterghem, Y.; Evenepoel, P. P-Cresyl Sulfate and Indoxyl Sulfate in Hemodialysis Patients. *Clin. J. Am. Soc. Nephrol.* **2009**, *4*, 1932–1938. [CrossRef]
23. Sakai, T.; Takadate, A.; Otagiri, M. Characterization of Binding Site of Uremic Toxins on Human Serum Albumin. *Biol. Pharm. Bull.* **1995**, *18*, 1755–1761. [CrossRef]
24. Zaidi, N.; Ahmad, E.; Rehan, M.; Rabbani, G.; Ajmal, M.R.; Zaidi, Y.; Subbarao, N.; Khan, R.H. Biophysical Insight into Furosemide Binding to Human Serum Albumin: A Study to Unveil Its Impaired Albumin Binding in Uremia. *J. Phys. Chem. B* **2013**, *117*, 2595–2604. [CrossRef] [PubMed]
25. Yamamoto, S.; Sasahara, K.; Domon, M.; Yamaguchi, K.; Ito, T.; Goto, S.; Goto, Y.; Narita, I. pH-Dependent Protein Binding Properties of Uremic Toxins In Vitro. *Toxins* **2021**, *13*, 116. [CrossRef] [PubMed]
26. Bulavin, L.A.; Khorolskyi, O.V. Concentration Dependences of Macromolecular Sizes in Aqueous Solutions of Albumins. *Ukr. J. Phys.* **2020**, *65*, 619. [CrossRef]
27. Liberi, S.; Linciano, S.; Moro, G.; De Toni, L.; Cendron, L.; Angelini, A. Structural Analysis of Human Serum Albumin in Complex with the Fibrate Drug Gemfibrozil. *Int. J. Mol. Sci.* **2022**, *23*, 1769. [CrossRef] [PubMed]
28. Lu, P.-H.; Yu, M.-C.; Wei, M.-J.; Kuo, K.-L. The Therapeutic Strategies for Uremic Toxins Control in Chronic Kidney Disease. *Toxins* **2021**, *13*, 573. [CrossRef]
29. Zhu, Y.-B.; Zhang, Y.-P.; Zhang, J.; Zhang, Y.-B. Evaluation of Vitamin C Supplementation on Kidney Function and Vascular Reactivity Following Renal Ischemic Injury in Mice. *Kidney Blood Press. Res.* **2016**, *41*, 460–470. [CrossRef]
30. Vila Cuenca, M.; van Bezu, J.; Beelen, R.H.J.; Vervloet, M.G.; Hordijk, P.L. Stabilization of Cell-Cell Junctions by Active Vitamin D Ameliorates Uraemia-Induced Loss of Human Endothelial Barrier Function. *Nephrol. Dial. Transplant.* **2019**, *34*, 252–264. [CrossRef]
31. Seliger, S.L.; Salimi, S.; Pierre, V.; Giffuni, J.; Katzel, L.; Parsa, A. Microvascular Endothelial Dysfunction Is Associated with Albuminuria and CKD in Older Adults. *BMC Nephrol.* **2016**, *17*, 82. [CrossRef]
32. Alexandrou, M.-E.; Gkaliagkousi, E.; Loutradis, C.; Dimitriadis, C.; Mitsopoulos, E.; Lazaridis, A.; Nikolaidou, B.; Dolgiras, P.; Douma, S.; Papagianni, A.; et al. Haemodialysis and Peritoneal Dialysis Patients Have Severely Impaired Post-Occlusive Skin Forearm Vasodilatory Response Assessed with Laser Speckle Contrast Imaging. *Clin. Kidney J.* **2021**, *14*, 1419–1427. [CrossRef]
33. Tumur, Z.; Niwa, T. Indoxyl Sulfate Inhibits Nitric Oxide Production and Cell Viability by Inducing Oxidative Stress in Vascular Endothelial Cells. *Am. J. Nephrol.* **2009**, *29*, 551–557. [CrossRef]
34. Gondouin, B.; Cerini, C.; Dou, L.; Sallée, M.; Duval-Sabatier, A.; Pletinck, A.; Calaf, R.; Lacroix, R.; Jourde-Chiche, N.; Poitevin, S.; et al. Indolic Uremic Solutes Increase Tissue Factor Production in Endothelial Cells by the Aryl Hydrocarbon Receptor Pathway. *Kidney Int.* **2013**, *84*, 733–744. [CrossRef]
35. Lekawanvijit, S. Cardiotoxicity of Uremic Toxins: A Driver of Cardiorenal Syndrome. *Toxins* **2018**, *10*, 352. [CrossRef] [PubMed]
36. Schroeder, J.C.; Dinatale, B.C.; Murray, I.A.; Flaveny, C.A.; Liu, Q.; Laurenzana, E.M.; Lin, J.M.; Strom, S.C.; Omiecinski, C.J.; Amin, S.; et al. The Uremic Toxin 3-Indoxyl Sulfate Is a Potent Endogenous Agonist for the Human Aryl Hydrocarbon Receptor. *Biochemistry* **2010**, *49*, 393–400. [CrossRef] [PubMed]
37. Dou, L.; Poitevin, S.; Sallée, M.; Addi, T.; Gondouin, B.; McKay, N.; Denison, M.S.; Jourde-Chiche, N.; Duval-Sabatier, A.; Cerini, C.; et al. Aryl Hydrocarbon Receptor Is Activated in Patients and Mice with Chronic Kidney Disease. *Kidney Int.* **2018**, *93*, 986–999. [CrossRef] [PubMed]
38. Lekawanvijit, S.; Krum, H. Cardiorenal Syndrome: Role of Protein-Bound Uremic Toxins. *J. Ren. Nutr.* **2015**, *25*, 149–154. [CrossRef] [PubMed]
39. Peng, Y.-S.; Ding, H.-C.; Lin, Y.-T.; Syu, J.-P.; Chen, Y.; Wang, S.-M. Uremic Toxin P-Cresol Induces Disassembly of Gap Junctions of Cardiomyocytes. *Toxicology* **2012**, *302*, 11–17. [CrossRef]
40. Azevedo, M.L.V.; Bonan, N.B.; Dias, G.; Brehm, F.; Steiner, T.M.; Souza, W.M.; Stinghen, A.E.M.; Barreto, F.C.; Elifio-Esposito, S.; Pecoits-Filho, R.; et al. P-Cresyl Sulfate Affects the Oxidative Burst, Phagocytosis Process, and Antigen Presentation of Monocyte-Derived Macrophages. *Toxicol. Lett.* **2016**, *263*, 1–5. [CrossRef] [PubMed]
41. Cohen, G.; Vanholder, R. Special Issue: Immune Dysfunction in Uremia. *Toxins* **2021**, *13*, 70. [CrossRef]
42. Fujii, H.; Goto, S.; Fukagawa, M. Role of Uremic Toxins for Kidney, Cardiovascular, and Bone Dysfunction. *Toxins* **2018**, *10*, 202. [CrossRef]
43. Niwa, T. Uremic Toxicity of Indoxyl Sulfate. *Nagoya J. Med. Sci.* **2010**, *72*, 1–11.
44. Sun, C.-Y.; Hsu, H.-H.; Wu, M.-S. P-Cresol Sulfate and Indoxyl Sulfate Induce Similar Cellular Inflammatory Gene Expressions in Cultured Proximal Renal Tubular Cells. *Nephrol. Dial. Transplant.* **2013**, *28*, 70–78. [CrossRef]
45. Watanabe, H.; Miyamoto, Y.; Honda, D.; Tanaka, H.; Wu, Q.; Endo, M.; Noguchi, T.; Kadowaki, D.; Ishima, Y.; Kotani, S.; et al. P-Cresyl Sulfate Causes Renal Tubular Cell Damage by Inducing Oxidative Stress by Activation of NADPH Oxidase. *Kidney Int.* **2013**, *83*, 582–592. [CrossRef]

46. Krieter, D.H.; Hackl, A.; Rodriguez, A.; Chenine, L.; Moragues, H.L.; Lemke, H.-D.; Wanner, C.; Canaud, B. Protein-Bound Uraemic Toxin Removal in Haemodialysis and Post-Dilution Haemodiafiltration. *Nephrol. Dial. Transplant.* **2010**, *25*, 212–218. [CrossRef]
47. Itoh, Y.; Ezawa, A.; Kikuchi, K.; Tsuruta, Y.; Niwa, T. Protein-Bound Uremic Toxins in Hemodialysis Patients Measured by Liquid Chromatography/Tandem Mass Spectrometry and Their Effects on Endothelial ROS Production. *Anal. Bioanal. Chem.* **2012**, *403*, 1841–1850. [CrossRef] [PubMed]
48. Carpi, A.; Donadio, C.; Tramonti, G. *Progress in Hemodialysis: From Emergent Biotechnology to Clinical Practice*; IntechOpen Ltd.: London, UK, 2011; ISBN 978-953-307-377-4. Available online: https://www.intechopen.com/books/353 (accessed on 4 December 2023).
49. Fagugli, R.M.; De Smet, R.; Buoncristiani, U.; Lameire, N.; Vanholder, R. Behavior of Non-Protein-Bound and Protein-Bound Uremic Solutes during Daily Hemodialysis. *Am. J. Kidney Dis.* **2002**, *40*, 339–347. [CrossRef] [PubMed]
50. van Gelder, M.K.; Middel, I.R.; Vernooij, R.W.M.; Bots, M.L.; Verhaar, M.C.; Masereeuw, R.; Grooteman, M.P.; Nubé, M.J.; van den Dorpel, M.A.; Blankestijn, P.J.; et al. Protein-Bound Uremic Toxins in Hemodialysis Patients Relate to Residual Kidney Function, Are Not Influenced by Convective Transport, and Do Not Relate to Outcome. *Toxins* **2020**, *12*, 234. [CrossRef]
51. Cupisti, A.; Bolasco, P.; D'Alessandro, C.; Giannese, D.; Sabatino, A.; Fiaccadori, E. Protection of Residual Renal Function and Nutritional Treatment: First Step Strategy for Reduction of Uremic Toxins in End-Stage Kidney Disease Patients. *Toxins* **2021**, *13*, 289. [CrossRef]
52. Tiong, M.K.; Krishnasamy, R.; Smith, E.R.; Hutchison, C.A.; Ryan, E.G.; Pascoe, E.M.; Hawley, C.M.; Hewitson, T.D.; Jardine, M.J.; Roberts, M.A.; et al. Effect of a Medium Cut-off Dialyzer on Protein-Bound Uremic Toxins and Mineral Metabolism Markers in Patients on Hemodialysis. *Hemodial. Int.* **2021**, *25*, 322–332. [CrossRef]
53. Maheshwari, V.; Thijssen, S.; Tao, X.; Fuertinger, D.H.; Kappel, F.; Kotanko, P. In Silico Comparison of Protein-Bound Uremic Toxin Removal by Hemodialysis, Hemodiafiltration, Membrane Adsorption, and Binding Competition. *Sci. Rep.* **2019**, *9*, 909. [CrossRef]
54. Tetali, S.D.; Jankowski, V.; Luetzow, K.; Kratz, K.; Lendlein, A.; Jankowski, J. Adsorption Capacity of Poly(Ether Imide) Microparticles to Uremic Toxins. *Clin. Hemorheol. Microcirc.* **2016**, *61*, 657–665. [CrossRef]
55. Falconi, C.A.; Junho, C.V.C.; Fogaça-Ruiz, F.; Vernier, I.C.S.; da Cunha, R.S.; Stinghen, A.E.M.; Carneiro-Ramos, M.S. Uremic Toxins: An Alarming Danger Concerning the Cardiovascular System. *Front. Physiol.* **2021**, *12*, 686249. [CrossRef]
56. Ronco, C.; Clark, W.R. Haemodialysis Membranes. *Nat. Rev. Nephrol.* **2018**, *14*, 394–410. [CrossRef] [PubMed]
57. Ronco, C.; Neri, M.; Lorenzin, A.; Garzotto, F.; Clark, W.R. Multidimensional Classification of Dialysis Membranes. *Contrib. Nephrol.* **2017**, *191*, 115–126. [CrossRef]
58. Deltombe, O.; Van Biesen, W.; Glorieux, G.; Massy, Z.; Dhondt, A.; Eloot, S. Exploring Protein Binding of Uremic Toxins in Patients with Different Stages of Chronic Kidney Disease and during Hemodialysis. *Toxins* **2015**, *7*, 3933–3946. [CrossRef]
59. Schulman, G.; Agarwal, R.; Acharya, M.; Berl, T.; Blumenthal, S.; Kopyt, N. A Multicenter, Randomized, Double-Blind, Placebo-Controlled, Dose-Ranging Study of AST-120 (Kremezin) in Patients with Moderate to Severe CKD. *Am. J. Kidney Dis.* **2006**, *47*, 565–577. [CrossRef]
60. Yamamoto, S.; Kazama, J.J.; Omori, K.; Matsuo, K.; Takahashi, Y.; Kawamura, K.; Matsuto, T.; Watanabe, H.; Maruyama, T.; Narita, I. Continuous Reduction of Protein-Bound Uraemic Toxins with Improved Oxidative Stress by Using the Oral Charcoal Adsorbent AST-120 in Haemodialysis Patients. *Sci. Rep.* **2015**, *5*, 14381. [CrossRef]
61. Meijers, B.K.; Weber, V.; Bammens, B.; Dehaen, W.; Verbeke, K.; Falkenhagen, D.; Evenepoel, P. Removal of the Uremic Retention Solute P-Cresol Using Fractionated Plasma Separation and Adsorption. *Artif. Organs* **2008**, *32*, 214–219. [CrossRef]
62. Brettschneider, F.; Tölle, M.; von der Giet, M.; Passlick-Deetjen, J.; Steppan, S.; Peter, M.; Jankowski, V.; Krause, A.; Kühne, S.; Zidek, W.; et al. Removal of Protein-Bound, Hydrophobic Uremic Toxins by a Combined Fractionated Plasma Separation and Adsorption Technique. *Artif. Organs* **2013**, *37*, 409–416. [CrossRef]
63. Pavlenko, D.; Giasafaki, D.; Charalambopoulou, G.; van Geffen, E.; Gerritsen, K.G.F.; Steriotis, T.; Stamatialis, D. Carbon Adsorbents With Dual Porosity for Efficient Removal of Uremic Toxins and Cytokines from Human Plasma. *Sci. Rep.* **2017**, *7*, 14914. [CrossRef]
64. Rocchetti, M.T.; Cosola, C.; di Bari, I.; Magnani, S.; Galleggiante, V.; Scandiffio, L.; Dalfino, G.; Netti, G.S.; Atti, M.; Corciulo, R.; et al. Efficacy of Divinylbenzenic Resin in Removing Indoxyl Sulfate and P-Cresol Sulfate in Hemodialysis Patients: Results From an In Vitro Study and An In Vivo Pilot Trial (Xuanro4-Nature 3.2). *Toxins* **2020**, *12*, 170. [CrossRef] [PubMed]
65. Sirich, T.L.; Plummer, N.S.; Gardner, C.D.; Hostetter, T.H.; Meyer, T.W. Effect of Increasing Dietary Fiber on Plasma Levels of Colon-Derived Solutes in Hemodialysis Patients. *Clin. J. Am. Soc. Nephrol. CJASN* **2014**, *9*, 1603–1610. [CrossRef] [PubMed]
66. Hai, X.; Landeras, V.; Dobre, M.A.; DeOreo, P.; Meyer, T.W.; Hostetter, T.H. Mechanism of Prominent Trimethylamine Oxide (TMAO) Accumulation in Hemodialysis Patients. *PLoS ONE* **2015**, *10*, e0143731. [CrossRef] [PubMed]
67. Krieter, D.H.; Kerwagen, S.; Rüth, M.; Lemke, H.-D.; Wanner, C. Differences in Dialysis Efficacy Have Limited Effects on Protein-Bound Uremic Toxins Plasma Levels over Time. *Toxins* **2019**, *11*, 47. [CrossRef] [PubMed]
68. Kim, Y.G.; Lee, S.H.; Jung, S.W.; Jung, G.T.; Lim, H.J.; Kim, K.P.; Jo, Y.-I.; Jin, K.; Moon, J.Y. The Medium Cut-Off Membrane Does Not Lower Protein-Bound Uremic Toxins. *Toxins* **2022**, *14*, 779. [CrossRef]
69. Magnani, S.; Atti, M. Uremic Toxins and Blood Purification: A Review of Current Evidence and Future Perspectives. *Toxins* **2021**, *13*, 246. [CrossRef]

70. Yamamoto, S.; Sato, M.; Sato, Y.; Wakamatsu, T.; Takahashi, Y.; Iguchi, A.; Omori, K.; Suzuki, Y.; Ei, I.; Kaneko, Y.; et al. Adsorption of Protein-Bound Uremic Toxins Through Direct Hemoperfusion With Hexadecyl-Immobilized Cellulose Beads in Patients Undergoing Hemodialysis. *Artif. Organs* **2018**, *42*, 88–93. [CrossRef]
71. Lee, S.; Sirich, T.L.; Meyer, T.W. Improving Clearance for Renal Replacement Therapy. *Kidney360* **2021**, *2*, 1188–1195. [CrossRef]
72. Bammens, B.; Evenepoel, P.; Verbeke, K.; Vanrenterghem, Y. Removal of the Protein-Bound Solute p-Cresol by Convective Transport: A Randomized Crossover Study. *Am. J. Kidney Dis. Off. J. Natl. Kidney Found.* **2004**, *44*, 278–285. [CrossRef]
73. Cornelis, T.; Eloot, S.; Vanholder, R.; Glorieux, G.; van der Sande, F.M.; Scheijen, J.L.; Leunissen, K.M.; Kooman, J.P.; Schalkwijk, C.G. Protein-Bound Uraemic Toxins, Dicarbonyl Stress and Advanced Glycation End Products in Conventional and Extended Haemodialysis and Haemodiafiltration. *Nephrol. Dial. Transplant.* **2015**, *30*, 1395–1402. [CrossRef] [PubMed]
74. Sirich, T.L.; Luo, F.J.-G.; Plummer, N.S.; Hostetter, T.H.; Meyer, T.W. Selectively Increasing the Clearance of Protein-Bound Uremic Solutes. *Nephrol. Dial. Transplant.* **2012**, *27*, 1574–1579. [CrossRef] [PubMed]
75. Sirich, T.L.; Funk, B.A.; Plummer, N.S.; Hostetter, T.H.; Meyer, T.W. Prominent Accumulation in Hemodialysis Patients of Solutes Normally Cleared by Tubular Secretion. *J. Am. Soc. Nephrol.* **2014**, *25*, 615–622. [CrossRef]
76. Sandeman, S.R.; Zheng, Y.; Ingavle, G.C.; Howell, C.A.; Mikhalovsky, S.V.; Basnayake, K.; Boyd, O.; Davenport, A.; Beaton, N.; Davies, N. A Haemocompatible and Scalable Nanoporous Adsorbent Monolith Synthesised Using a Novel Lignin Binder Route to Augment the Adsorption of Poorly Removed Uraemic Toxins in Haemodialysis. *Biomed. Mater.* **2017**, *12*, 035001. [CrossRef] [PubMed]
77. Meyer, T.W.; Peattie, J.W.T.; Miller, J.D.; Dinh, D.C.; Recht, N.S.; Walther, J.L.; Hostetter, T.H. Increasing the Clearance of Protein-Bound Solutes by Addition of a Sorbent to the Dialysate. *J. Am. Soc. Nephrol.* **2007**, *18*, 868–874. [CrossRef] [PubMed]
78. Madero, M.; Cano, K.B.; Campos, I.; Tao, X.; Maheshwari, V.; Brown, J.; Cornejo, B.; Handelman, G.; Thijssen, S.; Kotanko, P. Removal of Protein-Bound Uremic Toxins during Hemodialysis Using a Binding Competitor. *Clin. J. Am. Soc. Nephrol.* **2019**, *14*, 394–402. [CrossRef] [PubMed]
79. Lee, S.; Sirich, T.L.; Meyer, T.W. Improving Solute Clearances by Hemodialysis. *Blood Purif.* **2022**, *51*, 20–31. [CrossRef]
80. Tao, X.; Thijssen, S.; Kotanko, P.; Ho, C.-H.; Henrie, M.; Stroup, E.; Handelman, G. Improved Dialytic Removal of Protein-Bound Uraemic Toxins with Use of Albumin Binding Competitors: An in Vitro Human Whole Blood Study. *Sci. Rep.* **2016**, *6*, 23389. [CrossRef]
81. Carter, D.C.; Ho, J.X. Structure of Serum Albumin. *Adv. Protein Chem.* **1994**, *45*, 153–203. [CrossRef]
82. Maheshwari, V.; Tao, X.; Thijssen, S.; Kotanko, P. Removal of Protein-Bound Uremic Toxins Using Binding Competitors in Hemodialysis: A Narrative Review. *Toxins* **2021**, *13*, 622. [CrossRef]
83. Rodrigues, F.S.C.; Faria, M. Adsorption- and Displacement-Based Approaches for the Removal of Protein-Bound Uremic Toxins. *Toxins* **2023**, *15*, 110. [CrossRef]
84. Rodrigues, F.S.C.; Brilhante, D.; Macêdo, A.; Pires, R.F.; Faria, M. Ibuprofen-Immobilized Thin Films: A Novel Approach to Improve the Clearance of Protein-Bound Uremic Toxins. *ACS Appl. Mater. Interfaces* **2024**, *16*, 6589–6604. [CrossRef] [PubMed]
85. Bertuzzi, A.; Mingrone, G.; Gandolfi, A.; Greco, A.V.; Ringoir, S.; Vanholder, R. Binding of Indole-3-Acetic Acid to Human Serum Albumin and Competition with L-Tryptophan. *Clin. Chim. Acta* **1997**, *265*, 183–192. [CrossRef]
86. de Loor, H.; Meijers, B.K.I.; Meyer, T.W.; Bammens, B.; Verbeke, K.; Dehaen, W.; Evenepoel, P. Sodium Octanoate to Reverse Indoxyl Sulfate and P-Cresyl Sulfate Albumin Binding in Uremic and Normal Serum during Sample Preparation Followed by Fluorescence Liquid Chromatography. *J. Chromatogr. A* **2009**, *1216*, 4684–4688. [CrossRef]
87. Li, J.; Wang, Y.; Xu, X.; Cao, W.; Shen, Z.; Wang, N.; Leng, J.; Zou, N.; Shang, E.; Zhu, Z.; et al. Improved Dialysis Removal of Protein-Bound Uremic Toxins by Salvianolic Acids. *Phytomedicine* **2019**, *57*, 166–173. [CrossRef]
88. Saar-Kovrov, V.; Zidek, W.; Orth-Alampour, S.; Fliser, D.; Jankowski, V.; Biessen, E.A.L.; Jankowski, J. Reduction of Protein-Bound Uraemic Toxins in Plasma of Chronic Renal Failure Patients: A Systematic Review. *J. Intern. Med.* **2021**, *290*, 499–526. [CrossRef] [PubMed]
89. Florens, N.; Yi, D.; Juillard, L.; Soulage, C.O. Using Binding Competitors of Albumin to Promote the Removal of Protein-Bound Uremic Toxins in Hemodialysis: Hope or Pipe Dream? *Biochimie* **2018**, *144*, 1–8. [CrossRef] [PubMed]

Disclaimer/Publisher's Note: The statements, opinions and data contained in all publications are solely those of the individual author(s) and contributor(s) and not of MDPI and/or the editor(s). MDPI and/or the editor(s) disclaim responsibility for any injury to people or property resulting from any ideas, methods, instructions or products referred to in the content.

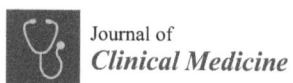

Systematic Review

Cannulation Technique of Vascular Access in Hemodialysis and the Impact on the Arteriovenous Fistula Survival: Systematic Review and Meta-Analysis

Ricardo Peralta [1,2,*], Luís Sousa [3,4] and António Filipe Cristovão [1]

1. Lisbon School of Nursing, University of Lisbon, 1600-096 Lisbon, Portugal; acristovao@esel.pt
2. NephroCare Portugal, Fresenius Medical Care Portugal, 1750-233 Lisbon, Portugal
3. School of Health Atlântica (ESSATLA), 2730-036 Oeiras, Portugal; luismmsousa@gmail.com
4. Comprehensive Health Research Centre (CHRC), 7000-811 Evora, Portugal
* Correspondence: ricardo.peralta@fmc-ag.com

Abstract: Adequate cannulation technique (CT) methods and successful puncture are essential for hemodialysis (HD) and arteriovenous fistula (AVF) maintenance. This systematic review and meta-analysis was designed to identify which CT allows better AVF primary patency and lower rates of complications in HD patients. The search was carried out on the CINAHL, MEDLINE, Cochrane Library, and Joanna Briggs Institute Library databases to identify all randomized controlled trials (RCTs) and observational studies comparing clinical outcomes of buttonhole (BH) versus rope ladder cannulation (RL) from 2010 to 2022. The Risk-of-Bias (Rob 2) tool was used for RCTs and the ROBINS-I was used for non-randomized studies. RevMan 5.4 was used for the meta-analysis. A total of five RCTs, one quasi-randomized controlled trial, and six observational studies were included. When compared with RL cannulation, BH cannulation significantly increased bacteremia (RR, 2.76, 95% CI (1.14, 6.67), $p = 0.02$) but showed no differences in AVF primary patency (HR, 1.06, 95% CI (0.45, 4.21), $p = 0.90$). There was no thrombosis reduction (RR, 0.51, 95% CI (0.23, 1.14), $p = 0.10$) or intervention number reduction (RR, 0.93, 95% CI (0.49, 1.80), $p = 0.84$) with BH. Outcomes like pain, hematoma, and aneurysm could not be merged due to a lack of data, reported as medians, as well as due to different definitions. The quality in general was poor and the heterogeneity among the studies prevented us from merging the outcomes.

Keywords: meta-analysis; end-stage renal disease; chronic kidney disease; hemodialysis; buttonhole; rope ladder; cannulation technique

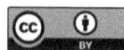

Citation: Peralta, R.; Sousa, L.; Cristovão, A.F. Cannulation Technique of Vascular Access in Hemodialysis and the Impact on the Arteriovenous Fistula Survival: Systematic Review and Meta-Analysis. *J. Clin. Med.* **2023**, *12*, 5946. https://doi.org/10.3390/jcm12185946

Academic Editor: Hiroshi Tanaka

Received: 10 August 2023
Revised: 30 August 2023
Accepted: 7 September 2023
Published: 13 September 2023

Copyright: © 2023 by the authors. Licensee MDPI, Basel, Switzerland. This article is an open access article distributed under the terms and conditions of the Creative Commons Attribution (CC BY) license (https://creativecommons.org/licenses/by/4.0/).

1. Introduction

With the increase in the number of elderly patients, the exhaustion of vascular territory, and the emergence of diabetes as the primary cause of renal etiology, the establishment and preservation of suitable vascular access (VA) is essential for the successful treatment of patients with end-stage kidney disease (ESKD) on hemodialysis (HD) programs. A functioning VA is the lifeline [1,2] that allows patients the undergoing of HD such as renal replacement therapy, allowing their survival and the maintenance of an acceptable quality of life. Conversely, the preservation and maintenance of a complication-free VA remains the Achilles' heel of this field [2,3]. Moreover, VA dysfunctions remain the major cause of comorbidities and hospitalizations [4–6] in ESKD patients. The selections of the most suitable cannulation technique (CT) and VA cannulation are the most important aspects in dialysis [7], and nurses have the responsibility for constantly updating their knowledge and skills in this area. Selection of the best technique is fundamental to the proper use of VA and allows effective treatment; the correct and appropriate choice of arteriovenous fistula (AVF) cannulation is the key to its preservation and the prevention of VA-related dysfunction [8]. The technique that has always been referenced and recommended as preferable for AVF cannulation is the rope ladder (RL) technique [9,10].

However, challenges have been identified in the use of this cannulation technique such as severe pain with an impact on treatment time [11,12] and an increased risk of hematomas [13]. However, nurses tend not to explore the entire length of the vessel due to the increased risk of infiltration, and even with a protocol for the use of the RL technique, they end up using area cannulation [14]. The area CT leads to a decreased vein wall and tissue thickening and consequent aneurysm formation, with the increased risk of vein wall rupture [8]. Despite this knowledge, it is the most commonly used technique in some European countries, being used in 65.8% (44% to 77%) of patients compared to 28.2% for RL and 6% for BH [15]. The BH technique has some limitations since it must be used exclusively in AVF and requires the cannulation to be performed by the same nurse until the tunnel is built, and it is time-consuming. Although some have reported the advantages of BH, others have reported increased risks of local infection and bacteremia [16,17], even after major re-education and asepsis technique campaigns [18].

In recent years, some studies have been published [17,19,20] that may contribute to clarifying which CT allows for greater fistula survival and fewer complications. Therefore, this study aims to identify which CT allows for greater AVF survival and a lower rate of complications and which CT causes less pain for patients who undergo regular hemodialysis.

2. Materials and Methods

2.1. Search Strategy

This systematic review and meta-analysis was conducted in accordance with Preferred Reporting Items for Systematic Reviews and Meta-Analysis (PRISMA) guidelines [21]. The protocol was registered in the PROSPERO database prior to commencement (registration number CRD42021237050).

We conducted searches on the EBSCO platform, accessing the Cumulative Index of Nursing and Allied Health Literature (CINAHL) and MEDLINE databases using the following Medical Subject Headings (MeSH) (2021) and strategy: ((MH "Dialysis") OR (MH "Renal Dialysis") OR (MH "Hemodialysis") OR (MH "Kidney Failure Chronic")) AND (((MH "Arteriovenous Fistula") OR (MH "Catheterization")) AND (("Buttonhole") OR (buttonhole) (OR constant site)) AND ((rope-ladder) OR (ropeladder) OR (rotating site))). We also considered other databases such as the Cochrane Library, ScienceDirect web, Joanna Briggs Institute Library Evidence-Based Practice Network (JBI), SCOPUS, ResearchGate, American Society of Nephrology (ASN), American Nephrology Nurses Association (ANNA), Sociedade Espanhola de Nefrologia (SEN), and Sociedade Brasileira de Nefrologia (SBN). We considered these databases because they publish randomized controlled trials (RCTs) and observational studies in the nephrology field. All the articles included in the review were available in full text. A flow chart is shown in Figure 1.

2.2. Inclusion and Exclusion Criteria

We included all RCTs and quasi-experimental and prospective observational studies published between January 2000 and January 2022 that satisfied the following criteria: studies that compare CTs and thus define the advantages and risks of each CT; primary and full studies, or abstracts that include one or some outcomes. We reviewed articles in English that enrolled adults aged 18 years and older who underwent hemodialysis using an autogenous AVF. Patients who underwent BH were considered the experimental group, and patients who underwent RL or other CT were considered the control group.

We excluded studies associating patient data from home hemodialysis with data from hospital or hemodialysis clinics and studies with incidents of patients on hemodialysis and qualitative studies.

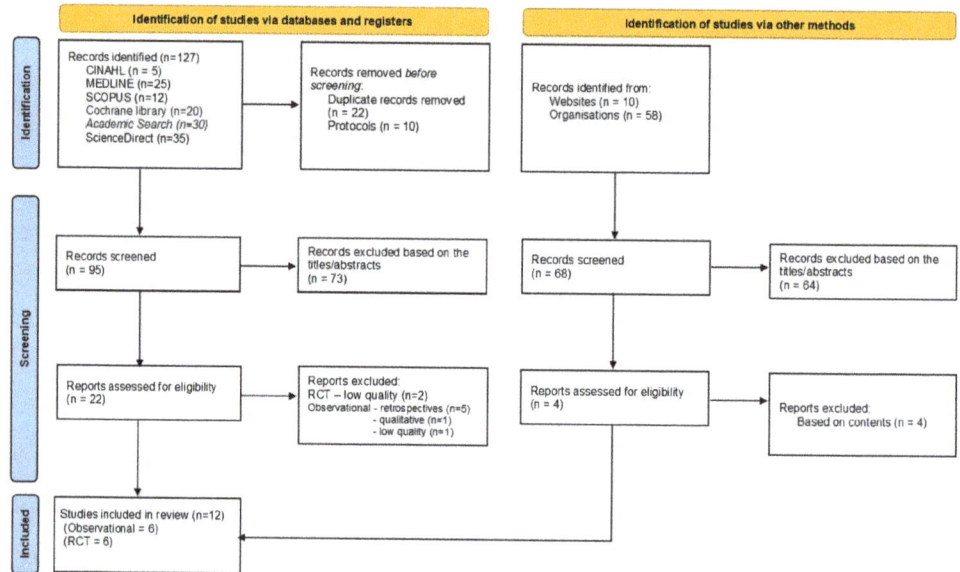

Figure 1. Study flow diagram.

2.3. Outcome Indicators

The primary outcome was the fistula primary patency, and according to Lee T. et al. [22], this was evaluated by the percentage of AVF in use from the study start to the time of the first clinical intervention for angioplasty or vascular surgery (unassisted patency).

The secondary outcome was considered fistula survival, for which failure was defined as AVF no longer used for successful HD. The numbers of interventions, thrombosis, bacteremia, cannulation pain related to CT, hematoma or infiltration, bleeding time, aneurysm, and unsuccessful cannulation were considered.

2.4. Data Extraction

First, the studies were independently selected by a reviewer (RP). The titles and content of the abstracts were assessed. Then, the second reviewer (AC) carried out the subsequent verification and validation. This selection was made strictly according to the inclusion and exclusion criteria defined in the protocol published elsewhere [23]. All duplicate studies were refused. When the title and abstract were not sufficiently enlightening, a new search was carried out for the full article. After this selection, the full versions of the potentially eligible studies were extracted.

2.5. Quality Assessment

To assess the risk of bias in RCT studies, we used the Revised Cochrane Risk-of-Bias Tool for Randomized Trials (RoB 2) tool [24]. According to the number of articles selected and the evidence found, studies with low methodological quality were excluded. Therefore, each study was categorized as presenting low risk, high risk, or unclear risk of bias. For non-randomized studies, the Risk of Bias In Non-Randomized Studies of Interventions (ROBINS-I) [25] was used.

2.6. Statistical Analysis

The studies selected for the systematic review were presented in a summary table with the following main attributes: the author's name, year of publication, country, study design, sample size (*n*), and outcome analysis method. Outcomes: participant's characteristics (average age, comorbidities), context of dialysis (hospital, clinic, or home), follow-up of the study (months), and primary and secondary outcomes obtained, including the pain scoring tool used to define the severity of pain. We performed a meta-analysis only when studies were sufficiently homogeneous in terms of participants, interventions, outcomes, measurement, and method of aggregation (e.g., mean, proportion). We presented the results in a narrative form when statistical comparisons were not possible. Tables and figures were included to facilitate the presentation of the data. Meta-analysis was performed with the generic inverse variance method using Cochrane Collaboration Review Manager software (RevMan 5.4) for Windows.

3. Results

3.1. Characteristics of the Included Studies

We selected five RCTs [13,16,19,26,27], one controlled clinical trial [28], and six observational studies [14,29–31]. Two were crossover studies [32,33], and the characteristics are shown in Tables 1 and S1. For the meta-analysis, only RCT studies and outcomes that could be merged were considered.

The studies were published between 2010 and 2022 with the inclusion of 717 patients in the RCT studies and 633 in the observational ones. The studies were mostly carried out in one clinic, with three in multiple clinics and one between a hospital and multicenter. The control group assumed a wide range of designations such as traditional RL [26] (TRL), standard needling [13,16] (SN), usual practice [27] (UP), traditional method [29] (TM), and area technique [31,32]. The remaining studies in the control group used the RL, but among the 12 studies, only 1 used a diagram [19] for guidance of puncture sites during follow-up. The follow-up period varied between 2 and 60 months.

3.2. Risk-of-Bias Assessment for RCT Studies

Figure 2 shows the risk-of-bias assessment that estimated the relative effect of the unassisted primary patency between BH and RL.

Only four studies evaluated this outcome [16,19,27,28] (Figure S1). Risk of bias was observed in the randomization process in one study [28], and no studies blinded personnel or participants due to the visibility and characteristics of the intervention. Some baseline characteristics that may influence the outcome were not evaluated or were significantly different between the two groups. The intended interventions were not illustrated in detail in the trial protocol, mainly cannulation in RL. In two studies, the control group was designated as the usual practice [27], and standard needling [16] and implementation of the CT were not described.

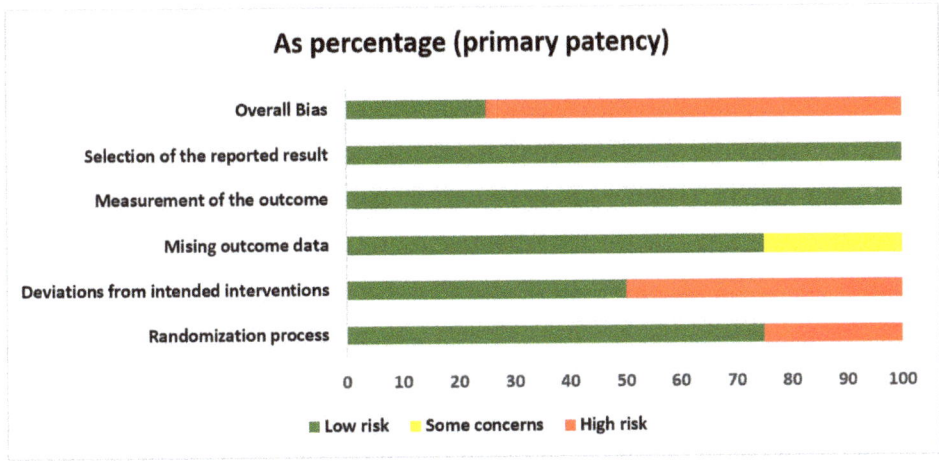

Figure 2. Risk of bias: review author judgments on each risk-of-bias item presented as percentages across the included RCTs.

Table 1. Characteristics of included randomized clinical trial.

First Author	Publication Year	Origin	Study Design	Context	Sample Size	Interventions		Protocol		Follow-Up (Months)	Outcomes
						Experimental Group	Control Group	Experimental Group	Control Group		
MacRae J. et al. [13]	2012	Canada	RCT	Center	140	BH	Standard needling	Specified	Not specified	12	①②③⑤
MacRae J. et al. [16]	2014	Canada	RCT	Center	139	BH	Standard needling	Specified	Not specified	19.2 vs. 17.2	⑤⑧⑨⑩
Peralta R. et al. [19]	2022	Portugal	RCT	Multicentric	172	MuST	BH and RL	Specified	Specified	12	④⑤⑨⑩
Struthers J. et al. [26]	2010	United Kingdom	RCT	Center	56	BH	Traditional RL	Specified	Not specified	6	①②③④⑤⑧
Vaux E. et al. [27]	2013	United Kingdom	RCT	Center	127	BH	Usual practice	Specified	Not specified	12	①②③④⑤⑨ ⑩
Chan M. et al. [28]	2014	USA	CCT	Center	83	BH	RL	Specified	Not specified	12	⑤⑨

Note: ① pain; ② hematoma; ③ bleeding time; ④ aneurism formation/development; ⑤ bacteremia related to vascular access; ⑧ thrombosis; ⑨ AVF survival; ⑩ number of interventions. Abbreviations: RCT: randomized clinical trial; CCT: controlled clinical trial; BH: buttonhole; MuST: multiple single cannulation technique; RL: rope ladder.

3.3. Risk-of-Bias Assessment for Observational Studies

All studies had a critical risk of bias in the first two domains (Figures 3 and S2). No baseline factors that could bias the outcomes were assessed, participant selection was not randomized, and no studies blinded personnel or participants. All involved participants had used AVF before the study began. Some studies had few participants [32,33], and in 50% of the studies, the follow-up was less than four months. Limitations were also identified in the remaining domains; no study described how it implemented the CT in the control group or used a diagram for the RL. Bias was due to missing data [30], and in another study [31], the participants in the control group used RL and area CT.

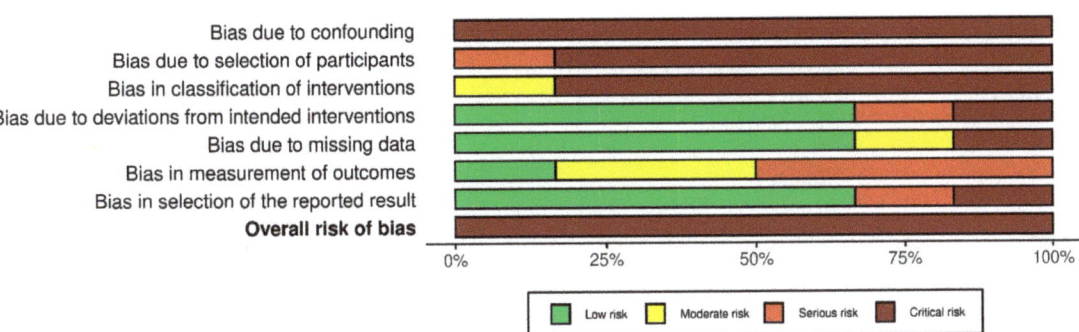

Figure 3. Risk of bias: review author judgments about the risk of bias in non-randomized studies of interventions.

3.4. Primary Outcome—Unassisted Primary Patency

Four RCTs reported this outcome, and the results are shown in Table S2. For the meta-analysis, three studies [19,27,28] were used that reported data in a hazard ratio, as shown in Figure 4. The test showed high heterogeneity among the studies, and using the random effects model ($p < 0.1$ e $I^2 = 81\%$), it was not possible to prove which CT allowed greater unassisted primary patency (HR, 1.06 (95% CI 0.45–2.50) $p = 0.90$).

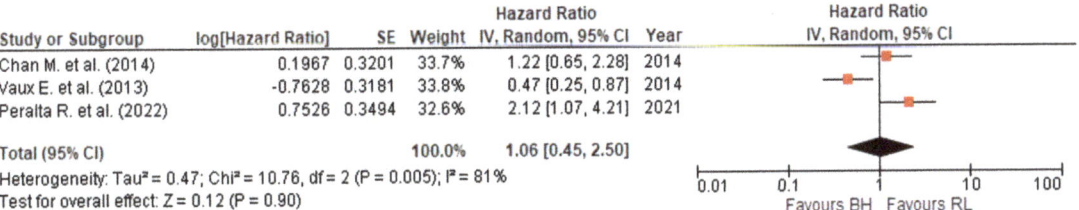

Figure 4. Result of unassisted primary survival rate between BH and RL. The hazard ratio of each study, Chan M. et al. (2014) [28], Vaux E. et al. (2013) [27], and Peralta R. et al. (2022) [19], is shown in red.

3.5. Number of Interventions in the Fistula

There were three studies (Table S3) that reported the number of interventions for AVF and after merging data (Figure 5) showed the existence of high heterogeneity. When using the random effects model ($p < 0.1$ e $I^2 = 78\%$), it was not possible to prove which CT allowed a lower rate of interventions (angioplasty or surgery) in AVF (RR, 0.93 (95% CI 0.49–1.80) $p = 0.84$).

3.6. Arteriovenous Fistula Thrombosis

In the four studies that reported AVF thrombosis [16,19,26,27] (Table S3), apparently, there was a higher incidence of thrombosis in the control group. At least one study [27] showed the highest frequency of thrombosis events related to usual CT (eight events) compared to BH (one event). After merging the data (Figure 6) of these four studies, they were shown to be homogeneous using the fixed effects model ($p > 0.1$ e $I^2 = 0\%$). However, it was not possible to confirm which CT allowed a lower frequency of AVF thrombosis (RR, 0.51 (95% CI 0.23–1.14) $p = 0.10$).

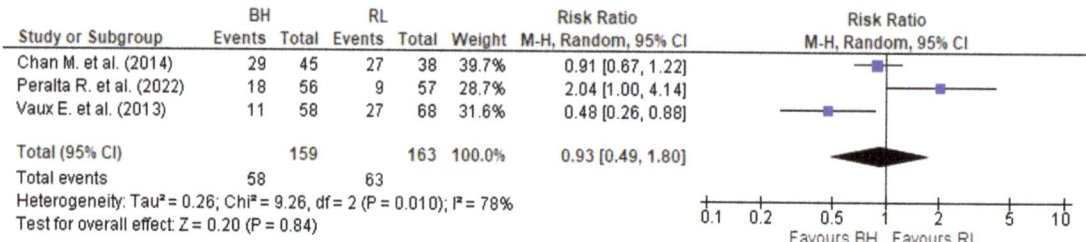

Figure 5. Result of the number of interventions in the AVF between the buttonhole and the rope ladder. The risk ratio of each study, Chan M. et al. (2014) [28], Peralta R. et al. (2022) [19], and Vaux E. et al. (2013) [27], is shown in blue.

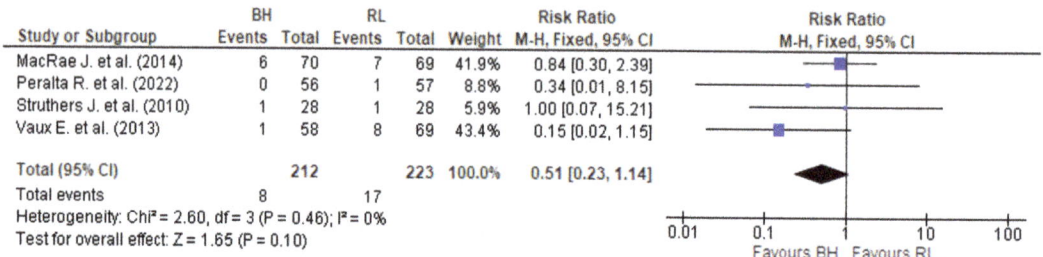

Figure 6. Result of the number of cases of thrombosis in the AVF between the buttonhole and the rope ladder. The risk ratio of each study, MacRae J. et al. (2014) [16], Peralta R. et al. (2022) [19], Struthers J. et al. (2010) [26], and Vaux E. et al. (2013) [27], is shown in blue.

3.7. Bacteremia and/or Localized Signs of Infection Related to Vascular Access

All six RCTs (Table S4) assessed the frequency of bacteremia and localized signs of infection related to vascular access. Three studies [13,16,28] reported a higher incidence of bacteremia associated with BH, and one [27] showed more infection rates associated with the usual-practice group (0.09/1000 AVF days).

Vascular access infection was reported by three observational studies [14,30,31] but with different methodologies for assessment and presentation of results. Even so, the studies by van Loon et al. [14] and Glerup R. et al. [31] showed a significantly higher rate of infection ($p < 0.001$) associated with BH (Table S5).

RCTs [13,16,27,28] were merged using the fixed effect model. The test showed homogeneity among studies, $p > 0.1$ and $I^2 = 47\%$. A significant difference was observed (Figure 7) in the incidence of bacteremia associated with BH (RR, 2.76 (95% CI 1.14–6.67) $p = 0.02$).

There also seemed to be a higher rate of localized infection in the BH group. MacRae J. et al. [13] showed a significant difference ($p = 0.003$) in local signs of infection associated with BH (50 per 1000/HD sessions) compared with the SN group (22.4/1000 HD sessions).

3.8. Cannulation Pain

There were three RCTs [13,26,27] (Table S6) that assessed cannulation pain and reported it as a median, but these data could not be merged. However, there seemed to be a marginal advantage in the Vaux et al. study [27] ($p = 0.05$) regarding pain reduction in the control group. In this study, eight patients asked to change to the usual practice because of pain associated with the BH. In contrast, three observational studies [29,32,33] (Table S7) showed a significant reduction in pain ($p = 0.0049$, and $p < 0.001$) when using BH. Of the eight studies evaluating cannulation pain, in five studies, the participants used analgesic cream.

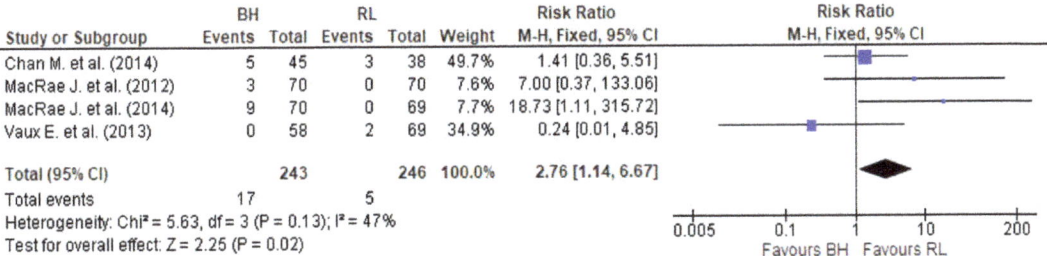

Figure 7. Result of the rate of bacteremia associated with cannulation techniques in arteriovenous fistulas. The risk ratio of each study, Chan M. et al. (2014) [28], MacRae J. et al. (2012) [13], MacRae J. et al. (2014) [16], and Vaux E. et al. (2013) [27], is shown in blue.

3.9. Hematoma Associated with Cannulation Techniques

There were two RCTs [13,26] (Table S8) and two observational studies [14,30] (Table S9) that reported a reduction in the rate of hematomas associated with BH. MacRae et al. [13] showed a significant reduction in the rate of hematomas using BH ($p = 0.003$) compared with SN. Van Loon et al. [14] also found that the patients in the BH group had lesser hematoma formation ($p < 0.0001$). Apparently, there was an advantage associated with BH in reducing hematomas, but it was not possible to merge data because the presentation of the results was different. We understand that further studies are needed to assess the frequency of hematomas associated with CT.

3.10. Bleeding Time Post-Dialysis

The three RCTs [13,26,27] (Table S8) failed to show the advantage of BH in bleeding time after needle removal. The data could not be merged because of the various definitions of hemostasis and because the data were presented differently. Contrarily, three observational studies [29,32,33] concluded that the bleeding time was significantly lower in patients in the BH group (Table S9).

3.11. Aneurysm Formation/Aneurysm Enlargement

There seemed to be unanimity of both RCTs (Table S10) and observational studies (Table S11) in finding that BH was associated with a reduction in aneurysms. The buttonhole significantly reduced existing aneurysm enlargement when it was compared with traditional rope ladder needling [26] and usual practice [27]. When assessing the prospect of aneurysm formation, only one study [19] reported that BH was advantageous over RL. The data could not be merged because of the various definitions of aneurysm enlargement and because the data were presented differently. Observational studies [14,29,30] reported that patients in the BH group had less aneurysm formation, but the follow-up in these studies was short, between 3 and 9 months.

3.12. Unsuccessful Cannulation

Nurses perceived significantly higher levels of difficulty with both arterial and venous cannulation in the BH [13] group ($p < 0.001$) compared to standard CT mainly after the fourth month. In another study [27], BH could not be implemented or there were subsequent problems with cannulation in four (6.89%) patients. There were two observational studies [14,30] (Table S11) that assessed unsuccessful cannulations and concluded that BH was associated with a significant increase in miscannulation [14] and where patients in the control group required more than two cannulation attempts [30]. The authors mentioned that miscannulation in the BH group may be attributed to the "trampoline" effect due to the wrong angle of cannulation when the needle is inserted in the tunnel; the needle encounters greater resistance because it does not have the same penetration capacity.

4. Discussion

The outcome measures used were numerous and heterogeneous at every level—measurement, metric, method of aggregation, time point of measurement, and follow-up—making it very difficult to reliably evaluate the comparative effectiveness of interventions. There were no attempts to standardize some definitions, mainly the CT used in the control group, which had implications for decisions in clinical practice and improvement in the quality of life of patients under hemodialysis. The different puncture classifications in the control group described above led us to think that they were different puncture methods, or we presumed that the studies used area CT instead of RL. Only one study used patients with incident AVF and described in detail how RL was implemented. They also used the multiple single cannulation technique (MuST) [19,34,35], recently described as a hybrid CT between the rope ladder and the buttonhole that incorporates the benefits from both with promising results. The experimental group and the control group used different CT methods, and therefore blinding could not be applied to patients, nurses, or researchers. Half of the observational studies had fewer than 50 participants, and two were clinical crossover studies with only 21 and 31 patients. Consequently, our comparative assessments of the meta-analysis results from RCTs to guide evidence-based clinical practice are likely to be problematic. The need to standardize outcome measures for vascular access complications has been recognized and several proposals have been published over the last two decades [8,22,36].

Other studies [37] also faced limitations. The outcome measures were assessed in dozens of different ways, and this made it impossible to compare the results across trials and determine that all trials contributed relevant and usable information.

The results of this meta-analysis indicated that BH did not show evidence of superiority in primary patency or in the reduction in the number of interventions when compared with RL. In the study by MacRae et al. [16], no significant differences ($p = 0.20$) were found in AVF survival, even with longer follow-up. These are very important outcome indicators, but there was limited research and the few selected studies revealed considerable heterogeneity ($I^2 = 81\%$). Therefore, it is recommended that future studies perform more analysis on fistula survival.

The results of this meta-analysis are inconclusive if BH reduces the number of cases of thrombosis; however, there was a clear trend toward a lower incidence of this event. Two previous systematic reviews [38,39] concluded that BH significantly reduced the occurrence of thrombosis. However, in our study, the higher incidence of thrombosis was associated with studies [16,26,27] in which BH was compared with other often ill-defined CTs such as standard needling, traditional rope ladder, and usual practice.

The results indicated that BH has a higher risk of AVF bacteremia than RL. These results are similar to those of another systematic review [40], which showed that infection risk was approximately threefold higher with BH cannulation (RR, 3.34; 95% CI, 0.91 to 12.20; $p = 0.07$). However, we must consider that there were only four trials with a small sample size (243 versus 246) and a small event size (17 versus 5), and these results showed a lack of statistical power. A retrospective observational study [17] using National Healthcare Safety Network (NHSN) surveillance data concluded that BH was associated with a significantly higher risk of access-related bloodstream infection (adjusted relative risk (aRR), 2.6; 95% CI, 2.4–2.8) and local access-site infection (aRR, 1.5; 95% CI, 1.4–1.6) than RL. Despite the re-education programs associated with a strict asepsis policy, audit cycles, and the active eradication of staphylococcus aureus bacteremia, infection rates remained high in BH [18].

However, other studies [38,39] did not find significant differences in the risk of infection between BH and RL. This complication may occur late and not be reported in studies with follow-ups of less than 12 months [16]. To support this inference, an observational [31] study with 60 months of follow-up concluded that bacteremia was significantly higher for buttonhole compared to stepladder/area needling.

This study showed that BH did not reduce the incidence of pain, despite the reduction in injury caused by blunt needles. However, this can be explained by the increase in miscannulation and the "trampoline" effect [14,30] using blunt needles. Two other studies drew the same conclusion [38,39].

There is a clear trend in favor of BH in reducing the rate of hematomas and aneurysm development in RCTs and observational studies. This is in accordance with other studies [38,39] that showed some results, but we should not forget that in these literature reviews, some studies used a CT that is different from RL. On the other hand, the significant increase in aneurysms when using RL, even with an implemented protocol, may be associated with the daily use of area cannulation by professionals [14].

As limitations of this study, we found some constraints on the quality of the included studies, especially the observational studies. The multiple definitions of RL in the control group limited the results, with implications for decisions in clinical practice. Also, the follow-up lengths of the studies were short, and outcomes such as infection and new aneurysms occurred late. Another limitation was the small number of studies and participants, so it would have been useful to conduct a sequential analysis of trials [41,42].

5. Conclusions

This meta-analysis demonstrated that BH is significantly associated with higher bacteremia; however, it found no differences in AVF primary patency, number of interventions, or thrombosis. Therefore, BH should be exclusively reserved for home dialysis patients or those with anatomical constraints, as described by some authors [10,43].

To select the best CT for each person, it is necessary to adopt a decision model [44,45] that also involves the patient. In this way, we recommend that VA care should be extended to the patient with education, promoting the development of self-care behaviors by providing the necessary knowledge to patients [46]. To avoid the indiscriminate use of area CT, RL must be implemented with a diagram adjusted to each patient.

Supplementary Materials: The following supporting information can be downloaded at: https://www.mdpi.com/article/10.3390/jcm12185946/s1, Figure S1: Summary of the risk of bias of the 5 domains assessed in each RCT; Figure S2: Summary of the risk of bias of the 7 domains assessed from the observational studies; Table S1: Characteristics of included observational studies; Table S2: Relative effect of the unassisted primary patency of arteriovenous fistula; Table S3: Number of interventions and thrombosis as the outcome of cannulation techniques in arteriovenous fistulas; Table S4: Bacteremia and local signs of infection as an outcome of the cannulation technique in arteriovenous fistulas in RCT studies; Table S5: Bacteremia and local signs of infection as an outcome of the cannulation technique in arteriovenous fistulas in observational studies; Table S6: Pain as an outcome of the cannulation technique in arteriovenous fistulas in RCT studies; Table S7: Pain as an outcome of the cannulation technique in arteriovenous fistulas in observational studies; Table S8: Hematoma and bleeding time as an outcome of the cannulation technique in arteriovenous fistulas in RCT studies; Table S9: Hematoma and bleeding time as an outcome of the cannulation technique in arteriovenous fistulas in observational studies; Table S10: Aneurism formation/development as an outcome of the cannulation technique in arteriovenous fistulas in RCT studies; Table S11: Aneurism formation/development and unsuccessful cannulation as an outcome of the cannulation technique in arteriovenous fistulas in observational studies.

Author Contributions: Conceptualization, R.P.; methodology, R.P. and A.F.C.; investigation R.P. and A.F.C.; writing—original draft preparation, R.P.; writing—review and editing, R.P., L.S. and A.F.C.; supervision, L.S. and A.F.C. All authors have read and agreed to the published version of the manuscript.

Funding: This research received no external funding.

Institutional Review Board Statement: Not applicable.

Informed Consent Statement: Not applicable.

Data Availability Statement: The data presented in this study are available on request from the corresponding author.

Conflicts of Interest: The authors declare no conflict of interest.

References

1. Lee, T. Novel paradigms for dialysis vascular access: Downstream vascular biology-is there a final common pathway? *Clin. J. Am. Soc. Nephrol.* **2013**, *8*, 2194–2201. [CrossRef] [PubMed]
2. Nath, K.A. Dialysis Vascular Access Intervention and the Search for Biomarkers. *J. Am. Soc. Nephrol.* **2016**, *27*, 970–972. [CrossRef] [PubMed]
3. Ethier, J.; Mendelssohn, D.C.; Elder, S.J.; Hasegawa, T.; Akizawa, T.; Akiba, T.; Canaud, B.J.; Pisoni, R.L. Vascular access use and outcomes: An international perspective from the dialysis outcomes and practice patterns study. *Nephrol. Dial. Transplant.* **2008**, *23*, 3219–3226. [CrossRef] [PubMed]
4. Feldman, H.I.; Held, P.J.; Hutchinson, J.T.; Stoiber, E.; Hartigan, M.F.; Berlin, J.A. Hemodialysis vascular access morbidity in the United States. *Kidney Int.* **1993**, *43*, 1091–1096. [CrossRef] [PubMed]
5. Roy-Chaudhury, P.; Sukhatme Vikas, P.; Cheung, A.K. Hemodialysis Vascular Access Dysfunction: A Cellular and Molecular Viewpoint. *J. Am. Soc. Nephrol.* **2006**, *17*, 1112–1127. [CrossRef]
6. Dhingra, R.K.; Young, E.W.; Hulbert-Shearon, T.E.; Leavey Sean, F.; Port, F.K. Type of vascular access and mortality in U.S. hemodialysis patients. *Kidney Int.* **2001**, *60*, 1443–1451. [CrossRef]
7. McCann, M.; Einarsdottir, H.; Waeleghem, J.P.V.; Murphy, F.; Sedgwick, J. Vascular access management II: AVF/AVG cannulation techniques and complications. *J. Ren. Care* **2009**, *35*, 90–98. [CrossRef]
8. Gallieni, M.; Hollenbeck, M.; Inston, N.; Kumwenda, M.; Powell, S.; Tordoir, J.; Al Shakarchi, J.; Berger, P.; Bolignano, D.; Cassidy, D.; et al. Clinical practice guideline on peri- and postoperative care of arteriovenous fistulas and grafts for haemodialysis in adults. *Nephrol. Dial. Transplant.* **2019**, *34*, II1–II42. [CrossRef]
9. Ibeas, J.; Roca-Tey, R.; Vallespín, J.; Moreno, T.; Moñux, G.; Martí-Monrós, A.; del Pozo, J.L.; Gruss, E.; de Arellano, M.R.; Fontseré, N.; et al. Spanish Clinical Guidelines on Vascular Access for Haemodialysis. *Nefrologia* **2017**, *37* (Suppl. S1), 1–191. [CrossRef]
10. Lok, C.E.; Huber, T.S.; Lee, T.; Shenoy, S.; Yevzlin, A.S.; Abreo, K.; Allon, M.; Asif, A.; Astor, B.C.; Glickman, M.H.; et al. KDOQI Clinical Practice Guideline for Vascular Access: 2019 Update. *Am. J. Kidney Dis.* **2020**, *75*, S1–S164. [CrossRef]
11. Aitken, E.; McLellan, A.; Glen, J.; Serpell, M.; Mactier, R.; Clancy, M. Pain resulting from arteriovenous fistulae: Prevalence and impact. *Clin. Nephrol.* **2013**, *80*, 328–333. [CrossRef] [PubMed]
12. da Silva, O.M.; Rigon, E.; Dalazen, J.; Bissoloti, A.; Rabelo-Silva, E.R. Pain during Arteriovenous Fistula Cannulation in Chronic Renal Patients on Hemodialysis. *Open J. Nurs.* **2016**, *06*, 1028–1037. [CrossRef]
13. MacRae, J.M.; Ahmed, S.B.; Atkar, R.; Hemmelgarn, B.R. A randomized trial comparing buttonhole with rope ladder needling in conventional hemodialysis patients. *Clin. J. Am. Soc. Nephrol.* **2012**, *7*, 1632–1638. [CrossRef] [PubMed]
14. Van Loon, M.M.; Goovaerts, T.; Kessels, A.G.H.; Van Der Sande, F.M.; Tordoir, J.H.M. Buttonhole needling of haemodialysis arteriovenous fistulae results in less complications and interventions compared to the rope-ladder technique. *Nephrol. Dial. Transplant.* **2010**, *25*, 225–230. [CrossRef]
15. Parisotto, M.T.; Schoder, V.U.; Miriunis, C.; Grassmann, A.H.; Scatizzi, L.P.; Kaufmann, P.; Stopper, A.; Marcelli, D. Cannulation technique influences arteriovenous fistula and graft survival. *Kidney Int.* **2014**, *86*, 790–797. [CrossRef]
16. MacRae, J.M.; Ahmed, S.B.; Hemmelgarn, B.R. Arteriovenous fistula survival and needling technique: Long-term results from a randomized buttonhole trial. *Am. J. Kidney Dis.* **2014**, *63*, 636–642. [CrossRef]
17. Lyman, M.; Nguyen Duc, B.; Shugart, A.; Gruhler, H.; Lines, C.; Patel, P.R. Risk of Vascular Access Infection Associated With Buttonhole Cannulation of Fistulas: Data From the National Healthcare Safety Network. *Am. J. Kidney Dis.* **2020**, *76*, 82–89. [CrossRef]
18. Collier, S.; Kandil, H.; Yewnetu, E.; Cross, J.; Caplin, B.; Davenport, A. Infection Rates Following Buttonhole Cannulation in Hemodialysis Patients. *Ther. Apher. Dial.* **2016**, *20*, 476–482. [CrossRef]
19. Peralta, R.; Fazendeiro Matos, J.; Pinto, B.; Gonçalves, P.; Sousa, R.; Felix, C.; Carvalho, H.; Vinhas, J.; Ponce, P. Multiple single cannulation technique of arteriovenous fistula: A randomized controlled trial. *Hemodial. Int.* **2022**, *26*, 4–12. [CrossRef]
20. Huang, S.H.S.; MacRae, J.; Ross, D.; Imtiaz, R.; Hollingsworth, N.; Nesrallah, G.E.; Copland, M.A.; McFarlane, P.A.; Chan, C.T.; Zimmerman, D. Buttonhole versus stepladder cannulation for home hemodialysis: A multicenter, randomized, pilot trial. *Clin. J. Am. Soc. Nephrol.* **2019**, *14*, 403–410. [CrossRef]
21. Page, M.J.; McKenzie, J.E.; Bossuyt, P.M.; Boutron, I.; Hoffmann, T.C.; Mulrow, C.D.; Shamseer, L.; Tetzlaff, J.M.; Akl, E.A.; Brennan, S.E.; et al. The PRISMA 2020 statement: An updated guideline for reporting systematic reviews. *BMJ* **2021**, *372*, n71. [CrossRef]
22. Lee, T.; Mokrzycki, M.; Moist, L.; Maya, I.; Vazquez, M.; Lok, C.E. Standardized Definitions for Hemodialysis Vascular Access. *Semin. Dial.* **2011**, *24*, 515–524. [CrossRef]

23. Peralta, R.; Sousa, L.; Cristóvão, A.F. Cannulation technique of vascular access in haemodialysis and the impact on the arteriovenous fistula survival: Protocol of systematic review. *Int. J. Environ. Res. Public Health* **2022**, *18*, 12554. [CrossRef]
24. Sterne, J.A.C.; Savović, J.; Page, M.J.; Elbers, R.G.; Blencowe, N.S.; Boutron, I.; Cates, C.J.; Cheng, H.-Y.; Corbett, M.S.; Eldridge, S.M.; et al. *Revised Cochrane Risk-of-Bias Tool for Randomized Trials (RoB 2)*; Cochrane: London, UK, 2019; pp. 1–24. Available online: https://methods.cochrane.org/risk-bias-2 (accessed on 1 March 2021).
25. Sterne, J.A.C.; Hernán, M.A.; Reeves, B.C.; Savović, J.; Berkman, N.D.; Viswanathan, M.; Henry, D.; Altman, D.G.; Ansari, M.T.; Boutron, I.; et al. ROBINS-I: A tool for assessing risk of bias in non-randomized studies of interventions. *BMJ* **2016**, *355*, i4919. Available online: http://www.riskofbias.info (accessed on 1 March 2021). [CrossRef] [PubMed]
26. Struthers, J.; Allan, A.; Peel, R.K.; Lambie, S.H. Buttonhole needling of ateriovenous fistulae: A randomized controlled trial. *ASAIO J.* **2010**, *56*, 319–322. [CrossRef] [PubMed]
27. Vaux, E.; King, J.; Lloyd, S.; Moore, J.; Bailey, L.; Reading, I.; Naik, R. Effect of buttonhole cannulation with a polycarbonate peg on in-center hemodialysis fistula outcomes: A randomized controlled trial. *Am. J. Kidney Dis.* **2013**, *62*, 81–88. [CrossRef] [PubMed]
28. Chan, M.R.; Shobande, O.; Vats, H.; Wakeen, M.; Meyer, X.; Bellingham, J.; Astor, B.C.; Yevzlin, A.S. The effect of buttonhole cannulation vs. rope-ladder technique on hemodialysis access patency. *Semin. Dial.* **2014**, *27*, 210–216. [CrossRef]
29. Pergolotti, A.; Rich, E.; Lock, K. The effect of the buttonhole method vs. the traditional method of AV fistula cannulation on hemostasis, needle stick pain, pre-needle stick anxiety, and presence of aneurysms in ambulatory patients on hemodialysis. *Nephrol. Nurs. J.* **2011**, *38*, 333–336.
30. Smyth, W.; Hartig, V.; Manickam, V. Outcomes of buttonhole and rope-ladder cannulation techniques in a tropical renal service. *J. Ren. Care* **2013**, *39*, 157–165. [CrossRef]
31. Glerup, R.; Svensson, M.; Jensen, J.D.; Christensen, J.H. Staphylococcus aureus Bacteremia Risk in Hemodialysis Patients Using the Buttonhole Cannulation Technique: A Prospective Multicenter Study. *Kidney Med.* **2019**, *1*, 263–270. [CrossRef]
32. Sukthinthai, N.; Sittipraneet, A.; Tummanittayangkoon, B.; Vasuvattakul, S.; Chanchairujira, T. Buttonhole technique better than area puncture technique on hemostasis and pain associated with needle cannulation. *J. Med. Assoc. Thai.* **2012**, *95* (Suppl. S2), S208–S212. [PubMed]
33. Kim, M.K.; Kim, H.S. Clinical effects of buttonhole cannulation method on hemodialysis patients. *Hemodial. Int.* **2013**, *17*, 294–299. [CrossRef] [PubMed]
34. Peralta, R.; Matos, J.F.; Carvalho, H. Safe Needling of Arteriovenous Fistulae in Patients on Hemodialysis: Literature Review and a New Approach. *Nephrol. Nurs. J.* **2021**, *48*, 169–177. [CrossRef]
35. Peralta, R.; Sousa, R.; Pinto, B.; Gonçalves, P.; Felix, C.; Fazendeiro Matos, J. Commentary on: "Multiple single cannulation technique of arteriovenous fistula: A randomized controlled trial". *Arch. Nephrol. Ren. Stud.* **2021**, *1*, 28–33.
36. Sidawy, A.N.; Gray, R.; Besarab, A.; Henry, M.; Ascher, E.; Silva, M., Jr.; Miller, A.; Scher, L.; Trerotola, S.; Gregory, R.T.; et al. Recommended standards for reports dealing with arteriovenous hemodialysis accesses. *J. Vasc. Surg.* **2002**, *35*, 603–610. [CrossRef] [PubMed]
37. Viecelli, A.K.; O'Lone, E.; Sautenet, B.; Craig, J.C.; Tong, A.; Chemla, E.; Hooi, L.S.; Lee, T.; Lok, C.; Polkinghorne, K.R.; et al. Vascular Access Outcomes Reported in Maintenance Hemodialysis Trials: A Systematic Review. *Am. J. Kidney Dis.* **2018**, *71*, 382–391. [CrossRef] [PubMed]
38. Ren, C.; Han, Y.; Huang, B.; Yuan, L.; Cao, Y.; Yang, X. Efficacy of buttonhole cannulation (BH) in hemodialysis patients with arteriovenous fistula: A meta-analysis. *Int. J. Clin. Exp. Med.* **2016**, *9*, 15363–15370.
39. Wang, L.-P.; Tsai, L.-H.; Huang, H.-Y.; Okoli, C.; Guo, S.-E. Effect of buttonhole cannulation versus rope- ladder cannulation in hemodialysis patients with vascular access: A systematic review and meta -analysis of randomized/clinical controlled trials. *Medicine* **2022**, *101*, e29597. [CrossRef]
40. Muir, C.A.; Kotwal, S.S.; Hawley, C.M.; Polkinghorne, K.; Gallagher, M.P.; Snelling, P.; Jardine, M.J. Buttonhole cannulation and clinical outcomes in a home hemodialysis cohort and systematic review. *Clin. J. Am. Soc. Nephrol.* **2014**, *9*, 110–119. [CrossRef]
41. Kang, H. Trial sequential analysis: Novel approach for meta-analysis. *Anesth. Pain Med.* **2021**, *16*, 138–150. [CrossRef]
42. Sanfilippo, F.; La Via, L.; Tigano, S.; Morgana, A.; La Rosa, V.; Astuto, M. Trial sequential analysis: The evaluation of the robustness of meta-analyses findings and the need for further research. *Euromediterranean Biomed. J.* **2021**, *16*, 104–107. [CrossRef]
43. Nesrallah, G.E. Pro: Buttonhole cannulation of arteriovenous fistulae. *Nephrol. Dial. Transplant.* **2016**, *31*, 520–523. [CrossRef] [PubMed]
44. Pinto, R.; Duarte, F.; Mata, F.; Sousa, C.; Salgueiro, A.; Fernandes, I. Construção e validação de um modelo de decisão para a canulação da fístula arteriovenosa em hemodiálise. *Rev. Enferm. Ref.* **2023**, *VI*, 1–8. [CrossRef]
45. Pinto, R.; Sousa, C.; Salgueiro, A.; Fernandes, I. Arteriovenous fistula cannulation in hemodialysis: A vascular access clinical practice guidelines narrative review. *J. Vasc. Access.* **2022**, *23*, 825–831. [CrossRef]
46. Sousa, C.N.; Apóstolo, J.L.A.; Figueiredo, M.H.J.S.; Dias, V.F.F.; Teles, P.; Martins, M.M. Construction and validation of a scale of assessment of self-care behaviors with arteriovenous fistula in hemodialysis. *Hemodial. Int.* **2015**, *19*, 306–313. [CrossRef] [PubMed]

Disclaimer/Publisher's Note: The statements, opinions and data contained in all publications are solely those of the individual author(s) and contributor(s) and not of MDPI and/or the editor(s). MDPI and/or the editor(s) disclaim responsibility for any injury to people or property resulting from any ideas, methods, instructions or products referred to in the content.

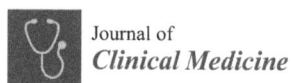

Communication

Recent Advances in the Nutritional Screening, Assessment, and Treatment of Japanese Patients on Hemodialysis

Junko Ishida [1,*] and Akihiko Kato [2]

1. Department of Food and Nutritional Environment, College of Human Life and Environment, Kinjo Gakuin University, Nagoya 463-8521, Japan
2. Blood Purification Unit, Hamamatsu University Hospital, Hamamatsu 431-3192, Japan
* Correspondence: ishida@kinjo-u.ac.jp; Tel.: +81-52-798-0180

Abstract: Patients on hemodialysis (HD) have a higher rate of protein-energy wasting (PEW) due to lower dietary intake of energy and protein (particularly on dialysis days) and greater loss of many nutrients in the dialysate effluent than other patients. The most well-known method of nutritional screening is the subjective global assessment. Moreover, the Global Leadership Initiative on MalnutIrition has developed the first internationally standardized method for diagnosing malnutrition; however, its use in patients on HD has not been established. In contrast, the nutritional risk index for Japanese patients on HD has recently been developed as a screening tool for malnutrition in patients on HD, based on the modified PEW criteria. These tools are beneficial for screening nutritional disorders, enabling registered dietitians to assess patients' dietary intake on dialysis and non-dialysis days and provide advice on dietary intake, especially immediately after dialysis cessation. Oral supplementation with enteral nutrients containing whey protein may also be administered when needed. In patients that experience adverse effects from oral supplementation, intradialytic parenteral nutrition (IDPN) should be combined with moderate dietary intake because IDPN alone cannot provide sufficient nutrition.

Keywords: protein-energy wasting (PEW); nutritional screening; nutritional assessment; hemodialysis

Citation: Ishida, J.; Kato, A. Recent Advances in the Nutritional Screening, Assessment, and Treatment of Japanese Patients on Hemodialysis. *J. Clin. Med.* **2023**, *12*, 2113. https://doi.org/10.3390/jcm12062113

Academic Editor: Ernesto Paoletti

Received: 15 January 2023
Revised: 19 February 2023
Accepted: 4 March 2023
Published: 8 March 2023

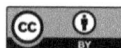

Copyright: © 2023 by the authors. Licensee MDPI, Basel, Switzerland. This article is an open access article distributed under the terms and conditions of the Creative Commons Attribution (CC BY) license (https://creativecommons.org/licenses/by/4.0/).

1. Introduction

Nutritional problems are prevalent in patients with chronic kidney disease (CKD). Malnutrition is closely associated with the risk of onset and progression of cardiovascular disease, sarcopenia, frailty, infection, and cognitive impairment. In addition, poor nutritional status is associated with poor healthy-longevity outcomes, such as the requirement of support and long-term care, institutionalization in nursing homes, and hospitalization [1]. Nutritional disorders in patients with kidney disease are termed as "protein-energy wasting" (PEW), a state of disordered catabolism resulting from metabolic and nutritional derangements. PEW is induced by both anorexia and decreased nutrient intake and various other factors such as uremic toxins, inflammation, oxidative stress, hyper-catabolism, metabolic acidosis, low testosterone levels, growth hormone resistance, insulin resistance, physical inactivity, loss of nutrients from urine and dialysate, and comorbidities [2,3]. Cachexia represents a very severe form of PEW that is often associated with profound physiological, metabolic, psychological, and immunological disorders [2].

Recently, the National Kidney Foundation and the Academy of Nutrition and Dietetics updated the National Kidney Foundation's Kidney Disease Outcomes Quality Initiative (NKF-KDOQI) Clinical Practice Guidelines for Nutrition in Chronic Kidney Disease [4]. The guidelines suggest that patients with CKD stages 3–5D should be screened for nutrition status biannually. The guidelines also provide direction for when a registered dietitian should perform a detailed nutrition assessment. However, many of the statements in the guidelines were based on expert opinion from U.S. nephrologists. Furthermore, the cut-off values for nutritional parameters such as body mass index (BMI) and creatinine index in the guidelines cannot apply to Japanese patients on HD due to the smaller body size and muscle mass volume in this population. The timing of blood sampling before HD is also different between Japan (at 2-day intervals) and USA (mid-week), leading to inconsistencies in laboratory measures. Thus, an individualized and specialized approach will be needed to screen and assess the nutritional status of Japanese patients on HD.

The Dialysis Outcomes and Practice Patterns Study (DOPPS) reported that the prevalence of serum C-reactive protein (CRP) >10 mg/L was much lower in Japan (10%) than in seven European countries (30 to 44%) and Australia/New Zealand (36%), where 57% of CRP measurements were ≤1 mg/L in Japan [5]. In contrast, when the association of nutritional parameters was compared with mortality risk in 12 DOPPS-joining countries, the impact of malnutrition on total death was most potent in Japan [6]. It is therefore likely that the nutritional problem has more impact than microinflammation-induced catabolism in Japanese patients on HD upon improving their survival prognosis.

In this review, we mainly focus on inadequate nutritional intake in Japanese patients on HD. We first introduce the methods of nutritional screening and assessment for patients undergoing HD. Thereafter, we outline the relationship between malnutrition and sarcopenia and frailty and discuss the usefulness of the Global Leadership Initiative on Malnutrition (GLIM) criteria, which are proposed as the first international standard criteria for malnutrition diagnosis. Third, the daily micronutrient intake among patients on dialysis is often deficient. Particularly, magnesium (Mg) intake is independently associated with serum Mg level [7]. Deficiencies in the daily intake of zinc (Zn) is also related to worse nutritional and body composition parameters and higher mortality risk in patients on HD [8]. Thus, we review the effect of Mg and Zn deficiencies on the clinical outcomes of patients on HD [9,10]. In addition, we demonstrate the usefulness of oral nutritional support (ONS) and intradialytic parenteral nutrition (IDPN) as nutritional supplements for PEW in Japan.

2. Nutritional Assessment Methods for Dialysis Patients

The prevalence of PEW is high in patients on chronic HD and is closely associated with morbidity and mortality. The subjective global assessment (SGA) has been validated as an objective screening tool for nutritional risk in patients on chronic HD. Other screening tools include the malnutrition-inflammation score (MIS), geriatric nutritional risk index (GNRI), mini-nutritional assessment short form (MNA-SF), and malnutrition universal screening tool (MUST). Thus, we reviewed the usefulness of these screening tools for assessing nutritional risk in patients on HD.

2.1. SGA

The SGA is a nutritional assessment method that includes medical history and physical examination sections. The SGA is the most widely used method for assessing subjective nutritional status worldwide [11].

The medical history section comprises five questions on (1) weight loss (during the preceding 6 months or changes over the past 2 weeks), (2) dietary intake (compared to normal conditions), (3) gastrointestinal symptoms (over the last 2 weeks), (4) functional capacity or energy level, and (5) metabolic demands (relationship between disease and nutritional requirements). The physical examination section includes five questions on (1) loss of subcutaneous fat, (2) muscle wasting, (3) edema formation at the ankle or (4) sacrum, and (5) ascites. These criteria are subjectively evaluated as either normal (0), mild (1+), moderate (2+), or severe (3+). Based on medical history and physical examination findings, clinicians rank SGA severity into three categories: (A) well nourished, (B) moderate or suspected malnutrition, and (C) severe malnutrition [11].

In the United States, the 7-point SGA scale is used to assess the nutritional status of patients with CKD. This scale comprises six questions on weight change, dietary intake, gastrointestinal symptoms, functional capacity, disease status/comorbidities as related to nutritional needs, and physical examination (used to evaluate weight change such as loss of subcutaneous fat, muscle wasting, and edema related to undernutrition). Answers are rated from 1 to 7 points. A rating of 6 or 7 indicates very mild risk to no risk (well-nourished status), while 3 to 5 indicates mild to moderate risk, and 1 or 2 in most categories indicates significant physical signs of malnutrition.

Nutritional assessment using the 7-point SGA scale in elderly patients with advanced CKD (mean body mass index (BMI): 28.4 kg/m^2) showed that 28% of the patients had moderate nutritional risk (SGA rating, 3 to 5) [12]. A study of 1601 Dutch patients on HD (mean age: 59 years) showed that 23% of the patients had moderate nutritional risk (SGA rating 4 to 5), and 5% had severe nutritional disorders (SGA rating, 1 to 3). Nutritional risk was also present in 55% of patients with BMI < 22 kg/m^2, 40% of patients with BMI 22–25 kg/m^2 (normal body weight), and 25% of patients with BMI > 30 kg/m^2 (obesity). Lower BMI was associated with more frequent complications. In addition, the 7-point SGA was useful for predicting the 7-year mortality risk [13].

Therefore, the nutritional guidelines of the 2020 NKF-KDOQI recommend the use of the 7-point SGA for assessing the nutritional status of patients on dialysis (Level 1, Recommendation B) [4].

2.2. MIS

The MIS was initially developed by Kalantar-Zadeh et al. to assess nutritional deficits in patients on HD [8]. It comprises 10 items and a combination of the 7-point SGA with dialysis vintage, BMI, and laboratory parameters (serum albumin level and total iron-binding capacity) [14]. Each item is rated from 0 to 3 points, with a total score of 30 points, with higher scores indicating worse nutritional status. The KDOQI guidelines suggest MIS use as an assessment tool (Level 2, Recommendation C) [4]. A higher MIS score over time is associated with reduction in dietary intake, body fat percentage, upper-arm muscle circumference, and a high risk of hospitalization and mortality [14]. It has also been reported that the survival prognosis is poor when the MIS score is ≥ 7 [15]. Moreover, a global review demonstrated that 28% to 54% of patients on dialysis had nutritional risk when assessed using either the SGA or MIS [16].

2.3. GNRI

The GNRI was initially designed to predict the risk of malnutrition-related complications and mortality in elderly, hospitalized French persons [17]. The GNRI is a simple and objective tool for assessing nutritional status based on only actual and ideal body weight (BW) and serum albumin levels. Ideal BW can be calculated using the Lorentz formula, which considers a patient's body height and sex. When body height measurement is difficult to perform, it is estimated using a formula based on knee height. When the actual BW exceeds the ideal BW, we set the actual/ideal BW ratio to 1 (Table 1) [18]. In Japan, BW corresponding to a BMI of 22 kg/m^2 is often used as an ideal BW, and in patients on HD, dry weight is used as the actual BW [18].

Table 1. Geriatric Nutritional Risk Index (GNRI).

GNRI formula	(14.89 × albumin (g/dL)) + (41.7 × (weight/ideal weight)) ideal weight is calculated from the Lorentz equations (WLo) or weight equivalent to BMI = 22 kg/m^2
The Lorentz equations (WLo) formula	For men: ideal weight = H − 100 − ([H − 150]/4) For women: ideal weight = H − 100 − ([H − 150]/2.5)
If height cannot be obtained	For men: H (cm) = (2.02 × KH (cm)) − (0.04 × age (y)) + 64.19 For women: H (cm) = (1.83 × KH (cm)) − (0.24 × age (y)) + 84.88

Modified from [18]. Abbreviations: albumin, serum albumin; weight, actual body weight; ideal weight, ideal body weight; H, height; KH, knee height. NOTE: When the body weight exceeds the ideal body weight, the ideal weight rather than the actual weight is used to calculate the index. In the original reference, four grades of nutritional-related risk are defined: major risk (GNRI: <82), moderate risk (GNRI: 82 to <92), low risk (GNRI: 92 to ≤98), and no risk (GNRI: >98). For patients on hemodialysis: risk of nutrition (GNRI ≤ 91), without risk (GNRI > 91).

The GNRI is frequently used for assessing nutritional conditions owing to its simplicity. However, this tool would likely reflect medium- to long-term nutritional status rather than short-term nutritional status because (1) the biological half-life of serum albumin is approximately 3 weeks, (2) albumin is mainly stored extravascularly, and (3) the variability of serum albumin level is less than its metabolic turnover rate. In addition, although the cut-off GNRI value for survival prognosis have been reported as 89.3 to 96.0 in patients on HD and 94.55 to 96.4 in patients on peritoneal dialysis (PD), there is no standard cut-off value for survival prognosis [19].

2.4. MNA-SF

The MNA-SF is a screening method for assessing the nutritional status of elderly individuals. The MNA-SF assesses six items to rate the nutritional state (0 to 14 points): (1) reduced dietary intake over the past 3 months (0 to 2 points), (2) weight loss over the past 3 months (0 to 3 points), (3) ambulation (0 to 2 points), (4) mental stress or acute illness over the past 3 months (0 to 2 points), (5) depression or dementia (0 to 2 points), and (6) BMI or calf circumference (0 to 3 points). A score of 7 or less indicates malnourishment, a score of 8–11 indicates the risk of malnutrition, and a score of 12–14 indicates a normal nutritional status [20].

When the MNA-SF was applied for patients on HD, 30.1% of the patients were classified as well nourished, 59.3% as being at risk of malnutrition, and 10.6% as malnourished [21]. In addition, there was a 2.50-fold higher risk of all-cause mortality in patients at risk of malnutrition and a 3.89-fold higher risk in malnourished patients compared with those with a normal nutritional status [21].

2.5. MUST

MUST is a nutritional screening method developed by the British Association for Parenteral and Enteral Nutrition for home-care patients. In MUST, assessment of nutritional risk is based on the total scores for BMI, weight loss, acute illness, and undernutrition (Table 2) [22]. In patients on HD, MUST can effectively screen for the presence of PEW, with a sensitivity of 100% and a specificity of 98% [23].

Table 2. Malnutrition Universal Screening Tool (MUST) diagnostic criteria.

Score	BMI (kg/m^2)	Unplanned Weight Loss in the Past 3–6 Months (%)	Acute Disease Effect + No Nutritional Intake for > 5 Days
0	>20.0	<5	None
1	18.5–20.0	5–10	
2	<18.5	>10	There has been or is likely

Modified from [22]. Total score of 6 points: 0, low risk (routine clinical care); 1, medium risk (observe); ≥2, high risk (active intervention of dietitian or nutrition support team).

2.6. New Indicators for Muscle Wasting

Myostatin is a myokine predominantly expressed in skeletal muscle, and it regulates muscle growth negatively. Myostatin is overexpressed in uremic sarcopenia [24]. Recently, blood myostatin was reported to be negatively related to muscle mass and muscle strength, as assessed by handgrip strength, in patients on peritoneal dialysis [25] and in those on HD [26]. However, this association is not a universal finding. This may be due to the influence of various factors such as age, gender, inflammatory state, physical activity, and the different assay techniques for myostatin measurement [27].

Brain-derived neurotrophic factor (BDNF) is another myokine produced by immune cells and skeletal muscle. BDNF is involved in the regulation of synaptic function and in the maintenance of the neuromuscular system as well as in muscle development and metabolism [28]. Deus et al. [29] showed that 6 months of resistance training just before HD sessions improved handgrip strength in line with increased BDNF. Serum BDNF levels were also positively associated with handgrip strength, role-emotional, and emotional well-being scales and negatively associated with the Beck depression inventory score [29]. Miyazaki et al. [30] evaluated the relationship between BDNF and sarcopenia and frailty in regular patients on HD. Plasma BDNF levels were significantly lower in patients with severe sarcopenia and was correlated with muscle strength and physical performance, such as in the 6 m walk test, short physical performance battery, and the 5-time chair stand test. BDNF was also positively correlated with body weight. Similarly, in recipients of kidney transplantation, serum BDNF levels were significantly higher, but serum myostatin levels were significantly lower in the group with low skeletal muscle mass index (SMI), as measured with dual-energy X-ray absorptiometry (DXA), compared with the normal group [31].

Creatinine kinetic modelling is also proposed as an indirect indicator of muscle mass volume in patients on HD. The creatinine generation rate (CGR) can be calculated by measuring the pre- and post-dialysis creatinine concentrations. Because age and gender are independent determinants of CGR, CGR is usually adjusted for age and gender using a previously reported equation (i.e., %CGR) [32]. A recent study demonstrated that the cut-off value of %CGR for detecting low muscle mass volume (SMI less than 7.0 kg/m^2 in men and less than 5.7 kg/m^2 in women) was 109.83, with a sensitivity of 68% and a specificity of 88% in Japanese HD patients [33]. The ratio of serum creatinine to cystatin C is also demonstrated to be useful in predicting skeletal muscle mass and strength in patients with non-dialysis CKD [34].

3. Diagnostic Criteria for PEW

3.1. International Diagnostic Criteria

The International Society of Renal Nutrition and Metabolism (ISRNM) Expert Committee reported diagnostic criteria for PEW in 2008 (Table 3) [2]. The criteria comprised four categories. PEW is diagnosed when at least three out of the four categories (and at least one test in each of the selected category) are satisfied.

Table 3. Protein energy wasting (PEW) diagnostic criteria.

Category	Criteria
Serum chemistry	• Serum albumin < 3.8 g per 100 mL (bromocresol green test) • Serum prealbumin (transthyretin) < 30 mg per 100 mL (for patients on hemodialysis alone) • Serum cholesterol < 100 mg per 100 mL
Body mass	• BMI < 23 kg/m^2 (Asians have low BMI) • Unintentional weight loss: 5% over 3 months or 10% over 6 months • Total body fat percentage < 10%
Muscle mass	• Reduced muscle mass: 5% over 3 months or 10% over 6 months • Reduced mid-arm muscle circumference area: reduction > 10% • In relation to 50th percentile of reference population • Creatinine appearance
Dietary intake	• Unintentional low DPI: <0.8 g/kg/day for at least 2 months for patients on dialysis or <0.6 g/kg/day for patients with CKD stages 2–5 • Unintentional low DEI: <25 kcal/kg/day for at least 2 months

Modified from [2]. Abbreviations: DPI, dietary protein intake; DEI, dietary energy intake. NOTE: At least three out of the four listed categories (and at least one test in each of the selected categories) must be satisfied for the diagnosis of kidney disease-related PEW. However, these diagnostic criteria have not been widely used because body composition and dietary intake need to be assessed over several months, and the validity of the cut-off values for Japanese patients with CKD is unknown.

PEW is caused by inadequate intake of nutrients and a hypercatabolic state in which skeletal muscle, visceral protein, and stored body fat are exhausted through various stimuli. The stimuli include inflammation, oxidative stress, accumulation of uremic toxins, insulin resistance, metabolic acidosis, and nutrient loss from effluent dialysate (Figure 1). In the category of low body mass, the BMI cut-off value was set at <23 kg/m^2 [2]. However, since

74.1% of Japanese patients on HD have a BMI of <24 kg/m², this cut-off is inappropriate for Japanese patients [35]. Therefore, the KDOQI guidelines state that diagnosing PEW using BMI is inappropriate unless the BMI is <18 kg/m² [4].

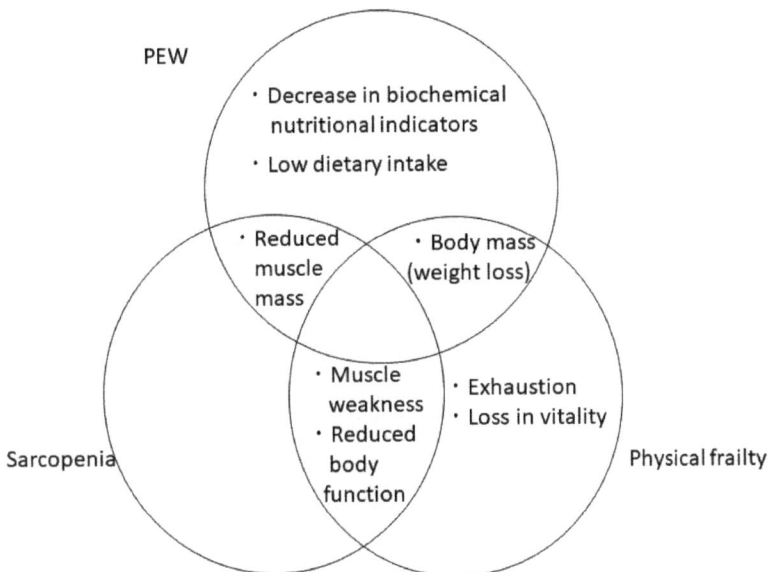

Figure 1. Association between protein-energy wasting (PEW) and sarcopenia and frailty.

3.2. Diagnostic Criteria for Japanese Patients on HD

The scientific committee of the Japanese Society for Dialysis Therapy (JSDT) developed a novel nutritional risk index, the Nutritional Risk Index for Japanese Hemodialysis (NRI-JH), after modifying the original PEW criteria (Table 4) [36]. The NRI-JH classifies patients on HD into three risk groups according to their total score, ranging from 0 to 13. The adjusted hazard ratio for 1-year survival was 1.96 (95% confidence interval (CI): 1.77–2.16) in the medium-risk group (score 8 to 10) and 3.91 (95% CI: 3.57–4.29) in the high-risk group (score 11 to 13), with the low-risk group (score 0 to 7) serving as a reference. The NRI-JH can stratify mortality risk in elderly patients on HD [36]. It is also useful for predicting long-term mortality [37].

Table 4. NRI-JH evaluation method.

Category	Criteria	Score
BMI	• ≥20 kg/m² • <20 kg/m²	3 0
Serum albumin (BCG)	• Age ≥ 65, <3.5 g/dL, age < 65, <3.7 g/dL • Age ≥ 65, ≥3.5 g/dL, age < 65, ≥3.7 g/dL	4 0
Serum creatinine	• Age ≥ 65, male < 9.7 mg/dL, female < 8.0 mg/dL • Age ≥ 65, male ≥ 9.7 mg/dL, female ≥ 8.0 mg/dL • Age < 65, male < 11.6 mg/dL, female < 9.7 mg/dL • Age < 65, male ≥ 11.6 mg/dL, female ≥ 9.7 mg/dL	4 0 4 0
Serum total cholesterol	• <130 mg/dL • ≥130 to <220 mg/dL • ≥220 mg/dL	1 0 2

Modified from [36]. Abbreviations: BCG, Bromocresol Green. NOTE: the sum of each point was calculated and divided into three risk groups: low-risk group (score, 0–7), medium-risk group (8–10), and high-risk group (11–13). BMI was calculated from weight measured after hemodialysis, and laboratory data were measured before hemodialysis.

4. Association of Malnutrition with Sarcopenia and Frailty

Malnutrition and sarcopenia/frailty are bidirectionally associated, but few studies have assessed the relationship between sarcopenia/frailty and nutritional status in the dialysis population.

4.1. SGA

Complications of nutritional risk by the 7-point SGA (≤5 points) in patients on HD were found in 66.7% of patients with sarcopenia, 65.7% of patients with pre-sarcopenia, and 51.2% of patients without sarcopenia [38]. There was a 2.99-fold higher risk of all-cause mortality when the patients had complications of malnutrition and sarcopenia, indicating that sarcopenia and malnutrition may additively worsen survival prognosis [38].

4.2. MIS

The MIS was inversely correlated with muscle power as assessed by handgrip strength in patients on HD (mean age: 58.3 years). The MIS was significantly associated with the risk of low handgrip strength (below the cut-off value for sarcopenia; odds ratio (OR) 1.202; 95% CI 1.073–1.347; $p < 0.01$) and with mortality (OR 1.322; 95% CI 1.192–1.467; $p < 0.01$), indicating that a worse nutritional status increases the risk of sarcopenia and mortality [39]. Among patients on PD, there was a significantly higher MIS in those with physical frailty than in those without (7.13 ± 3.22 vs. 5.12 ± 2.30, $p < 0.01$). In addition, patients with physical frailty and depressive symptoms had worse MIS scores (9.48 ± 3.97) [40].

4.3. GNRI

In Japanese patients on HD, the GNRI cut-off value for mortality (=91.5) [18] was related to the risk of a handgrip strength below the cut-off value associated with sarcopenia (based on the criteria of the Asian Working Group for Sarcopenia (AWGS) 2019 (male < 28 kg, female < 18 kg)) [41]. However, the sensitivity of the cut-off value for GNRI indicating possible sarcopenia by handgrip strength was 46%, and the specificity was 61% [41]. In addition, there was no difference in GNRI according to frailty status in Japanese patients on HD [42]. Therefore, further studies are needed to clarify the cut-off value of GNRI for the early detection of sarcopenia and frailty.

4.4. MNA-SF

Among malnourished patients on HD (MNA-SF score: 0 to 7), 43.5% of the patients were frail, and 34.8% were pre-frail. In addition, risk of malnutrition (MNA-SF score: 8 to 11) was complicated by frailty and pre-frailty in 30.1% and 50.0% of the patients, respectively. In contrast, frailty was found in only 12.4% of the patients with a normal nutritional status (MNA-SF score: 12 to 14) [40]. Patients on HD with MNA-SF ≤ 11 also had a 7.1-fold higher risk of frailty than those with good nourishment [42].

4.5. PEW

Muscle mass loss is included in the diagnostic criteria for PEW and sarcopenia. Body weight loss is also a common criterion for PEW and physical frailty (Figure 1). Therefore, PEW is expected to be closely related to sarcopenia and frailty.

4.6. GLIM Criteria

The GLIM criteria are the first internationally standardized diagnostic criteria for malnutrition in adults. They are applied using a two-step method involving risk screening and diagnostic assessment. First, nutritional risk screening is performed using validated screening tools (MNA-SF, SGA, MUST, GNRI, etc.). If the patient is considered at risk of malnutrition, the presence and severity of malnutrition are evaluated based on two categories: "phenotypic" and "etiologic" [43]. Body weight loss, reduced BMI, and reduced muscle mass are categorized as phenotypic criteria, whereas reduced food intake/assimilation and disease burden/inflammation are classified as etiologic criteria. For the diagnosis of malnutrition, the GLIM recommends the use of a combination of at least one phenotypic criterion and one etiologic criterion (Figure 2). Severity grading is determined using these three phenotypic items. If at least one of the criteria was classified as moderate or severe, we diagnosed moderate or severe malnutrition.

Phenotypic criterion			Etiologic criteria	
Non-volitional weight loss (%)	Low body mass index (kg/m^2)	Reduced muscle mass	Reduced food intake or assimilation	Disease burden/ inflammation
• > 5% within past 6 mo • > 10% beyond 6 mo	• < 20 if < 70 yr • < 22 if > 70 yr Asia • < 18.5 if < 70 yr • < 20 if > 70 yr	• Reduced by validated body composition measuring techniques Asia • thresholds for reduced muscle mass need to be adapted to race (mid-arm muscle or CC may be used)	• ≤ 50% of ER > 1 week or • any reduction for > 2 weeks • any chronic GI condition that adversely impacts food assimilation or absorption	• acute disease/ injury or • chronic disease-related
Requires at least 1 phenotypic criterion			Requires at least 1 etiologic criterion	

malnutrition			
severity grading			
Phenotypic	weight loss (%)	Low BMI (kg/m^2)	Reduced muscle mass
Stage 1 moderate	• 5-10% within the past 6 mo • 10-20% beyond 6 mo	• < 20 if < 70 yr • < 22 if ≥70 yr	• Mild to moderate deficit
Stage 2 Severe	• > 10% within the past 6 mo • > 20% beyomd 6 mo	• < 18.5 if < 70 yr • < 20 if ≥70 yr	• Severe deficit
Etiology: 4 categories of malnutrition associated with low nutrition and inflammation, malnutrition related to:			
• chronic disease with inflammation	• acute disease or injury with severe inflammation	• chronic disease with minimal or no perceived inflammation	• starvation including hunger/food shortage associated with socio-economic or environmental factors

Figure 2. Malnutrition diagnosis using Global Leadership Initiative on Malnutrition (GLIM) standards. Abbreviations: CC, calf circumference; ER, emergency requirements; GI, gastrointestinal; mo, month; yr, year. Modified from [43].

The criteria for loss of muscle mass were not described in the GLIM categories. However, in elderly Japanese inpatients, mild to moderate muscle mass loss corresponds to a maximal calf circumference of ≤30 cm in men and ≤29 cm in women, and severe loss corresponds to ≤28 cm in men and ≤26 cm in women [44]. Therefore, muscle mass loss can be substituted by calf circumference measurement.

Presently, the usefulness of the GLIM criteria for diagnosing malnutrition in patients on dialysis is unclear. A recent study demonstrated that the sensitivity of the GLIM criteria in detecting malnutrition diagnosed by a well-established method (either 7-point SGA or MIS) was low (61 to 72%), indicating that the GLIM score did not perform better than the 7-point SGA and MIS. In addition, its predictive ability for survival prognosis was inferior to that of the 7-point SGA and MIS [45]. In contrast, a Korean study showed that malnutrition diagnosed using the GLIM criteria was significantly associated with the risk of all-cause mortality and hospitalization due to infection in patients on chronic HD [46].

5. Anorexia and Nutritional Deficiencies in Dialysis Patients

5.1. Anorexia

Approximately 40% of patients on HD were aware of loss of appetite when asked about their appetite in the past 4 weeks [47]. In particular, appetite tended to decrease during lunch and dinner on dialysis days. The suggested causes of anorexia are (1) suppression of appetite signaling to the hypothalamus by increased inflammatory cytokines; (2) increased tryptophan transport across the blood–brain barrier due to decreased blood levels of branched-chain amino acids, which enhance serotonin synthesis in the brain and suppress appetite; (3) decreased ghrelin production from gastric endocrine cells with appetite-promoting effects; and (4) dysgeusia due to poor oral environment or zinc deficiency.

5.2. Insufficient Nutritional Intake

Achieving adequate dietary energy and protein intake remains a challenge for patients on HD. A recent review including eight studies with more than 100 patients on HD reported that dietary energy inadequacy (<35 kcal/kg BW/day) was found in 52 to 92% of the patients, whereas dietary protein inadequacy (<0.8 g/kg BW/day) was found in 32.3 to 81% [48].

5.3. Nutrient Loss during Dialysis

Approximately 6–12 g of amino acids and 7–8 g of protein are lost during each dialysis session [48]. In addition, water-soluble vitamins and trace elements such as zinc and carnitine are removed by diffusion and filtration. Furthermore, online hemodiafiltration removes more water-soluble vitamins and larger protein molecules than conventional HD [49].

5.4. Zn Deficiency

Because Zn is a trace element that is essential for maintaining the structure and functional expression of many proteins including enzymes, various symptoms occur in its deficiency. Serum Zn levels decrease with the progression of CKD stage, and approximately 70% of patients on HD and 60% of patients on PD have Zn deficiency (blood Zn < 60 µg/dL) [50].

Zn deficiency induces inflammation in muscle cells and increases oxidative stress by decreasing the activity of Zn-dependent antioxidant enzymes. In addition, Zn deficiency may contribute to the onset and progression of sarcopenia by decreasing the synthesis and increasing the degradation of muscle proteins, destabilizing neuromuscular transmitter sites and impairing neurotransmitter release. Zn deficiency also damages taste bud cells, leading to taste abnormalities.

In patients with CKD, there is a negative correlation between serum Zn concentration and salt taste-perception threshold; thus, the amount of daily salt intake is higher in Zn-deficient patients [51]. In addition, patients on HD with inadequate Zn intake (men < 10, women < 8 mg/day) had a 4.1-fold higher risk of all-cause mortality than those with adequate Zn intake [52].

In the general population, the relationship between blood Zn levels and dietary Zn intake was weak [53,54], although it is known that an association exists between zinc deficiency and reduced taste thresholds [55]. Similarly, there was no relationship between serum Zn and dietary Zn intake in patients on HD [56]. However, oral Zn supplementation is useful for mitigating taste disorders in patients on HD [56,57]. For example, a dose of Zn acetate (50 mg/day) for 6 months improved taste sensations such as salty, sweet, and bitter along with an increase in serum Zn concentration from 75 ± 8 to 97 ± 10 µg/dL [58]. We also preliminary observed improvement in salty taste thresholds in 28 patients on HD following oral Zn administration for 6 months (Figure 3, unpublished data). However, long-term Zn acetate administration should be avoided because Zn can directly prevent copper absorption from the intestinal tract, which may cause leukopenia and pancytopenia due to severe copper deficiency [59].

5.5. Mg Deficiency

Mg is the second most abundant intracellular cation. It performs various functions such as membrane stabilization, nerve conduction, ion transport, and intracellular energy metabolism and is involved in all reactions that require adenosine triphosphate (ATP). Mg is abundant in seaweed, seafood, sesame seeds, and nuts and is absorbed through the small intestine. Hypomagnesemia (<1.8 mg/dL) is one of the most common electrolyte disorders. The prevalence of hypomagnesemia did not decline even in CKD stages G4 and G5, where the prevalence rate was approximately 15% [60]. Since potassium-rich foods are rich in Mg, dietary restriction of potassium may lead to a lower intake of Mg. Moreover, hypomagnesemia may be induced by proton pump inhibitors, which are known to inhibit the passive/active transport of Mg from the small intestine [61].

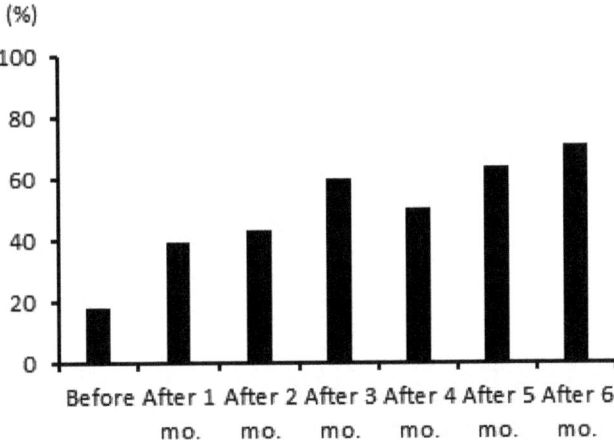

Figure 3. Taste thresholds during 6 months of zinc replacement therapy. Subjects: Twenty-eight patients on hemodialysis with serum zinc levels < 80 µg/dL (male: 19, female: 9). Methods: Nobelzin® tablets (zinc acetate dihydrate) were orally administered to maintain serum zinc levels within 70–120 µg/dL, and salty taste thresholds were measured with the "SALSAVE® impregnated paper test". Those who could taste salt in the salt-impregnated filter paper with the lowest salt concentration were considered to have normal taste, the percentage of whom is shown.

Mg inhibits the formation of calcium protein particles (CPP) associated with the development of vascular calcification [62]. Among patients on HD, there is a J-curve relationship between hyperphosphatemia and mortality in patients with serum Mg concentration < 2.7 mg/dL, while the risk disappeared in patients with serum Mg > 3.1 mg/dL, implying that Mg may protective against hyperphosphatemia [62].

In patients on HD, Mg can be supplied by increasing the Mg concentration in the dialysate or administering oral Mg preparations. When the Mg concentration of the dialysate was increased from 1 to 2 mEq/L, secondary CPP formed after a significantly long period (after 28 days), suggesting that Mg supplementation may slow vascular calcification [63]. A meta-analysis of eight studies demonstrated that oral Mg supplementation also decreased serum parathyroid hormone levels and the intima-media thickness of the common carotid artery [64].

5.6. Oral Dysfunction

Oral function declines with age. Oral dysfunction is closely related to poor food intake, which can easily lead to dysphagia and malnutrition. Oral problems also affect the development of sarcopenia and frailty [65–67].

In Japan, a large-scale cohort study on the oral condition of elderly individuals was conducted in 2012, with a follow-up study lasting up to 4 years. The study reported that decline in ≥3 of six oral indicators (number of remaining teeth, chewing ability, tongue movement, gliding tongue, increase in food not chewed, and munching) was associated with a higher risk of physical frailty, sarcopenia, admission to nursing care, and death. Therefore, the appearance of such trivial deterioration in oral function is called "oral frailty" [68]. In 2018, "oral hypofunction" was added to Japan's healthcare fee list. Oral cavity dysfunction is evaluated by seven examination items: poor oral hygiene, oral dryness, reduced occlusal force, decreased tongue-lip motor function, decreased tongue pressure, decreased masticatory function, and deterioration of swallowing function (Table 5). Thus, oral hypofunction is defined as a state where three or more of these diagnostic criteria are met [69]. The Japanese Society of Gerodontology Academic Committee classified the process from health to oral dysfunction into four stages: the 1st stage of population approach, the 2nd stage of oral frailty, the 3rd stage of oral hypofunction, and the 4th stage of oral dysfunction. In addition, "oral frailty" is widely used in public campaigns to raise awareness regarding oral function.

Table 5. Measurements of clinical signs/symptoms of oral hypofunction.

Clinical Signs	Measurements
Poor oral hygiene	The total number of microorganisms (CFU/mL) is ≥106.5, or the revised tongue coating index is ≤50%
Oral dryness	The measured value obtained by a recommended moisture checker is less than 27.0
Reduced occlusal force	The occlusal force is less than 200 N, or the number of remaining teeth is <20
Decreased tongue-lip motor function	The number of any counts of /pa/, /ta/, or /ka/ produced per second is <6
Decreased tongue pressure	The maximum tongue pressure is less than 30 kPa
Decreased masticatory function	The glucose concentration obtained by chewing gelatin gummies is <100 mg/dL
Deterioration of swallowing function	The total score of the Eating Assessment Tool (EAT-10) is ≥3

Modified from [69].

Although patients on dialysis experience oral diseases more frequently than healthy individuals, dental care is limited. We preliminarily assessed the presence of sarcopenia, based on the AWGS 2019 cut-off values and oral hypofunction, in 141 patients on HD. We found that there was no difference in oral hygiene and swallowing function between the sarcopenia and non-sarcopenia groups, while the other items were significantly lower in the sarcopenia group (Table 6, unpublished data). Since oral frailty is detected at the pre-frail stage, it is important to objectively evaluate the oral condition and preserve oral function to prevent the development of PEW, sarcopenia, and frailty.

Table 6. Association between sarcopenia and oral hypofunction.

Oral Hypofunction	Dysfunction-Criteria	Sarcopenia Groups	Non-Sarcopenia Groups	p
Poor oral hygiene [1] (%)	≥50	17 (0–89)	22 (0–67)	N.S.
Oral dryness [2]	<27	25 (6–38)	26 (17–70)	<0.05
Reduced occlusal force (teeth number) [3]	<20	16 (0–31)	24 (0–32)	<0.05
Decreased tongue-lip motor function [4] (times/sec)	Any of them <6	5 (2–7)	6 (1–8)	<0.05
Decreased tongue pressure (kPa)	<30	25 (7–48)	33 (15–55)	<0.05
Decreased masticatory function [5] (mg/dL)	<100	106 (22–266)	124 (25–340)	<0.05
Deterioration of swallowing function [6] (point)	≥3	0 (0–10)	0 (0–32)	N.S.

Subjects: A total of 141 patients on hemodialysis (male: 96, female: 45). Variables were expressed as the median (range). Data were analyzed by the Mann–Whitney U-test. Note: [1] The measured revised tongue coating index (TCI); [2] the measured value obtained by a recommended moisture checker; [3] number of remaining teeth; [4] the number of any counts of /pa/, /ta/, or /ka/; [5] the glucose concentration obtained by chewing gelatin gummies; [6] the total score of the Eating Assessment Tool (EAT 10) questionnaires.

6. Nutritional Supplementation for PEW

6.1. Meal Supply at Dialysis Facilities

As large amounts of protein and amino acids are lost during HD sessions, it is reasonable to encourage patients to eat meals during or just after the dialysis procedure. Comparative studies showed that dietary energy and protein intake were lower during the dialysis-on days than during the dialysis-off days, indicating that in-central patients on HD may skip three meals per week during dialysis treatment. Therefore, the supply of intradialytic meals may be a therapeutic opportunity to improve PEW and health-related quality of life, particularly in malnourished patients, unless there is a low risk of postprandial hypotension, digestive symptoms, or aspiration. Recently, it was reported that the intake of milk protein (40 g) 1 h after the start of dialysis compensates for amino acid loss from the dialysate effluent and maintains plasma amino acid concentrations until the end of the dialysis session [70].

Many dialysis facilities have stopped providing meals due to the ongoing coronavirus disease (COVID-19) pandemic in Japan. A retrospective study demonstrated that because of the discontinuation of meal provision for 10 months, dry weight gradually decreased from 53.6 to 52.6 kg, and GNRI decreased from 91.5 to 89.5 in elderly patients on HD [71].

6.2. Home Nutrition Care for Patients on Dialysis

In patients on dialysis, weighted mean adherence rates of the recommended energy, protein, and fat intakes were 23.1%, 45.5%, and 41.4%, respectively [72]. Below are some tips for increasing energy and protein intake at home:

1. Increase energy intake: Fat contains high energy (9 kcal/g); thus, dietary fat intake is useful for increasing energy levels. Dietary fat is present in oils, fatty meats, dairy products, nuts, etc., which are present in beef or pork ribs, chicken thighs with skin, bacon, fried tofu, and cream cheese eaten with bread. In particular, medium-chain triglycerides (MCTs) are useful as energy sources because they do not form micelles, enter the general circulation system rapidly through the portal vein, and are transported to the liver for β-oxidization. Octane, a medium-chain fatty acid, activates ghrelin, which has appetite-promoting effects. In a study on healthy subjects, an intake of 45 mL/day of MCT oil increased the blood levels of active ghrelin by approximately two-fold [73]. Since MCT oil is tasteless and odorless, it can be easily added to main foods and side dishes;

2. Increase in protein intake: To increase protein intake, it is crucial to eat well on dialysis day. Eating a meal at the time of dialysis visit improves nutritional status and quality of life and reduces inflammatory reactions and mortality [74]. Although proteins are abundant in meat, fish, eggs, beans, and dairy products, it is important to consume a well-balanced diet rather than one rich in only one food group. In elderly Japanese patients on HD (70 years or older), amino acid supplementation may also be useful because oral administration of 12 g/day of amino acid preparations for 6 months improves appetite and increases protein intake and body weight [75].

6.3. Oral Nutritional Supplement: ONS

When dietary counseling is insufficient to achieve the planned nutritional requirements, ONS is recommended as the first step of nutritional support for patients on HD. ONS can add up to 10 kcal/kg and 0.3–0.4 g of protein/kg daily to spontaneous intake, helping the achievement of nutritional targets [76]. Intradialytic intake of protein-rich food or oral supplements appears to be effective in mitigating the catabolism associated with hemodialysis procedures and increasing the total protein intake.

ONS should be initiated with a daily protein intake of >1.2 g/kg/day [76]. The goals of ONS are achieving (1) serum albumin > 4.0 g/dL, (2) serum transthyretin (prealbumin) > 30 mg/dL, and (3) energy intake > 30–35 kcal/kg/day [76]. The K/DOQI guidelines [4] recommend that ONS be continued for at least 3 months. A meta-analysis of previous studies found that ONS increased serum albumin by an average of 0.22 g/dL in patients on HD [77].

Whey protein has several advantages such as fast absorption speed, high body retention rate, and a 26% content of branched-chain amino acids (14% leucine). In patients on PD, daily intake of whey protein powder (27.4 g, 116 kcal) ensured target protein intake and improved body indices such as body weight and body composition [78]. In patients on HD, an oral intake of 15 g of whey protein (plus 6000 IU of vitamin E) weekly for 8 weeks improved SGA and MIS [79]. Thus, enteral nutrients containing whey proteins are useful nutritional supplements.

A randomized clinical trial (RCT) was conducted in patients on HD, without diabetes, and with energy intakes of <30 kcal/kg/day. The subjects were divided into the two groups: one group ingested fat mainly from ONS (300 kcal, 97% energy from fats) added once daily after a meal, and the other group consumed only the routine diet [80]. After 12 weeks, although BMI, serum albumin, and body fat ratio increased slightly with the addition of ONS, the bioelectrical impedance analysis-derived phase angle did not differ between the two groups, indicating that energy supplementation with lipids is nutritionally inadequate.

6.4. IDPN

If nutritional requirements cannot be met with meals or ONS, IDPN should be considered [81]. IDPN is usually administered for 4 h throughout the dialysis session thrice a week. However, IDPN during dialysis three times a week cannot provide sufficient nutritional requirements; therefore, patients with IDPN should receive at least energy $\geq$ 20 kcal/kg/day and protein $\geq$ 0.8 to 0.9 g/kg/day from meals. With the revision of the package insert in June 2020, patients on dialysis in Japan can also use amino acid infusion preparations for general use and liver failure as well as general-use kit infusion products containing amino acids and glucose [81]. If oral intake combined with IDPN does not provide the required nutrients, total parenteral nutrition (TPN) should be considered.

Because of the risk of hyperglycemia, IDPN begins with a low concentration of glucose and then changes to a higher concentration after confirming that blood glucose levels do not increase. According to the guidelines of the European Society for Clinical Nutrition and Metabolism (ESPEN), the first week should be started at no more than 8 mL/kg/IDPN (500 mL at 60 kg) and up to 16 mL/kg/IDPN at the maximum, and then, the dosage per dialysis should not exceed 1000 mL [82]. In a recent RCT on patients with HD, IDPN was administered to a group of patients who had adequate dietary intake (energy $\geq$ 20 kcal/kg/day, protein $\geq$ 0.8 g/kg/day) but were unable to continue ONS due to digestive symptoms [83], while the control group only received weekly nutritional counseling. At three months, serum albumin increased from 3.6 to 3.8 g/dL, and energy intake and body weight increased in the IDPN group (total energy: 1100 kcal, water: 986 mL, continuous administration over 4 h on dialysis) compared to the control group. Therefore, IDPN may be useful in patients who cannot continue ONS because of their digestive symptoms.

6.5. New Medical Treatments

Ghrelin is an endogenous hormone that decreases acute and chronic inflammation, enhances the immune system, stimulates appetite, and causes physiologic pulsatile release of GH. Low ghrelin values in HD patients with PEW are linked to a markedly increased mortality risk, especially due to cardiovascular causes [84]. Because these wasted patients are so anorectic, ghrelin therapies may be useful in the treatment of PEW. A randomized crossover double-blind study [85] demonstrated that treatment with an oral ghrelin agonist, MK-0677, for 30 days provided a positive effect on IGF-1 in patients in HD. Anamorelin hydrochloride, a ghrelin receptor agonist, was firstly approved for gastric, pancreatic, and colorectal cancer patients with cachexia in Japan. Thus, this oral ghrelin agonist is expected to bring new advancements into the field of clinical nutrition as an effective therapeutic drug for cachexia.

Chronic *Helicobacter pylori* (*H. pylori*) infection in the gastric mucosa is associated with abnormal ghrelin levels. Therefore, eradication of *H. pylori* by proton-pump inhibitor and antibiotics may be useful to mitigate the progress of gastric atrophy and prevent a decline of plasma ghrelin and subsequent PEW [86].

Myostatin is an important therapeutic target for treating CKD-related sarcopenia. There are two strategies to inhibit myostatin pathways: one is a blockade by direct binding to myostatin itself, and the other is inhibition of the myostatin–ActRIIB complex. However, clinical studies in sarcopenic patients demonstrated that the anabolic intervention is likely better if a block of ActRII receptors is used. It is also becoming clear that myostatin-targeted therapies should not be seen as a substitute for physical activity and nutritional supplementation [87].

Insulin has a critical role in both glucose metabolism and in the maintenance of skeletal muscle mass. Activation of dipeptidyl peptidase 4 is associated with impairment of insulin signaling in skeletal muscle, presumably leading to loss of muscle function. Therefore, dipeptidyl peptidase 4 inhibitors (DPP4-I) are good candidates for sarcopenia treatment. In elderly patients with type 2 diabetes, the DPP4-I group showed greater muscle mass as well as better muscle strength and physical performance as compared with the sulfonylurea group [88]. A retrospective observational study also demonstrated that a DPP-4 inhibitor prevented the progressive loss of muscle mass, as evaluated by DXA, with ageing in elderly diabetic patients [89]. Sencan et al. [90] also found out that adding a DPP-4 inhibitor to the patients' treatments could effectively and significantly result in a positive effect on muscle strength during a 6-month follow-up period.

DPP-4 inhibitors are available for HD patients. Although there was no report to test the efficacy of DPP4-I on sarcopenia in advanced CKD patients, this agent may be a candidate in the prevention of muscle mass loss in diabetic patients on HD.

7. Conclusions

In this paper, we show a novel nutritional screening and assessment tool for Japanese patients on HD. The NRI-JH, a composite score of BMI, serum creatinine, albumin, and total cholesterol, is useful for screening the nutritional risk of Japanese patients on HD. When the total NRI-JH score exceeds 8 of 13 points, it is important to apply the GLIM criteria to diagnose the presence of malnutrition. Zn deficiency is very common in patients on HD and is associated with a lower threshold of salty taste. In addition, Mg deficiency is related to the progression of vascular calcification. Thus, when a patient on HD is diagnosed with malnutrition, Zn and Mg deficiencies should be evaluated.

When poor dietary intake is likely to be associated with the development of PEW, the first step is to review the daily diet and, if necessary, start ONS with enteral nutritional supplements. Enteral nutrition, particularly including whey proteins, is beneficial. Although IDPN is useful for nutritional supplementation in patients on HD who can eat to some extent, it should always be used in combination with oral intake of food or ONS since IDPN alone cannot replace deficient nutrients.

Author Contributions: All authors contributed to the conceptualization, writing, original draft preparation, review, and editing of the manuscript. All authors have read and agreed to the published version of the manuscript.

Funding: This work was supported by JSPS KAKENHI (Grant Number JP20K10391).

Institutional Review Board Statement: The study was conducted in accordance with the Declaration of Helsinki and was approved by the Institutional Ethics Committee of Kinjo Gakuin University (H18014, R21022).

Informed Consent Statement: Informed consent was obtained from all the subjects involved in our cited studies.

Data Availability Statement: Not applicable.

Acknowledgments: The authors would like to thank the Taiseikai Medical Clinic for their technical assistance in measuring oral dysfunction in dialysis patients on dialysis.

Conflicts of Interest: The authors declare no conflict of interest. The funders had no role in the study design; collection, analyses, or interpretation of data; writing of the manuscript; or decision to publish the results.

References

1. Kalantar-Zadeh, K.; Block, G.; McAllister, C.J.; Humphreys, M.H.; Kopple, J.D. Appetite and inflammation, nutrition, anemia, and clinical outcome in hemodialysis patients. *Am. J. Clin. Nutr.* **2004**, *80*, 299–307. [CrossRef]
2. Fouque, D.; Kalantar-Zadeh, K.; Kopple, J.; Cano, N.; Chauveau, P.; Cuppari, L.; Franch, H.; Guarnieri, G.; Ikizler, T.A.; Kaysen, G.; et al. A proposed nomenclature and diagnostic criteria for protein-energy wasting in acute and chronic kidney disease. *Kidney Int.* **2008**, *73*, 391–398. [CrossRef]
3. Hanna, R.M.; Ghobry, L.; Wassef, O.; Rhee, C.M.; Kalantar-Zadeh, K. A Practical Approach to Nutrition, Protein-Energy Wasting, Sarcopenia, and Cachexia in Patients with Chronic Kidney Disease. *Blood Purif.* **2020**, *49*, 202–211. [CrossRef]
4. Ikizler, T.A.; Burrowes, J.D.; Byham-Gray, L.D.; Campbell, K.L.; Carrero, J.J.; Chan, W.; Fouque, D.; Friedman, A.N.; Ghaddar, S.; Goldstein-Fuchs, D.J.; et al. KDOQI Clinical practice guideline for nutrition in CKD: 2020 update. *Am. J. Kidney Dis.* **2020**, *76*, S1–S107. [CrossRef]
5. Karaboyas, A.; Morgenstern, H.; Fleischer, N.L.; Vanholder, R.C.; Dhalwani, N.N.; Schaeffner, E.; Schaubel, D.E.; Akizawa, T.; James, G.; Sinsakul, M.V.; et al. Inflammation and Erythropoiesis-Stimulating Agent Response in Hemodialysis Patients: A Self-matched Longitudinal Study of Anemia Management in the Dialysis Outcomes and Practice Patterns Study (DOPPS). *Kidney Med.* **2020**, *2*, 286–296. [CrossRef]
6. Lopes, A.A.; Bragg-Gresham, J.L.; Elder, S.J.; Ginsberg, N.; Goodkin, D.A.; Pifer, T.; Lameire, N.; Marshall, M.R.; Asano, Y.; Akizawa, T.; et al. Independent and joint associations of nutritional status indicators with mortality risk among chronic hemodialysis patients in the Dialysis Outcomes and Practice Patterns Study (DOPPS). *J. Ren. Nutr.* **2010**, *20*, 224–234. [CrossRef]
7. Kitabayashi, K.; Yamamoto, S.; Narita, I. Magnesium intake by enteral formulation affects serum magnesium concentration in patients undergoing hemodialysis. *Ther. Apher. Dial.* **2022**, *26*, 749–755. [CrossRef]
8. Roozbeh, J.; Hedayati, P.; Sagheb, M.M.; Sharifian, M.; Hamidian Jahromi, A.; Shaabani, S.; Jalaeian, H.; Raeisjalali, G.A.; Behzadi, S. Effect of zinc supplementation on triglyceride, cholesterol, LDL, and HDL levels in zinc-deficient hemodialysis patients. *Ren. Fail.* **2009**, *31*, 798–801. [CrossRef]
9. Sakaguchi, Y.; Fujii, N.; Shoji, T.; Hayashi, T.; Rakugi, H.; Isaka, Y. Hypomagnesemia is a significant predictor of cardiovascular and non-cardiovascular mortality in patients undergoing hemodialysis. *Kidney Int.* **2014**, *85*, 174–181. [CrossRef]
10. Nakatani, S.; Mori, K.; Shoji, T.; Emoto, M. Association of Zinc Deficiency with Development of CVD Events in Patients with CKD. *Nutrients* **2021**, *13*, 1680. [CrossRef]
11. Detsky, A.S.; McLaughlin, J.R.; Baker, J.P.; Johnston, N.; Whittaker, S.; Mendelson, R.A.; Jeejeebhoy, K.N. What is subjective global assessment of nutritional status? *JPEN J. Parenter. Enter. Nutr.* **1987**, *11*, 8–13. [CrossRef]
12. Windahl, K.; Faxén Irving, G.; Almquist, T.; Lidén, M.K.; van de Luijtgaarden, M.; Chesnaye, N.C.; Voskamp, P.; Stenvinkel, P.; Klinger, M.; Szymczak, M.; et al. Prevalence and Risk of Protein-Energy Wasting Assessed by Subjective Global Assessment in Older Adults With Advanced Chronic Kidney Disease: Results From the EQUAL Study. *J. Ren. Nutr.* **2018**, *28*, 165–174. [CrossRef]
13. de Mutsert, R.; Grootendorst, D.C.; Boeschoten, E.W.; Brandts, H.; van Manen, J.G.; Krediet, R.T.; Dekker, F.W. Subjective global assessment of nutritional status is strongly associated with mortality in chronic dialysis patients. *Am. J. Clin. Nutr.* **2009**, *89*, 787–793. [CrossRef]
14. Kalantar-Zadeh, K.; Kopple, J.D.; Block, G.; Humphreys, M.H. A malnutrition-inflammation score is correlated with morbidity and mortality in maintenance hemodialysis patients. *Am. J. Kidney Dis.* **2001**, *38*, 1251–1263. [CrossRef]
15. Borges, M.C.; Vogt, B.P.; Martin, L.C.; Caramori, J.C. Malnutrition inflammation score cut-off predicting mortality in maintenance hemodialysis patients. *Clin. Nutr. ESPEN* **2017**, *17*, 63–67. [CrossRef]
16. Carrero, J.J.; Thomas, F.; Nagy, K.; Arogundade, F.; Avesani, C.M.; Chan, M.; Chmielewski, M.; Cordeiro, A.C.; Espinosa-Cuevas, A.; Fiaccadori, E.; et al. Global prevalence of protein-energy wasting in kidney disease: A meta-analysis of contemporary observational studies from the international society of renal nutrition and metabolism. *J. Ren. Nutr.* **2018**, *28*, 380–392. [CrossRef]
17. Bouillanne, O.; Morineau, G.; Dupont, C.; Coulombel, I.; Vincent, J.P.; Nicolis, I.; Benazeth, S.; Cynober, L.; Aussel, C. Geriatric nutritional risk index: A new index for evaluating at-risk elderly medical patients. *Am. J. Clin. Nutr.* **2005**, *82*, 777–783. [CrossRef]
18. Yamada, K.; Furuya, R.; Takita, T.; Maruyama, Y.; Yamaguchi, Y.; Ohkawa, S.; Kumagai, H. Simplified nutritional screening tools for patients on maintenance hemodialysis. *Am. J. Clin. Nutr.* **2008**, *87*, 106–113. [CrossRef] [PubMed]
19. Nakagawa, N.; Maruyama, K.; Hasebe, N. Utility of geriatric nutritional risk index in patients with chronic kidney disease: A mini-review. *Nutrients* **2021**, *13*, 3688. [CrossRef]
20. Rubenstein, L.Z.; Harker, J.O.; Salvà, A.; Guigoz, Y.; Vellas, B. Screening for undernutrition in geriatric practice: Developing the short-form mini-nutritional assessment (MNA-SF). *J. Gerontol. A Biol. Sci. Med. Sci.* **2001**, *56*, M366–M372. [CrossRef]

21. Holvoet, E.; Vanden Wyngaert, K.; Van Craenenbroeck, A.H.; Van Biesen, W.; Eloot, S. The screening score of Mini Nutritional Assessment (MNA) is a useful routine screening tool for malnutrition risk in patients on maintenance dialysis. *PLoS ONE* **2020**, *15*, e0229722. [CrossRef]
22. Stratton, R.J.; King, C.L.; Stroud, M.A.; Jackson, A.A.; Elia, M. "Malnutrition universal screening tool" predicts mortality and length of hospital stay in acutely ill elderly. *Br. J. Nutr.* **2006**, *95*, 325–330. [CrossRef]
23. Sohrabi, Z.; Kohansal, A.; Mirzahosseini, H.; Naghibi, M.; Zare, M.; Haghighat, N.; Akbarzadeh, M. Comparison of the nutritional status assessment methods for hemodialysis patients. *Clin. Nutr. Res.* **2021**, *10*, 219–229. [CrossRef]
24. Fahal, I.H. Uraemic sarcopenia: Aetiology and implications. *Nephrol. Dial. Transplant.* **2014**, *29*, 1655–1665. [CrossRef] [PubMed]
25. Yamada, S.; Tsuruya, K.; Yoshida, H.; Tokumoto, M.; Ueki, K.; Ooboshi, H.; Kitazono, T. Factors Associated with the Serum Myostatin Level in Patients Undergoing Peritoneal Dialysis: Potential Effects of Skeletal Muscle Mass and Vitamin D Receptor Activator Use. *Calcif. Tissue Int.* **2016**, *99*, 13–22. [CrossRef] [PubMed]
26. Delanaye, P.; Bataille, S.; Quinonez, K.; Buckinx, F.; Warling, X.; Krzesinski, J.M.; Pottel, H.; Burtey, S.; Bruyère, O.; Cavalier, E. Myostatin and Insulin-Like Growth Factor 1 Are Biomarkers of Muscle Strength, Muscle Mass, and Mortality in Patients on Hemodialysis. *J. Ren. Nutr.* **2019**, *29*, 511–520. [CrossRef]
27. Baczek, J.; Silkiewicz, M.; Wojszel, Z.B. Myostatin as a Biomarker of Muscle Wasting and other Pathologies-State of the Art and Knowledge Gaps. *Nutrients* **2020**, *12*, 2401. [CrossRef]
28. Hurtado, E.; Cilleros, V.; Nadal, L.; Simó, A.; Obis, T.; Garcia, N.; Santafé, M.M.; Tomàs, M.; Halievski, K.; Jordan, C.L.; et al. Muscle Contraction Regulates BDNF/TrkB Signaling to Modulate Synaptic Function through Presynaptic cPKCα and cPKCβI. *Front. Mol. Neurosci.* **2017**, *10*, 147. [CrossRef] [PubMed]
29. Deus, L.A.; Corrêa, H.L.; Neves, R.V.P.; Reis, A.L.; Honorato, F.S.; Silva, V.L.; Souza, M.K.; de Araújo, T.B.; de Gusmão Alves, L.S.; Sousa, C.V.; et al. Are Resistance Training-Induced BDNF in Hemodialysis Patients Associated with Depressive Symptoms, Quality of Life, Antioxidant Capacity, and Muscle Strength? An Insight for the Muscle-Brain-Renal Axis. *Int. J. Environ. Res. Public Health.* **2021**, *18*, 11299. [CrossRef] [PubMed]
30. Miyazaki, S.; Iino, N.; Koda, R.; Narita, I.; Kaneko, Y. Brain-derived neurotrophic factor is associated with sarcopenia and frailty in Japanese hemodialysis patients. *Geriatr. Gerontol. Int.* **2021**, *21*, 27–33. [CrossRef]
31. Koito, Y.; Yanishi, M.; Kimura, Y.; Tsukaguchi, H.; Kinoshita, H.; Matsuda, T. Serum Brain-Derived Neurotrophic Factor and Myostatin Levels Are Associated With Skeletal Muscle Mass in Kidney Transplant Recipients. *Transplant. Proc.* **2021**, *53*, 1939–1944. [CrossRef]
32. Shinzato, T.; Nakai, S.; Miwa, M.; Iwayama, N.; Takai, I.; Matsumoto, Y.; Morita, H.; Maeda, K. New method to calculate creatinine generation rate using pre- and postdialysis creatinine concentrations. *Artif. Organs* **1997**, *21*, 864–872. [CrossRef]
33. Mae, Y.; Takata, T.; Yamada, K.; Hamada, S.; Yamamoto, M.; Iyama, T.; Isomoto, H. Creatinine generation rate can detect sarcopenia in patients with hemodialysis. *Clin. Exp. Nephrol.* **2022**, *26*, 272–277. [CrossRef]
34. Lin, Y.L.; Chen, S.Y.; Lai, Y.H.; Wang, C.H.; Kuo, C.H.; Liou, H.H.; Hsu, B.G. Serum creatinine to cystatin C ratio predicts skeletal muscle mass and strength in patients with non-dialysis chronic kidney disease. *Clin. Nutr.* **2020**, *39*, 2435–2441. [CrossRef]
35. Nitta, K. 2019 Annual Dialysis Data Report, JSDT Renal Data Registry. *Nihon Toseki Igakkai Zasshi* **2020**, *53*, 579–632. [CrossRef]
36. Kanda, E.; Kato, A.; Masakane, I.; Kanno, Y. A new nutritional risk index for predicting mortality in hemodialysis patients: Nationwide cohort study. *PLoS ONE* **2019**, *14*, e0214524. [CrossRef]
37. Shimamoto, S.; Yamada, S.; Hiyamuta, H.; Arase, H.; Taniguchi, M.; Tsuruya, K.; Nakano, T.; Kitazono, T. Association of the nutritional risk index for Japanese hemodialysis patients with long-term mortality: The Q-Cohort Study. *Clin. Exp. Nephrol.* **2022**, *26*, 59–67. [CrossRef]
38. Macedo, C.; Amaral, T.F.; Rodrigues, J.; Santin, F.; Avesani, C.M. Malnutrition and sarcopenia combined increases the risk for mortality in older adults on hemodialysis. *Front. Nutr.* **2021**, *8*, 721941. [CrossRef]
39. Xavier, J.S.; Góes, C.R.; Borges, M.C.C.; Caramori, J.C.T.; Vogt, B.P. Handgrip strength thresholds are associated with malnutrition inflammation score (MIS) in maintenance hemodialysis patients. *J. Ren. Nutr.* **2022**, *32*, 739–743. [CrossRef]
40. Szeto, C.C.; Chan, G.C.; Ng, J.K.; Chow, K.M.; Kwan, B.C.; Cheng, P.M.; Kwong, V.W.; Law, M.C.; Leung, C.B.; Li, P.K. Depression and physical frailty have additive effect on the nutritional status and clinical outcome of chinese peritoneal dialysis. *Kidney Blood Press. Res.* **2018**, *43*, 914–923. [CrossRef]
41. Kono, K.; Moriyama, Y.; Yabe, H.; Hara, A.; Ishida, Y.; Yamada, T.; Nishida, Y. Relationship between malnutrition and possible sarcopenia in the AWGS 2019 consensus affecting mortality in hemodialysis patients: A prospective cohort study. *BMC Nephrol.* **2021**, *22*, 378. [CrossRef] [PubMed]
42. Takeuchi, H.; Uchida, H.A.; Kakio, Y.; Okuyama, Y.; Okuyama, M.; Umebayashi, R.; Wada, K.; Sugiyama, H.; Sugimoto, K.; Rakugi, H.; et al. The prevalence of frailty and its associated factors in japanese hemodialysis patients. *Aging Dis.* **2018**, *9*, 192–207. [CrossRef]
43. Cederholm, T.; Jensen, G.L.; Correia, M.I.T.D.; Gonzalez, M.C.; Fukushima, R.; Higashiguchi, T.; Baptista, G.; Barazzoni, R.; Blaauw, R.; Coats, A.; et al. GLIM criteria for the diagnosis of malnutrition—A consensus report from the global clinical nutrition community. *J. Cachexia Sarcopenia Muscle* **2019**, *10*, 207–217. [CrossRef] [PubMed]
44. Maeda, K.; Koga, T.; Nasu, T.; Takaki, M.; Akagi, J. Predictive accuracy of calf circumference measurements to detect decreased skeletal muscle mass and european society for clinical nutrition and metabolism-defined malnutrition in hospitalized older patients. *Ann. Nutr. Metab.* **2017**, *71*, 10–15. [CrossRef]

45. Avesani, C.M.; Sabatino, A.; Guerra, A.; Rodrigues, J.; Carrero, J.J.; Rossi, G.M.; Garibotto, G.; Stenvinkel, P.; Fiaccadori, E.; Lindholm, B. A comparative analysis of nutritional assessment using global leadership initiative on malnutrition versus subjective global assessment and malnutrition inflammation score in maintenance hemodialysis patients. *J. Ren. Nutr.* **2022**, *32*, 476–482. [CrossRef]
46. Song, H.C.; Shin, J.; Hwang, J.H.; Kim, S.H. Utility of the global leadership initiative on malnutrition criteria for the nutritional assessment of patients with end-stage renal disease receiving chronic hemodialysis. *J. Hum. Nutr. Diet.* **2023**, *36*, 97–107. [CrossRef]
47. Oliveira, C.M.; Kubrusly, M.; Lima, A.T.; Torres, D.M.; Cavalcante, N.M.; Jerônimo, A.L.; Oliveira, T.C. Correlation between nutritional markers and appetite self-assessments in hemodialysis patients. *J. Ren. Nutr.* **2015**, *25*, 301–307. [CrossRef]
48. Sahathevan, S.; Khor, B.H.; Ng, H.M.; Gafor, A.H.A.; Mat Daud, Z.A.; Mafra, D.; Karupaiah, T. Understanding development of malnutrition in hemodialysis patients: A narrative review. *Nutrients* **2020**, *12*, 3147. [CrossRef]
49. Schwotzer, N.; Kanemitsu, M.; Kissling, S.; Darioli, R.; Benghezal, M.; Rezzi, S.; Burnier, M.; Pruijm, M. Water-soluble vitamin levels and supplementation in chronic online hemodiafiltration patients. *Kidney Int. Rep.* **2020**, *5*, 2160–2167. [CrossRef]
50. Shimizu, S.; Tei, R.; Okamura, M.; Takao, N.; Nakamura, Y.; Oguma, H.; Maruyama, T.; Takashima, H.; Abe, M. Prevalence of zinc deficiency in japanese patients on peritoneal dialysis: Comparative study in patients on hemodialysis. *Nutrients* **2020**, *12*, 764. [CrossRef]
51. Kusaba, T.; Mori, Y.; Masami, O.; Hiroko, N.; Adachi, T.; Sugishita, C.; Sonomura, K.; Kimura, T.; Kishimoto, N.; Nakagawa, H.; et al. Sodium restriction improves the gustatory threshold for salty taste in patients with chronic kidney disease. *Kidney Int.* **2009**, *76*, 638–643. [CrossRef] [PubMed]
52. Garagarza, C.; Valente, A.; Caetano, C.; Ramos, I.; Sebastião, J.; Pinto, M.; Oliveira, T.; Ferreira, A.; Sousa Guerreiro, C. Zinc deficient intake in hemodialysis patients: A path to a high mortality risk. *J. Ren. Nutr.* **2022**, *32*, 87–93. [CrossRef] [PubMed]
53. Lowe, N.M.; Medina, M.W.; Stammers, A.L.; Patel, S.; Souverein, O.W.; Dullemeijer, C.; Serra-Majem, L.; Nissensohn, M.; Hall Moran, V. The relationship between zinc intake and serum/plasma zinc concentration in adults: A systematic review and dose-response meta-analysis by the EURRECA Network. *Br. J. Nutr.* **2012**, *108*, 1962–1971. [CrossRef]
54. Hennigar, S.R.; Lieberman, H.R.; Fulgoni, V.L., 3rd; McClung, J.P. Serum zinc concentrations in the US population are related to sex, age, and time of blood draw but not dietary or supplemental zinc. *J. Nutr.* **2018**, *148*, 1341–1351. [CrossRef]
55. Ueda, C.; Takaoka, T.; Sarukura, N.; Matsuda, K.; Kitamura, Y.; Toda, N.; Tanaka, T.; Yamamoto, S.; Takeda, N. Zinc nutrition in healthy subjects and patients with taste impairment from the view point of zinc ingestion, serum zinc concentration and angiotensin converting enzyme activity. *Auris Nasus Larynx* **2006**, *33*, 283–288. [CrossRef]
56. Argani, H.; Mahdavi, R.; Ghorbani-haghjo, A.; Razzaghi, R.; Nikniaz, L.; Gaemmaghami, S.J. Effects of zinc supplementation on serum zinc and leptin levels, BMI, and body composition in hemodialysis patients. *J. Trace Elem. Med. Biol.* **2014**, *28*, 35–38. [CrossRef]
57. Mariak, I.; Grzegorzewska, A.E. Serum zinc concentration with reference to other markers of continuous ambulatory peritoneal dialysis patients status. *Pol. Merkur. Lek.* **2002**, *12*, 282–287.
58. Mahajan, S.K.; Prasad, A.S.; Lambujon, J.; Abbasi, A.A.; Briggs, W.A.; McDonald, F.D. Improvement of uremic hypogeusia by zinc: A double-blind study. *Am. J. Clin. Nutr.* **1980**, *33*, 1517–1521. [CrossRef]
59. Marumo, A.; Yamamura, T.; Mizuki, T.; Tanosaki, S.; Suzuki, K. Copper deficiency-induced pancytopenia after taking an excessive amount of zinc formulation during maintenance hemodialysis. *J. Res. Med. Sci.* **2021**, *26*, 42. [CrossRef] [PubMed]
60. Oka, T.; Hamano, T.; Sakaguchi, Y.; Yamaguchi, S.; Kubota, K.; Senda, M.; Yonemoto, S.; Shimada, K.; Matsumoto, A.; Hashimoto, N.; et al. Proteinuria-associated renal magnesium wasting leads to hypomagnesemia: A common electrolyte abnormality in chronic kidney disease. *Nephrol. Dial. Transplant.* **2019**, *34*, 1154–1162. [CrossRef]
61. Srinutta, T.; Chewcharat, A.; Takkavatakarn, K.; Praditpornsilpa, K.; Eiam-Ong, S.; Jaber, B.L.; Susantitaphong, P. Proton pump inhibitors and hypomagnesemia: A meta-analysis of observational studies. *Medicine* **2019**, *98*, e17788. [CrossRef] [PubMed]
62. Sakaguchi, Y. The emerging role of magnesium in CKD. *Clin. Exp. Nephrol.* **2022**, *26*, 379–384. [CrossRef]
63. Bressendorff, I.; Hansen, D.; Schou, M.; Pasch, A.; Brandi, L. The effect of increasing dialysate magnesium on serum calcification propensity in subjects with end stage kidney disease: A randomized, controlled clinical trial. *Clin. J. Am. Soc. Nephrol.* **2018**, *13*, 1373–1380. [CrossRef] [PubMed]
64. Guo, G.; Zhou, J.; Xu, T.; Sheng, Z.; Huang, A.; Sun, L.; Yao, L. Effect of magnesium supplementation on chronic kidney disease-mineral and bone disorder in hemodialysis patients: A meta-analysis of randomized controlled trials. *J. Ren. Nutr.* **2022**, *32*, 102–111. [CrossRef]
65. Iwasaki, M.; Yoshihara, A.; Sato, M.; Minagawa, K.; Shimada, M.; Nishimuta, M.; Ansai, T.; Yoshitake, Y.; Miyazaki, H. Dentition status and frailty in community-dwelling older adults: A 5-year prospective cohort study. *Geriatr. Gerontol. Int.* **2018**, *18*, 256–262. [CrossRef]
66. Iwasaki, M.; Yoshihara, A.; Sato, N.; Sato, M.; Minagawa, K.; Shimada, M.; Nishimuta, M.; Ansai, T.; Yoshitake, Y.; Ono, T.; et al. A 5-year longitudinal study of association of maximum bite force with development of frailty in community-dwelling older adults. *J. Oral Rehabil.* **2018**, *45*, 17–24. [CrossRef]
67. Kikutani, T.; Yoshida, M.; Enoki, H.; Yamashita, Y.; Akifusa, S.; Shimazaki, Y.; Hirano, H.; Tamura, F. Relationship between nutrition status and dental occlusion in community-dwelling frail elderly people. *Geriatr. Gerontol. Int.* **2013**, *13*, 50–54. [CrossRef]
68. Tanaka, T.; Takahashi, K.; Hirano, H.; Kikutani, T.; Watanabe, Y.; Ohara, Y.; Furuya, H.; Tetsuo, T.; Akishita, M.; Iijima, K. Oral Frailty as a Risk Factor for Physical Frailty and Mortality in Community-Dwelling Elderly. *J. Gerontol. A Biol. Sci. Med. Sci.* **2018**, *73*, 1661–1667. [CrossRef]

69. Minakuchi, S.; Tsuga, K.; Ikebe, K.; Ueda, T.; Tamura, F.; Nagao, K.; Furuya, J.; Matsuo, K.; Yamamoto, K.; Kanazawa, M.; et al. Oral hypofunction in the older population: Position paper of the Japanese Society of Gerodontology in 2016. *Gerodontology* **2018**, *35*, 317–324. [CrossRef]
70. Hendriks, F.K.; Smeets, J.S.J.; van Kranenburg, J.M.X.; Broers, N.J.H.; van der Sande, F.M.; Verdijk, L.B.; Kooman, J.P.; van Loon, L.J.C. Amino acid removal during hemodialysis can be compensated for by protein ingestion and is not compromised by intradialytic exercise: A randomized controlled crossover trial. *Am. J. Clin. Nutr.* **2021**, *114*, 2074–2083. [CrossRef]
71. Notomi, S.; Kitamura, M.; Yamaguchi, K.; Harada, T.; Nishino, T.; Funakoshi, S.; Kuno, K. Impact of cafeteria service discontinuation at a dialysis facility on medium-term nutritional status of elderly patients undergoing hemodialysis. *Nutrients* **2022**, *14*, 1628. [CrossRef] [PubMed]
72. Lambert, K.; Mullan, J.; Mansfield, K. An integrative review of the methodology and findings regarding dietary adherence in end stage kidney disease. *BMC Nephrol.* **2017**, *18*, 318. [CrossRef]
73. Yoshimura, Y.; Shimazu, S.; Shiraishi, A.; Nagano, F.; Tominaga, S.; Hamada, T.; Kudo, M.; Yamasaki, Y.; Noda, S.; Bise, T. Ghrelin activation by ingestion of medium-chain triglycerides in healthy adults: A pilot trial. *J. Aging Res. Lifestyle* **2018**, *7*, 42–46. [CrossRef]
74. Kistler, B.M.; Benner, D.; Burrowes, J.D.; Campbell, K.L.; Fouque, D.; Garibotto, G.; Kopple, J.D.; Kovesdy, C.P.; Rhee, C.M.; Steiber, A.; et al. Eating during hemodialysis treatment: A consensus statement from the international society of renal nutrition and metabolism. *J. Ren. Nutr.* **2018**, *28*, 4–12. [CrossRef] [PubMed]
75. Hiroshige, K.; Sonta, T.; Suda, T.; Kanegae, K.; Ohtani, A. Oral supplementation of branched-chain amino acid improves nutritional status in elderly patients on chronic haemodialysis. *Nephrol. Dial. Transplant.* **2001**, *16*, 1856–1862. [CrossRef]
76. Sabatino, A.; Regolisti, G.; Karupaiah, T.; Sahathevan, S.; Sadu Singh, B.K.; Khor, B.H.; Salhab, N.; Karavetian, M.; Cupisti, A.; Fiaccadori, E. Protein-energy wasting and nutritional supplementation in patients with end-stage renal disease on hemodialysis. *Clin. Nutr.* **2017**, *36*, 663–671. [CrossRef] [PubMed]
77. Liu, P.J.; Ma, F.; Wang, Q.Y.; He, S.L. The effects of oral nutritional supplements in patients with maintenance dialysis therapy: A systematic review and meta-analysis of randomized clinical trials. *PLoS ONE* **2018**, *13*, e0203706. [CrossRef]
78. Sahathevan, S.; Se, C.H.; Ng, S.; Khor, B.H.; Chinna, K.; Goh, B.L.; Gafor, H.A.; Bavanandan, S.; Ahmad, G.; Karupaiah, T. Clinical efficacy and feasibility of whey protein isolates supplementation in malnourished peritoneal dialysis patients: A multicenter, parallel, open-label randomized controlled trial. *Clin. Nutr. ESPEN* **2018**, *25*, 68–77. [CrossRef]
79. Sohrabi, Z.; Eftekhari, M.H.; Eskandari, M.H.; Rezaianzadeh, A.; Sagheb, M.M. Intradialytic oral protein supplementation and nutritional and inflammation outcomes in hemodialysis: A randomized controlled trial. *Am. J. Kidney Dis.* **2016**, *68*, 122–130. [CrossRef]
80. Yang, Y.; Qin, X.; Chen, J.; Wang, Q.; Kong, Y.; Wan, Q.; Tao, H.; Liu, A.; Li, Y.; Lin, Z.; et al. The effects of oral energy-dense supplements on nutritional status in nondiabetic maintenance hemodialysis patients: A randomized controlled trial. *Clin. J. Am. Soc. Nephrol.* **2021**, *16*, 1228–1236. [CrossRef]
81. Yasukawa, R.; Hosojima, M.; Kabasawa, H.; Takeyama, A.; Ugamura, D.; Suzuki, Y.; Saito, A.; Narita, I. Intradialytic parenteral nutrition using a standard amino acid solution not for renal failure in maintenance hemodialysis patients with malnutrition: A multicenter pilot study. *Ren. Replace. Ther.* **2022**, *8*, 41. [CrossRef]
82. Cano, N.J.; Aparicio, M.; Brunori, G.; Carrero, J.J.; Cianciaruso, B.; Fiaccadori, E.; Lindholm, B.; Teplan, V.; Fouque, D.; Guarnieri, G.; et al. ESPEN Guidelines on parenteral nutrition: Adult renal failure. *Clin. Nutr.* **2009**, *28*, 401–414. [CrossRef]
83. Kittiskulnam, P.; Banjongjit, A.; Metta, K.; Tiranathanagul, K.; Avihingsanon, Y.; Praditpornsilpa, K.; Tungsanga, K.; Eiam-Ong, S. The beneficial effects of intradialytic parenteral nutrition in hemodialysis patients with protein energy wasting: A prospective randomized controlled trial. *Sci. Rep.* **2022**, *12*, 4529. [CrossRef]
84. Carrero, J.J.; Nakashima, A.; Qureshi, A.R.; Lindholm, B.; Heimbürger, O.; Bárány, P.; Stenvinkel, P. Protein-energy wasting modifies the association of ghrelin with inflammation, leptin, and mortality in hemodialysis patients. *Kidney Int.* **2011**, *79*, 749–756. [CrossRef]
85. Campbell, G.A.; Patrie, J.T.; Gaylinn, B.D.; Thorner, M.O.; Bolton, W.K. Oral ghrelin receptor agonist MK-0677 increases serum insulin-like growth factor 1 in hemodialysis patients: A randomized blinded study. *Nephrol. Dial. Transplant.* **2018**, *33*, 523–530. [CrossRef]
86. Sugimoto, M.; Yasuda, H.; Andoh, A. Nutrition status and Helicobacter pylori infection in patients receiving hemodialysis. *World J. Gastroenterol.* **2018**, *24*, 1591–1600. [CrossRef]
87. Verzola, D.; Barisione, C.; Picciotto, D.; Garibotto, G.; Koppe, L. Emerging role of myostatin and its inhibition in the setting of chronic kidney disease. *Kidney Int.* **2019**, *95*, 506–517. [CrossRef]
88. Rizzo, M.R.; Barbieri, M.; Fava, I.; Desiderio, M.; Coppola, C.; Marfella, R.; Paolisso, G. Sarcopenia in Elderly Diabetic Patients: Role of Dipeptidyl Peptidase 4 Inhibitors. *J. Am. Med. Dir. Assoc.* **2016**, *17*, 896–901. [CrossRef]
89. Bouchi, R.; Fukuda, T.; Takeuchi, T.; Nakano, Y.; Murakami, M.; Minami, I.; Izumiyama, H.; Hashimoto, K.; Yoshimoto, T.; Ogawa, Y. Dipeptidyl peptidase 4 inhibitors attenuates the decline of skeletal muscle mass in patients with type 2 diabetes. *Diabetes/Metab. Res. Rev.* **2018**, *34*, e2957. [CrossRef]
90. Sencan, C.; Dost, F.S.; Ates Bulut, E.; Isik, A.T. DPP4 inhibitors as a potential therapeutic option for sarcopenia: A 6-month follow-up study in diabetic older patients. *Exp. Gerontol.* **2022**, *164*, 111832. [CrossRef]

Disclaimer/Publisher's Note: The statements, opinions and data contained in all publications are solely those of the individual author(s) and contributor(s) and not of MDPI and/or the editor(s). MDPI and/or the editor(s) disclaim responsibility for any injury to people or property resulting from any ideas, methods, instructions or products referred to in the content.

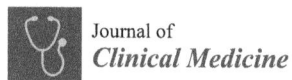

Communication

Clinical Significance of Trace Element Zinc in Patients with Chronic Kidney Disease

Hirotaka Fukasawa [1,*], Ryuichi Furuya [1], Mai Kaneko [1], Daisuke Nakagami [1], Yuri Ishino [1], Shuhei Kitamoto [1], Kyosuke Omata [1] and Hideo Yasuda [2]

1 Renal Division, Department of Internal Medicine, Iwata City Hospital, Iwata 438-8550, Shizuoka, Japan
2 First Department of Medicine, Hamamatsu University School of Medicine, Hamamatsu 431-3192, Shizuoka, Japan
* Correspondence: hfukasawaucsd@gmail.com

Abstract: The trace element zinc is essential for diverse physiological processes in humans. Zinc deficiency can impair growth, skin reproduction, immune function, maintenance of taste, glucose metabolism, and neurological function. Patients with chronic kidney disease (CKD) are susceptible to zinc deficiency, which is associated with erythropoiesis-stimulating agent (ESA) hypo-responsive anemia, nutritional problems, and cardiovascular diseases as well as non-specific symptoms such as dermatitis, prolonged wound healing, taste disturbance, appetite loss, or cognitive decline. Thus, zinc supplementation may be useful for the treatment of its deficiency, although it often causes copper deficiency, which is characterized by several severe disorders including cytopenia and myelopathy. In this review article, we mainly discuss the significant roles of zinc and the association between zinc deficiency and the pathogenesis of complications in patients with CKD.

Keywords: anemia; cardiovascular disease; chronic kidney disease; copper; nutrition; zinc

1. Introduction

Zinc (Zn^{2+}) is an essential trace element and the second most abundant divalent cation in the body next to iron (1.5–2.5 g in human body) [1]. Zinc plays an important role as a cofactor of more than 300 enzymes including alcohol dehydrogenase, alkaline phosphatase (ALP), angiotensin converting enzyme, carbonic anhydrase, collagenase, lactate dehydrogenase (LDH), and DNA and RNA polymerases (Table 1). Therefore, zinc is involved in the regulation of alcohol metabolism, bone metabolism, blood pressure control, cellular energy production, and nucleic acid synthesis [2–5]. Zinc also plays significant roles in the regulation of immune functions, genital functions, glucose metabolism, cognitive performance, and the structural maintenance of proteins, which are called zinc finger proteins including tumor necrosis factor (TNF)-α-induced protein 3 (TNFAIP3, also known as A20), nuclear factor-κB (NF-κB), nuclear factor erythroid 2-related factor 2 (Nrf2), and peroxisome proliferator-activated receptors (PPARs) [4,6–8]. In addition, zinc is essential in the active site of superoxide dismutase (SOD), an important antioxidant enzyme that catalyzes the dismutation of superoxide (O^-) [9,10]. Thus, zinc acts as an antioxidant agent and zinc deficiency is associated with an increased risk of cardiovascular disease [11,12].

On the other hand, zinc deficiency is characterized by non-specific symptoms including weight loss, growth retardation, alopecia, dermatitis, prolonged wound healing, taste disturbance, appetite loss, and cognitive decline [13,14]. Therefore, zinc deficiency is often overlooked.

According to the recommended dietary zinc intakes from practical guidelines, the ideal daily dose for adults is 8 mg/day for women and 11 mg/day for men [15]. The dietary zinc content and its bioavailability can influence the efficiency of zinc absorption as well as an individual's zinc status. Dietary zinc is actively absorbed throughout the small intestine; the main dietary sources of zinc include seafood (especially oysters), crustaceans,

Citation: Fukasawa, H.; Furuya, R.; Kaneko, M.; Nakagami, D.; Ishino, Y.; Kitamoto, S.; Omata, K.; Yasuda, H. Clinical Significance of Trace Element Zinc in Patients with Chronic Kidney Disease. *J. Clin. Med.* **2023**, *12*, 1667. https://doi.org/10.3390/jcm12041667

Academic Editor: Dong Zhou

Received: 21 December 2022
Revised: 2 February 2023
Accepted: 18 February 2023
Published: 20 February 2023

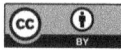

Copyright: © 2023 by the authors. Licensee MDPI, Basel, Switzerland. This article is an open access article distributed under the terms and conditions of the Creative Commons Attribution (CC BY) license (https:// creativecommons.org/licenses/by/ 4.0/).

red meat, and poultry, although zinc's bioavailability is lower in beans, nuts, and vegetables due to the presence of phytates [1]. Therefore, vegetarian or vegan diets may be a risk of zinc deficiency, especially in CKD patients. In the human body, 60% of zinc is stored in skeletal muscle and 20% in bones, while the circulating zinc accounts for only 0.1% of total body zinc [16]. In circulation, 80% of zinc is distributed in erythrocytes and 20% in serum, which is predominantly bound to several proteins such as albumin, α-macroglobulin, and transferrin [17]. In healthy populations, the major route of zinc excretion is via the gastrointestinal tract [18], although urinary excretion of zinc increases in patients with chronic kidney disease (CKD) [19].

Table 1. Main enzymes containing zinc, existing organs, and their functions.

Enzyme	Existing Organs	Functions
Alkaline phosphatase (ALP)	liver, bone, placenta, small intestine	dephosphorylation, bone metabolism
Alcohol dehydrogenase	liver, stomach, intestinal tract, kidney	alcohol metabolism
Aldolase	muscle, liver	glucose metabolism
Alkaline protease	small intestine	protein metabolism
Amylase	salivary gland, pancreas, small intestine	protein metabolism
Angiotensin coverting enzyme	lung, kidney, brain	regulation of blood pressure
Carbonic anhydrase	red blood cell	exchange between carbon dioxide and bicarbonate ion
Carboxypeptidase	pancreas, liver, kidney, small intestine	protein metabolism
Collagenase	all organs	hydrolysis of collagen
Dipeptidase	small intestine	protein metabolism
DNA polymerase	all organs	DNA synthesis
Glutamate dehydrogenase	liver	protein metabolism
Lactate dehydrogenase (LDH)	most organs	glucose metabolism
Leucine aminopeptidase	liver, kidney, intestinal tract, pancreas	protein metabolism
Ornithine transcarbamylase	liver	protein metabolism, nitrogen metabolism
Phospholipase C	all organs	lipid metabolism
RNA polymerase	all organs	RNA synthesis
Superoxide dismutase (SOD)	all organs	anti-oxidative stress, reactive oxygen suppression

Abbreviations: ALP, alkaline phosphatase; DNA, deoxyribonucleic acid; LDH, lactate dehydrogenase; RNA, ribonucleic acid; SOD, superoxide dismutase.

In this review article, we mainly discuss the clinical significance of zinc and the association between zinc deficiency and the pathogenesis of complications in patients with CKD.

2. Zinc Levels in CKD

Zinc deficiency can be caused by nutritional problems and, therefore, it is very common in developing countries, mainly in children and the elderly. On the other hand, it can be complicated with chronic diseases such as diabetes mellitus, inflammatory bowel disease, CKD, or cancer [20].

Several studies have demonstrated that plasma zinc levels were lower in non-dialysis dependent CKD patients than those of healthy individuals and these levels decreased along the progression of CKD stages [19,21,22].

In patients undergoing hemodialysis (HD) treatment, previous studies have demonstrated that circulating zinc levels were lower than those of healthy individuals [23,24].

Toida et al. [25] have also reported that serum zinc levels in most of incident hemodialysis patients (99.2%) were under the normal range (serum zinc level < 80 mg/dL) and 70.4% patients exhibited hypozincemia (serum zinc level < 60 mg/dL).

In patients undergoing peritoneal dialysis (PD) treatment, Panorchan et al. [26] have reported that mean plasma zinc levels were relatively low, with 57.2% of the patients under the normal range. Recently, Shimizu et al. [27] have reported that serum zinc levels in all PD patients (n = 47) were under the normal range and that there was no significant difference in the prevalence of zinc deficiency between PD and HD patients.

Thus, CKD patients are susceptible to zinc deficiency, which may be caused by an inadequate dietary intake due to uremia-related anorexia and dietary restriction, reduced gastrointestinal zinc absorption, adsorption of zinc by phosphate binders, and removal of zinc by dialysis procedure, which usually uses zinc-free dialysate (Figure 1) [24,28]. In addition, it is possible that CKD patients have variable susceptibility to zinc deficiency on the basis of several factors including genetic variation in the zinc transporter genes and relevant transcription factors, long-term diuretic use, and the original disease of CKD such as diabetes mellitus. However, Batista et al. [29] have reported that there was no significant difference in plasma zinc levels in hemodialysis patients with or without diabetes mellitus.

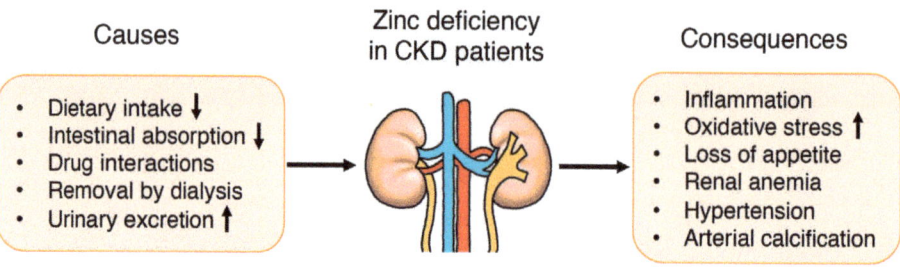

Figure 1. Causes and consequences of zinc deficiency in patients with CKD.

On the other hand, previous studies have demonstrated that zinc levels in erythrocytes were higher in non-dialysis dependent CKD patients than those in healthy individuals, while zinc levels in plasma were lower in the aforementioned patients [29,30]. These results suggest that zinc in circulation is differently distributed between CKD patients and healthy individuals.

3. Zinc and Renal Anemia

Renal anemia is a common complication in patients with CKD [31,32]. Until quite recently, the main therapeutic options for renal anemia were treatment with an erythropoiesis-stimulating agent (ESA) and iron supplementation. On the other hand, a problem in treating renal anemia is that the ESA dosage required to achieve the target hemoglobin level widely varies among CKD patients, so called as ESA hypo-responsiveness. Although several factors were reported to contribute to ESA hypo-responsiveness, including iron deficiency, inflammation, infection, inadequate dialysis procedure, and severe hyperparathyroidism [33,34], recent studies have demonstrated that zinc deficiency could also cause ESA hypo-responsiveness, particularly in patients undergoing HD [35,36].

In fact, Fukushima et al. [35] have showed that serum zinc levels were positively correlated with anemic parameters such as red blood cell (RBC) counts, hemoglobin (Hb), or hematocrit (Ht) levels in HD patients with lower zinc levels than the reference value (<80 mg/dL), and that zinc supplementation with polaprezinc (as 34 mg/day of zinc) could improve anemia and reduce ESA doses in those patients. Kobayashi et al. [36] have also showed that zinc supplementation with polaprezinc reduced serum ferritin levels, required ESA dosage, and erythropoietin responsiveness index, although it didn't change anemic parameters (RBC and Hb) in HD patients.

Although no previous studies have directly shown a relationship between zinc levels and Hb production or erythropoiesis, some experimental studies have reported that zinc finger proteins including BTB and CNC homology-1 (Bach-1), GATA-1, and growth factor independence-1B (Gfi-1B) play important roles in Hb synthesis and erythroid proliferation or differentiation [37–39]. Therefore, it is speculated that the improvement of renal anemia following zinc supplementation is caused by Hb synthesis and erythropoiesis via the functional modification of those transcription factors containing zinc, although the precise mechanism for how zinc deficiency affects those transcription factors in vivo remains unclear. Further studies are needed to clarify its mechanism.

4. Zinc and Nutrition in CKD

CKD patients are often suffering from nutritional problems, which are associated with increased morbidity and mortality [40]. In fact, body mass index (BMI [reference range; $18.5 \leq$ to <25.0]) in CKD patients exhibits lower than age- and sex-matched control subjects [41]. Several studies have demonstrated that higher BMI contributed to a survival advantage in CKD patients [42,43]. Since higher BMI is related to an increased risk of cardiovascular diseases and a higher mortality in the general population [44], this reverse relationship observed in CKD patients is known as the "risk factor paradox" or "reverse epidemiology" [45,46]. On the other hand, it is unclear whether this survival advantage associated with higher BMI in CKD patients is caused by increased muscle mass, fat mass, or both. One possible reason for why this question remains unclear is because BMI does not distinguish between muscle mass and adipose tissue [43]. In this regard, Beddhu et al. [47] have attempted to answer this question using 24-h urinary creatinine excretion as a marker for muscle mass in conjunction with BMI and proposed that muscle mass might be more important in this survival advantage than fat mass. Besides, Caetano et al. [48] have demonstrated that fat mass might be more important than muscle mass in predicting 1-year mortality with bioimpedance analysis.

Previously, El-Shazly et al. [49] have reported that serum zinc levels were positively correlated with body weights and BMIs, but negatively correlated with serum leptin levels in pediatric patients on dialysis. Several studies have also demonstrated that zinc supplementation resulted in a significant increase in body weights and BMIs, but a significant decrease in serum leptin levels in HD patients [49,50]. Therefore, it is suggested that zinc levels are associated with body composition in CKD patients, at least partially, although it remains uncertain whether muscle mass or fat mass was increased by zinc supplementation.

Recently, we have reported that serum zinc levels were positively correlated with the abdominal fat areas of HD patients [51]. In the experimental study, it has been reported that zinc stimulated the differentiation of pre-adipocytes to adipocytes in vitro [52]. Another report has demonstrated that zinc supplementation caused the increased size of adipocytes resulting in the adipose tissue hypertrophy in mice [53]. Zhang et al. [54] have reported that dietary zinc supplementation increased intramuscular adipose deposition in piglets. Chen et al. [55] have also reported that zinc supplementation for 6 weeks caused fat accumulation in the body of genetically obese mice and dietary-obese mice. These reports support the idea that zinc mainly affects adipose tissue in CKD patients, although further studies are needed to clarify the mechanism for how circulating zinc levels affect body composition.

5. Zinc and Cardiovascular Diseases in CKD

At present, it has become clearer that zinc deficiency is associated with oxidative stress, inflammation, and the development of cardiovascular diseases in CKD patients [12].

Lobo et al. [53,54] have reported that plasma zinc levels were negatively correlated with electronegative low-density lipoprotein [LDL(-), a lipid peroxidation and pro-atherosclerotic marker] and TNF-α levels in hemodialysis patients and have proposed that zinc deficiency may cause oxidative stress, inflammation, and subsequently, atherosclerosis.

Vascular calcification is a common complication in CKD patients and is a significant predictor of cardiovascular mortality [55]. Several studies have demonstrated that abdominal aortic calcification is significantly associated with cardiovascular events in CKD patients [56,57]. The pathophysiology of vascular calcification in CKD patients involves several factors including oxidative stress, inflammation, changes in extracellular matrix metabolism, and imbalances in calcium-phosphate metabolism referred to as CKD-mineral and bone disorder (CKD-MBD) [58,59]. Voelkl et al. [6] have reported that serum zinc levels were negatively correlated with a propensity for serum calcification in CKD patients and that zinc sulfate supplementation suppressed vascular calcification in CKD model mice via the increased aortic expression of TNFAIP3, which is a suppressor of the NF-κB transcription factor pathway. Zinc deficiency also activated the NACHT, LRR, and PYD domains-containing protein 3 (NLRP3) inflammasome and induced interleukin-1β (IL-1β) secretion in an animal model of acute kidney injury [60], although zinc treatment inhibited the activation of the NLRP3 inflammasome by the attenuation of reactive oxygen species (ROS) production in human peritoneal mesothelial cells [61].

Nrf2 is a transcription factor that regulates the cellular defense against oxidative stress by reducing ROS overproduction. Nrf2 also blocks inflammation by directly inhibiting transcription of the proinflammatory cytokine genes or inhibiting the activity of NF-κB signaling [8,62]. Previous study has demonstrated that CKD patients exhibited both downregulation of Nrf2 mRNA and upregulation of NF-κB mRNA expression, and that zinc supplementation caused increased Nrf2 expression as well as enhanced SOD synthesis, improved antioxidant defense, and reduced cardiovascular risk in CKD patients [63].

Systematic review and meta-analysis have reported the benefits of zinc supplementation on oxidative stress and inflammation, which resulted from the increase in SOD levels and the decrease in malonaldehyde and C-reactive protein (CRP) levels [64].

6. Zinc Supplementation and Risk of Copper Deficiency in CKD

Besides zinc, copper is also an essential trace element in physiological processes such as the regulation of oxidative stress, catecholamine metabolism, or hematopoiesis [22,65], although zinc supplementation can induce acquired copper deficiency known as zinc-induced copper deficiency (ZICD) [66]. ZICD can induce severe disorders including ESA hypo-responsive anemia, pseudo-myelodysplastic syndrome, or myelopathy [67–69], and several cases of ZICD have been reported in hemodialysis patients [70–72]. On the other hand, ZICD is relatively uncommon and, therefore, is often overlooked as a cause of anemia, pancytopenia, or myelopathy in patients with CKD.

Absorption of both zinc and copper occurs in the small intestine and is dependent on the relative concentrations of each element. The pathophysiology for ZICD may be explained by the interaction of copper and zinc with metallothionein (MT) proteins in the enterocytes of the small intestine. MT proteins form disulfide bonds with metals such as cadmium, zinc, and copper, and help maintain stable metal ion levels in the body [73]. The increased zinc concentration stimulates an increased synthesis of MT proteins, which results in more binding sites for both copper and zinc on MT proteins. Since copper has a greater binding affinity to MT proteins than zinc and the turnover rate of enterocytes is relatively rapid, copper bound to MT proteins is unable to be absorbed in the small intestine and is finally lost in the stool. Thus, ZICD can occur in CKD patients if zinc levels are remarkably high after zinc supplementation [70–72].

7. Conclusions and Future Perspectives

CKD patients are susceptible to zinc deficiency, which may often cause ESA hypo-responsive anemia, nutritional problems, or cardiovascular diseases as well as non-specific symptoms including dermatitis, prolonged wound healing, taste disturbance, and appetite loss. Although zinc supplementation is a useful treatment for CKD patients with its deficiency, risk of ZICD should be noted. Further studies are needed to determine how to manage zinc deficiency in CKD patients.

Author Contributions: Conceptualization, H.F., R.F. and H.Y.; writing—original draft preparation, H.F., M.K., D.N., Y.I., S.K. and K.O.; writing—review and editing, H.F. and R.F.; supervision, H.Y. All authors have read and agreed to the published version of the manuscript.

Funding: This research received no external funding.

Institutional Review Board Statement: Not applicable.

Informed Consent Statement: Not applicable.

Data Availability Statement: Not applicable.

Acknowledgments: We thank Takayasu Ohtake and Shuzo Kobayashi (Shonan Kamakura General Hospital, Kamakura, Japan) for giving us the opportunity to write this article.

Conflicts of Interest: The authors declare no conflict of interest.

References

1. Kenneth, H.; Brown, K.H.; Wuehler, S.E.; Peerson, J.M. The importance of zinc in human nutrition and estimation of the global prevalence of zinc deficiency. *Food Nutr. Bull.* **2001**, *22*, 113–125.
2. MacDonald, R.S. The role of zinc in growth and cell proliferation. *J. Nutr.* **2000**, *130*, 1500S–1508S. [CrossRef]
3. Roohani, N.; Hurrell, R.; Kelishadi, R.; Schulin, R. Zinc and its importance for human health: An integrative review. *J. Res. Med. Sci.* **2013**, *18*, 144–157. [PubMed]
4. Shi, Y.; Zou, Y.; Shen, Z.; Xiong, Y.; Zhang, W.; Liu, C.; Chen, S. Trace Elements, PPARs, and Metabolic Syndrome. *Int. J. Mol. Sci.* **2020**, *21*, 2612. [CrossRef] [PubMed]
5. Hou, R.; He, Y.; Yan, G.; Hou, S.; Xie, Z.; Liao, C. Zinc enzymes in medicinal chemistry. *Eur. J. Med. Chem.* **2021**, *226*, 113877. [CrossRef]
6. Voelkl, J.; Tuffaha, R.; Luong, T.T.D.; Zickler, D.; Masyout, J.; Feger, M.; Verheyen, N.; Blaschke, F.; Kuro, O.M.; Tomaschitz, A.; et al. Zinc Inhibits Phosphate-Induced Vascular Calcification through TNFAIP3-Mediated Suppression of NF-kappaB. *J. Am. Soc. Nephrol.* **2018**, *29*, 1636–1648. [CrossRef]
7. Jarosz, M.; Olbert, M.; Wyszogrodzka, G.; Mlyniec, K.; Librowski, T. Antioxidant and anti-inflammatory effects of zinc. Zinc-dependent NF-kappaB signaling. *Inflammopharmacology* **2017**, *25*, 11–24. [CrossRef]
8. He, F.; Ru, X.; Wen, T. NRF2, a Transcription Factor for Stress Response and Beyond. *Int. J. Mol. Sci.* **2020**, *21*, 4777. [CrossRef]
9. Prasad, A.S. Zinc: Role in immunity, oxidative stress and chronic inflammation. *Curr. Opin. Clin. Nutr. Metab. Care* **2009**, *12*, 646–652. [CrossRef]
10. Prasad, A.S.; Bao, B. Molecular Mechanisms of Zinc as a Pro-Antioxidant Mediator: Clinical Therapeutic Implications. *Antioxidants* **2019**, *8*, 164. [CrossRef]
11. Braun, L.A.; Ou, R.; Kure, C.; Trang, A.; Rosenfeldt, F. Prevalence of Zinc Deficiency in Cardiac Surgery Patients. *Heart Lung Circ.* **2018**, *27*, 760–762. [CrossRef] [PubMed]
12. Choi, S.; Liu, X.; Pan, Z. Zinc deficiency and cellular oxidative stress: Prognostic implications in cardiovascular diseases. *Acta Pharmacol. Sin.* **2018**, *39*, 1120–1132. [CrossRef] [PubMed]
13. Prasad, A.S. Recognition of zinc-deficiency syndrome. *Nutrition* **2001**, *17*, 67–69. [CrossRef]
14. Prasad, A.S. Zinc deficiency: Its characterization and treatment. *Met. Ions Biol. Syst.* **2004**, *41*, 103–137. [PubMed]
15. Kodama, H.; Tanaka, M.; Naito, Y.; Katayama, K.; Moriyama, M. Japan's Practical Guidelines for Zinc Deficiency with a Particular Focus on Taste Disorders, Inflammatory Bowel Disease, and Liver Cirrhosis. *Int. J. Mol. Sci.* **2020**, *21*, 2941. [CrossRef]
16. Iyengar, G.V. Reevaluation of the trace element content in reference man. *Radiat. Phys. Chem.* **1998**, *51*, 545–560. [CrossRef]
17. Krebs, N.F. Overview of zinc absorption and excretion in the human gastrointestinal tract. *J. Nutr.* **2000**, *130*, 1374S–1377S. [CrossRef]
18. Damianaki, K.; Lourenco, J.M.; Braconnier, P.; Ghobril, J.P.; Devuyst, O.; Burnier, M.; Lenglet, S.; Augsburger, M.; Thomas, A.; Pruijm, M. Renal handling of zinc in chronic kidney disease patients and the role of circulating zinc levels in renal function decline. *Nephrol. Dial. Transplant.* **2020**, *35*, 1163–1170. [CrossRef]
19. Shrimpton, R.; Gross, R.; Darnton-Hill, I.; Young, M. Zinc deficiency: What are the most appropriate interventions? *BMJ* **2005**, *330*, 347–349. [CrossRef]
20. Shih, C.T.; Shiu, Y.L.; Chen, C.A.; Lin, T.Y.; Huang, Y.L.; Lin, C.C. Changes in levels of copper, iron, zinc, and selenium in patients at different stages of chronic kidney disease. *Genom. Med. Biomark. Health Sci.* **2012**, *4*, 128–130. [CrossRef]
21. Lin, C.C.; Shih, C.T.; Lee, C.H.; Huang, Y.L. Changes in Trace Elements During Early Stages of Chronic Kidney Disease in Type 2 Diabetic Patients. *Biol. Trace Elem. Res.* **2018**, *186*, 330–336. [CrossRef] [PubMed]
22. Kiziltas, H.; Ekin, S.; Erkoc, R. Trace element status of chronic renal patients undergoing hemodialysis. *Biol. Trace Elem. Res.* **2008**, *124*, 103–109. [CrossRef] [PubMed]
23. Tonelli, M.; Wiebe, N.; Hemmelgarn, B.; Klarenbach, S.; Field, C.; Manns, B.; Thadhani, R.; Gill, J.; Alberta Kidney Disease, N. Trace elements in hemodialysis patients: A systematic review and meta-analysis. *BMC Med.* **2009**, *7*, 25. [CrossRef] [PubMed]

24. Toida, T.; Toida, R.; Ebihara, S.; Takahashi, R.; Komatsu, H.; Uezono, S.; Sato, Y.; Fujimoto, S. Association between Serum Zinc Levels and Clinical Index or the Body Composition in Incident Hemodialysis Patients. *Nutrients* **2020**, *12*, 3187. [CrossRef]
25. Takagi, K.; Masuda, K.; Yamazaki, M.; Kiyohara, C.; Itoh, S.; Wasaki, M.; Inoue, H. Metal ion and vitamin adsorption profiles of phosphate binder ion-exchange resins. *Clin. Nephrol.* **2010**, *73*, 30–35. [CrossRef]
26. Mafra, D.; Cuppari, L.; Cozzolino, S.M. Iron and zinc status of patients with chronic renal failure who are not on dialysis. *J. Ren. Nutr.* **2002**, *12*, 38–41. [CrossRef]
27. Batista, M.N.; Cuppari, L.; de Fatima Campos Pedrosa, L.; Almeida, M.; de Almeida, J.B.; de Medeiros, A.C.; Canziani, M.E. Effect of end-stage renal disease and diabetes on zinc and copper status. *Biol. Trace Elem. Res.* **2006**, *112*, 1–12. [CrossRef]
28. Iseki, K.; Ikemiya, Y.; Iseki, C.; Takishita, S. Haematocrit and the risk of developing end-stage renal disease. *Nephrol. Dial. Transplant.* **2003**, *18*, 899–905. [CrossRef]
29. Robinson, B.M.; Joffe, M.M.; Berns, J.S.; Pisoni, R.L.; Port, F.K.; Feldman, H.I. Anemia and mortality in hemodialysis patients: Accounting for morbidity and treatment variables updated over time. *Kidney Int.* **2005**, *68*, 2323–2330. [CrossRef]
30. Yamamoto, H.; Nishi, S.; Tomo, T.; Masakane, I.; Saito, K.; Nangaku, M.; Motoshi Hattori, M.; Suzuki, T.; Morita, S.; Ashida, A.; et al. 2015 Japanese Society for Dialysis Therapy: Guidelines for Renal Anemia in Chronic Kidney Disease. *Renal. Replace. Ther.* **2017**, *3*, 36. [CrossRef]
31. Babitt, J.L.; Eisenga, M.F.; Haase, V.H.; Kshirsagar, A.V.; Levin, A.; Locatelli, F.; Malyszko, J.; Swinkels, D.W.; Tarng, D.C.; Cheung, M.; et al. Controversies in optimal anemia management: Conclusions from a Kidney Disease: Improving Global Outcomes (KDIGO) Conference. *Kidney Int.* **2021**, *99*, 1280–1295. [CrossRef] [PubMed]
32. Fukushima, T.; Horike, H.; Fujiki, S.; Kitada, S.; Sasaki, T.; Kashihara, N. Zinc deficiency anemia and effects of zinc therapy in maintenance hemodialysis patients. *Ther. Apher. Dial.* **2009**, *13*, 213–219. [CrossRef] [PubMed]
33. Kobayashi, H.; Abe, M.; Okada, K.; Tei, R.; Maruyama, N.; Kikuchi, F.; Higuchi, T.; Soma, M. Oral zinc supplementation reduces the erythropoietin responsiveness index in patients on hemodialysis. *Nutrients* **2015**, *7*, 3783–3795. [CrossRef]
34. Suzuki, H.; Tashiro, S.; Hira, S.; Sun, J.; Yamazaki, C.; Zenke, Y.; Ikeda-Saito, M.; Yoshida, M.; Igarashi, K. Heme regulates gene expression by triggering Crm1-dependent nuclear export of Bach1. *EMBO J.* **2004**, *23*, 2544–2553. [CrossRef] [PubMed]
35. Anguita, E.; Hughes, J.; Heyworth, C.; Blobel, G.A.; Wood, W.G.; Higgs, D.R. Globin gene activation during haemopoiesis is driven by protein complexes nucleated by GATA-1 and GATA-2. *EMBO J.* **2004**, *23*, 2841–2852. [CrossRef] [PubMed]
36. Randrianarison-Huetz, V.; Laurent, B.; Bardet, V.; Blobe, G.C.; Huetz, F.; Dumenil, D. Gfi-1B controls human erythroid and megakaryocytic differentiation by regulating TGF-beta signaling at the bipotent erythro-megakaryocytic progenitor stage. *Blood* **2010**, *115*, 2784–2795. [CrossRef]
37. Bergstrom, J. Nutrition and mortality in hemodialysis. *J. Am. Soc. Nephrol.* **1995**, *6*, 1329–1341. [CrossRef]
38. Kopple, J.D.; Zhu, X.; Lew, N.L.; Lowrie, E.G. Body weight-for-height relationships predict mortality in maintenance hemodialysis patients. *Kidney Int.* **1999**, *56*, 1136–1148. [CrossRef]
39. Degoulet, P.; Legrain, M.; Reach, I.; Aime, F.; Devries, C.; Rojas, P.; Jacobs, C. Mortality risk factors in patients treated by chronic hemodialysis. Report of the Diaphane collaborative study. *Nephron* **1982**, *31*, 103–110. [CrossRef]
40. Leavey, S.F.; McCullough, K.; Hecking, E.; Goodkin, D.; Port, F.K.; Young, E.W. Body mass index and mortality in 'healthier' as compared with 'sicker' haemodialysis patients: Results from the Dialysis Outcomes and Practice Patterns Study (DOPPS). *Nephrol. Dial. Transplant.* **2001**, *16*, 2386–2394. [CrossRef]
41. Calle, E.E.; Thun, M.J.; Petrelli, J.M.; Rodriguez, C.; Heath, C.W., Jr. Body-mass index and mortality in a prospective cohort of U.S. adults. *N. Engl. J. Med.* **1999**, *341*, 1097–1105. [CrossRef] [PubMed]
42. Fleischmann, E.H.; Bower, J.D.; Salahudeen, A.K. Risk factor paradox in hemodialysis: Better nutrition as a partial explanation. *ASAIO J.* **2001**, *47*, 74–81. [CrossRef]
43. Kalantar-Zadeh, K.; Block, G.; Humphreys, M.H.; Kopple, J.D. Reverse epidemiology of cardiovascular risk factors in maintenance dialysis patients. *Kidney Int.* **2003**, *63*, 793–808. [CrossRef] [PubMed]
44. Beddhu, S.; Pappas, L.M.; Ramkumar, N.; Samore, M. Effects of body size and body composition on survival in hemodialysis patients. *J. Am. Soc. Nephrol.* **2003**, *14*, 2366–2372. [CrossRef] [PubMed]
45. Caetano, C.; Valente, A.; Oliveira, T.; Garagarza, C. Body Composition and Mortality Predictors in Hemodialysis Patients. *J. Ren. Nutr.* **2016**, *26*, 81–86. [CrossRef]
46. El-Shazly, A.N.; Ibrahim, S.A.; El-Mashad, G.M.; Sabry, J.H.; Sherbini, N.S. Effect of zinc supplementation on body mass index and serum levels of zinc and leptin in pediatric hemodialysis patients. *Int. J. Nephrol. Renovasc. Dis.* **2015**, *8*, 159–163.
47. Argani, H.; Mahdavi, R.; Ghorbani-haghjo, A.; Razzaghi, R.; Nikniaz, L.; Gaemmaghami, S.J. Effects of zinc supplementation on serum zinc and leptin levels, BMI, and body composition in hemodialysis patients. *J. Trace Elem. Med. Biol.* **2014**, *28*, 35–38. [CrossRef]
48. Fukasawa, H.; Niwa, H.; Ishibuchi, K.; Kaneko, M.; Iwakura, T.; Yasuda, H.; Furuya, R. The Impact of Serum Zinc Levels on Abdominal Fat Mass in Hemodialysis Patients. *Nutrients* **2020**, *12*, 656. [CrossRef]
49. Ghosh, C.; Yang, S.H.; Kim, J.G.; Jeon, T.I.; Yoon, B.H.; Lee, J.Y.; Lee, E.Y.; Choi, S.G.; Hwang, S.G. Zinc-chelated Vitamin C Stimulates Adipogenesis of 3T3-L1 Cells. *Asian-Australas J. Anim. Sci.* **2013**, *26*, 1189–1196. [CrossRef]
50. Huang, X.; Jiang, D.; Zhu, Y.; Fang, Z.; Che, L.; Lin, Y.; Xu, S.; Li, J.; Huang, C.; Zou, Y.; et al. Chronic High Dose Zinc Supplementation Induces Visceral Adipose Tissue Hypertrophy without Altering Body Weight in Mice. *Nutrients* **2017**, *9*, 1138. [CrossRef]

51. Zhang, H.B.; Wang, M.S.; Wang, Z.S.; Zhou, A.M.; Zhang, X.M.; Dong, X.W.; Peng, Q.H. Supplementation dietary zinc levels on growth performance, carcass traits, and intramuscular fat deposition in weaned piglets. *Biol. Trace Elem. Res.* **2014**, *161*, 69–77. [CrossRef]
52. Chen, M.D.; Lin, P.Y.; Cheng, V.; Lin, W.H. Zinc supplementation aggravates body fat accumulation in genetically obese mice and dietary-obese mice. *Biol. Trace Elem. Res.* **1996**, *52*, 125–132. [CrossRef]
53. Lobo, J.C.; Torres, J.P.; Fouque, D.; Mafra, D. Zinc deficiency in chronic kidney disease: Is there a relationship with adipose tissue and atherosclerosis? *Biol. Trace Elem. Res.* **2010**, *135*, 16–21. [CrossRef] [PubMed]
54. Lobo, J.C.; Stockler-Pinto, M.B.; Farage, N.E.; Faulin Tdo, E.; Abdalla, D.S.; Torres, J.P.; Velarde, L.G.; Mafra, D. Reduced plasma zinc levels, lipid peroxidation, and inflammation biomarkers levels in hemodialysis patients: Implications to cardiovascular mortality. *Ren. Fail.* **2013**, *35*, 680–685. [CrossRef] [PubMed]
55. Gorriz, J.L.; Molina, P.; Cerveron, M.J.; Vila, R.; Bover, J.; Nieto, J.; Barril, G.; Martinez-Castelao, A.; Fernandez, E.; Escudero, V.; et al. Vascular calcification in patients with nondialysis CKD over 3 years. *Clin. J. Am. Soc. Nephrol.* **2015**, *10*, 654–666. [CrossRef] [PubMed]
56. Peeters, M.J.; van den Brand, J.A.; van Zuilen, A.D.; Koster, Y.; Bots, M.L.; Vervloet, M.G.; Blankestijn, P.J.; Wetzels, J.F.; Group, M.S. Abdominal aortic calcification in patients with CKD. *J. Nephrol.* **2017**, *30*, 109–118. [CrossRef]
57. Furusawa, K.; Takeshita, K.; Suzuki, S.; Tatami, Y.; Morimoto, R.; Okumura, T.; Yasuda, Y.; Murohara, T. Assessment of abdominal aortic calcification by computed tomography for prediction of latent left ventricular stiffness and future cardiovascular risk in pre-dialysis patients with chronic kidney disease: A single center cross-sectional study. *Int. J. Med. Sci.* **2019**, *16*, 939–948. [CrossRef]
58. Paloian, N.J.; Giachelli, C.M. A current understanding of vascular calcification in CKD. *Am. J. Physiol. Renal. Physiol.* **2014**, *307*, F891–F900. [CrossRef]
59. Ketteler, M.; Block, G.A.; Evenepoel, P.; Fukagawa, M.; Herzog, C.A.; McCann, L.; Moe, S.M.; Shroff, R.; Tonelli, M.A.; Toussaint, N.D.; et al. Executive summary of the 2017 KDIGO Chronic Kidney Disease-Mineral and Bone Disorder (CKD-MBD) Guideline Update: What's changed and why it matters. *Kidney Int.* **2017**, *92*, 26–36. [CrossRef]
60. Summersgill, H.; England, H.; Lopez-Castejon, G.; Lawrence, C.B.; Luheshi, N.M.; Pahle, J.; Mendes, P.; Brough, D. Zinc depletion regulates the processing and secretion of IL-1beta. *Cell Death Dis.* **2014**, *5*, e1040. [CrossRef]
61. Fan, Y.; Zhang, X.; Yang, L.; Wang, J.; Hu, Y.; Bian, A.; Liu, J.; Ma, J. Zinc inhibits high glucose-induced NLRP3 inflammasome activation in human peritoneal mesothelial cells. *Mol. Med. Rep.* **2017**, *16*, 5195–5202. [CrossRef]
62. Kim, J.; Cha, Y.N.; Surh, Y.J. A protective role of nuclear factor-erythroid 2-related factor-2 (Nrf2) in inflammatory disorders. *Mutat. Res.* **2010**, *690*, 12–23. [CrossRef] [PubMed]
63. Pedruzzi, L.M.; Cardozo, L.F.; Daleprane, J.B.; Stockler-Pinto, M.B.; Monteiro, E.B.; Leite, M., Jr.; Vaziri, N.D.; Mafra, D. Systemic inflammation and oxidative stress in hemodialysis patients are associated with down-regulation of Nrf2. *J. Nephrol.* **2015**, *28*, 495–501. [CrossRef] [PubMed]
64. Wang, L.J.; Wang, M.Q.; Hu, R.; Yang, Y.; Huang, Y.S.; Xian, S.X.; Lu, L. Effect of Zinc Supplementation on Maintenance Hemodialysis Patients: A Systematic Review and Meta-Analysis of 15 Randomized Controlled Trials. *Biomed. Res. Int.* **2017**, *2017*, 1024769. [CrossRef]
65. Tahir, N.; Ashraf, A.; Waqar, S.H.B.; Rafae, A.; Kantamneni, L.; Sheikh, T.; Khan, R. Copper deficiency, a rare but correctable cause of pancytopenia: A review of literature. *Expert. Rev. Hematol.* **2022**, *15*, 999–1008. [CrossRef]
66. Nishime, K.; Kondo, M.; Saito, K.; Miyawaki, H.; Nakagawa, T. Zinc Burden Evokes Copper Deficiency in the Hypoalbuminemic Hemodialysis Patients. *Nutrients* **2020**, *12*, 577. [CrossRef] [PubMed]
67. Prasad, A.S.; Brewer, G.J.; Schoomaker, E.B.; Rabbani, P. Hypocupremia induced by zinc therapy in adults. *JAMA* **1978**, *240*, 2166–2168. [CrossRef] [PubMed]
68. Hoffman, H.N., 2nd; Phyliky, R.L.; Fleming, C.R. Zinc-induced copper deficiency. *Gastroenterology* **1988**, *94*, 508–512. [CrossRef] [PubMed]
69. Kumar, N. Copper deficiency myelopathy (human swayback). *Mayo Clin. Proc.* **2006**, *81*, 1371–1384. [CrossRef]
70. Higuchi, T.; Matsukawa, Y.; Okada, K.; Oikawa, O.; Yamazaki, T.; Ohnishi, Y.; Fujita, T.; Fukuda, N.; Soma, M.; Matsumoto, K. Correction of copper deficiency improves erythropoietin unresponsiveness in hemodialysis patients with anemia. *Intern. Med.* **2006**, *45*, 271–273. [CrossRef]
71. Rissardo, J.P.; Caprara, A.L. Copper deficiency myelopathy secondary to parenteral zinc supplementation during chronic dialysis. *Neurol. Asia* **2019**, *24*, 79–82.
72. Munie, S.; Pintavorn, P. Erythropoietin-Resistant Anemia Secondary to Zinc-Induced Hypocupremia in a Hemodialysis Patient. *Case Rep. Nephrol. Dial.* **2021**, *11*, 167–175. [CrossRef] [PubMed]
73. Si, M.; Lang, J. The roles of metallothioneins in carcinogenesis. *J. Hematol. Oncol.* **2018**, *11*, 107. [CrossRef] [PubMed]

Disclaimer/Publisher's Note: The statements, opinions and data contained in all publications are solely those of the individual author(s) and contributor(s) and not of MDPI and/or the editor(s). MDPI and/or the editor(s) disclaim responsibility for any injury to people or property resulting from any ideas, methods, instructions or products referred to in the content.

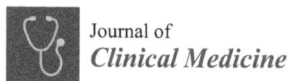

Communication

The Impact and Treatment of COVID-19 in Hemodialysis Patients

Daisuke Katagiri [1,*] and Kan Kikuchi [2]

1 Department of Nephrology, National Center for Global Health and Medicine, Tokyo 162-8655, Japan
2 Division of Nephrology, Shimoochiai Clinic, Tokyo 161-0033, Japan
* Correspondence: dkatagiri@hosp.ncgm.go.jp; Tel.: +81-3-3202-7181

Abstract: Background: Patients with coronavirus disease 2019 (COVID-19) undergoing maintenance hemodialysis have a poor prognosis and limited treatment options. Methods: This paper outlines the impact of COVID-19, its treatment, and the efficacy of vaccines in Japanese patients undergoing hemodialysis with a review of the literature. Results: Patients undergoing dialysis in dialysis facilities are at greater risk of exposure to severe acute respiratory syndrome coronavirus 2 than the general population due to limited isolation capabilities. Therefore, vaccines are expected to be effective for patients undergoing dialysis. In addition, effective use of available medications is important because treatment options are limited. Conclusions: Efforts should be made to prevent the spread of the infection to high-risk patients undergoing dialysis while ensuring the effective use of vaccines.

Keywords: COVID-19; hemodialysis; vaccination

Citation: Katagiri, D.; Kikuchi, K. The Impact and Treatment of COVID-19 in Hemodialysis Patients. *J. Clin. Med.* **2023**, *12*, 838. https://doi.org/10.3390/jcm12030838

Academic Editor: Magdi Yaqoob

Received: 21 December 2022
Revised: 11 January 2023
Accepted: 18 January 2023
Published: 20 January 2023

Copyright: © 2023 by the authors. Licensee MDPI, Basel, Switzerland. This article is an open access article distributed under the terms and conditions of the Creative Commons Attribution (CC BY) license (https://creativecommons.org/licenses/by/4.0/).

1. Introduction

In December 2019, an outbreak of unknown viral pneumonia was reported among patients in Wuhan, Hubei Province, People's Republic of China. Over a short period, infection by a novel severe acute respiratory syndrome coronavirus 2 (SARS-CoV-2) spread worldwide. SARS-CoV-2 has been identified as an animal-derived coronavirus and is the same pathogen responsible for severe acute respiratory syndrome (SARS) and Middle East respiratory syndrome (MERS). On 11 March 2020, the World Health Organization (WHO) declared a pandemic status, and SARS-CoV-2 was linked to a severe acute respiratory condition. SARS-CoV-2 has been reported to be stable on environmental surfaces for approximately 3 days. Therefore, preventing infection among staff is crucial in medical institutions.

Initial coronavirus disease 2019 (COVID-19) symptoms are similar to those of influenza, including fever, cough, malaise, and dyspnea. The median hospitalization time was 7 days. Diarrhea and taste and smell disorders may occur; however, they are not inevitable. Data from the COVID-19 Registry Japan (COVIREGI-JP), which is a Japanese registry of patients with COVID-19, showed that 60% of hospitalized patients did not require oxygen administration, whereas 30% required oxygen administration, 9% required ventilation or extracorporeal membrane oxygenation (ECMO), and 7.5% died [1]. Therefore, predicting which patients will become critically ill is important for using limited medical resources [2].

In severe cases, COVID-19 causes respiratory tract infection symptoms, such as acute respiratory distress syndrome and cytokine release syndrome (CRS)-like symptoms because of excessive inflammation. Endothelial cell damage and disruption of the immunomodulatory system lead to multiple organs failure. During the COVID-19 pandemic, the number of dialysis cases in the hospital was also reported to have increased greatly, partly due to the involvement of acute kidney injury [3]. Therefore, in addition to antiviral drugs, various therapies have been investigated to suppress excess cytokines, such as steroids, neutralizing antibody therapy, and some blood purification therapies [4,5]. However, patients undergoing dialysis are prone to severe disease, and their treatment options are limited because of renal dysfunction. This manuscript outlines the current impact of COVID-19 and its treatment in Japanese patients undergoing dialysis.

2. Number and Severity of Patients with COVID-19 Undergoing Dialysis in Japan

The first case of COVID-19 in a patient undergoing dialysis was reported in Japan on 1 March 2020 [6]. The Japanese Association of Dialysis Physicians, the Japanese Society for Dialysis Therapy, and the Japanese Society of Nephrology established the Joint Committee on Countermeasures against SARS-CoV-2 infection in Dialysis Patients to monitor the infection status of patients undergoing dialysis in Japan. As shown in Figure 1, the number of infected patients on dialysis continues to increase in Japan. Although the number of deaths appears to have decreased compared with the past, partly due to the spread of vaccines, continued attention should be given in the future. As of November 2022, the total number of infected patients was 12,978, and the infection rate was 3.8% of the total number of patients on maintenance dialysis in Japan (approximately 340,000). Overall, 658 confirmed deaths have been recorded due to COVID-19 among patients undergoing dialysis, with a mortality rate of 5.1% higher than that in the general population (0.2%). Figure 2 shows that even after the virus mutated to Omicron, the mortality rate among patients undergoing dialysis remained higher than that of the general population, particularly among those aged <60 years.

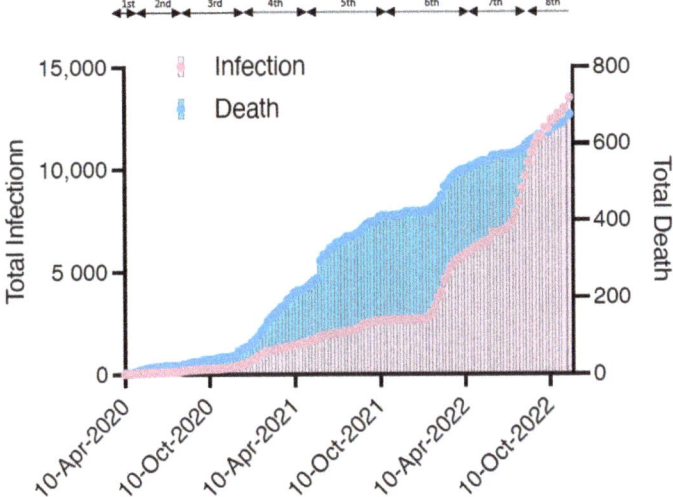

Figure 1. The total number of infected patients undergoing dialysis in Japan and the number of deaths. The periods of the first to eighth waves (the 8th wave is ongoing) are also shown. Data were taken from the website of the Japanese Association of Dialysis Physicians (http://www.touseki-ikai.or.jp/, accessed on 7 December 2022) and plotted.

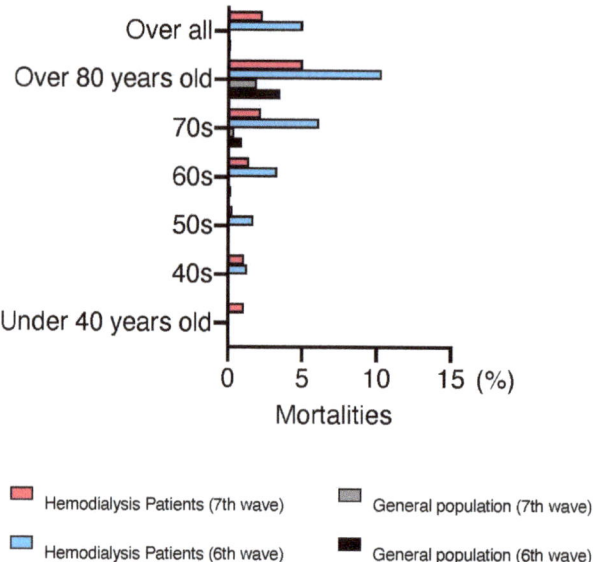

Figure 2. Mortalities in the general population and patients undergoing dialysis after the sixth wave. This figure was drawn from the 9 November 2022 report of the Advisory Board for New Coronavirus Infections (https://www.mhlw.go.jp/content/10900000/001010896.pdf, accessed on 7 December 2022) and the "Report on COVID-19 Infection Cases at Dialysis Facilities" jointly published by the Japanese Association of Dialysis Physicians, the Japanese Society for Dialysis Therapy, and the Japanese Society of Nephrology. This figure is accurate as of 7 December 2022.

3. Efficacy of COVID-19 Vaccination in Patients with End-Stage Renal Disease

During the first to fourth waves, vaccines had not yet been developed and disseminated in Japan; however, they became widespread during the fifth wave. The weakening of the virus may have played a role in the significant decrease in severe cases and deaths among patients undergoing dialysis. However, these patients remain at high risk compared with the general population, as shown above.

Several studies have analyzed the efficacy and safety of the COVID-19 vaccine among patients undergoing hemodialysis [7,8]. A study of 148 and 20 patients undergoing hemodialysis and peritoneal dialysis, respectively, reported similar efficacy of COVID-19 mRNA vaccination [9]. Although caution must be exercised during interpretation due to the heterogeneous study design, in most studies, humoral responses were lower than that in the control group. In contrast, seroconversion rates and the number of patients in whom S-protein reactive T-cell immunity was detected, were very high [10]. On 15 October 2021, the American Society of Nephrology released a statement on the need for vaccines for patients undergoing dialysis [11]. The report emphasizes the importance of vaccination in patients with end-stage renal disease (ESRD) to reduce the increased risk of complications and death secondary to COVID-19 infection. In addition, patients with end-stage kidney disease and kidney transplantation have a reduced antibody response to the COVID-19 vaccine; however, antibody production has been shown to increase with the third and fourth doses [12]. Multivariate logistic regression analysis was used to examine post-infection oxygen demand in patients with post-vaccinated infection and breakthrough infection in Japan [13]. The odds ratio (OR) 0.197 (95% confidence interval [CI]: 0.120–0.322), $p < 0.001$, showed that patients with breakthrough infection had lower oxygen demand. The prognosis of breakthrough-infected patients was also better than that of unvaccinated patients.

4. Infection Control and Hospitalization of Patients Undergoing Dialysis in Japan

Patients receiving dialysis at the center were at greater risk of exposure to SARS-CoV-2 than the general population because of their limited isolation capabilities [14]. They were initially required by national policy to be hospitalized because of the high mortality rate associated with COVID-19 [6]. A report from Canada showed that the rate of hospitalization, 30-day mortality, and overall mortality were all significantly lower in patients receiving home dialysis, including patients undergoing peritoneal dialysis, than in those undergoing outpatient hemodialysis [15]. However, an analysis by Kikuchi et al. based on Japanese registries comparing patients receiving peritoneal dialysis and hemodialysis in terms of overall survival and length of hospitalization showed no significant difference between the two groups [16]. Therefore, caution should be exercised because overly strict infection precautions increase the burden on staff, increase healthcare costs, and make compliance more challenging. Infection control in patients undergoing dialysis has traditionally been well-established in Japan, and the 5th edition of the guidelines was issued in 2020 [17]. The following is a list of infection control measures that are in place at dialysis facilities in Japan regularly:

(1) Personal protective equipment (PPE) is recommended for the medical staff in the dialysis unit.

Before performing procedures such as puncture, hemostasis, catheter access and management, and wound care, hand hygiene should be performed by washing hands with soap and running water or using a quick-drying hand sanitizer, and unused disposable gloves should be worn. In addition, wear a disposable nonpermeable gown or plastic apron, surgical mask, goggles, or face shield when performing procedures such as puncture, hemostasis, catheter access and management, and wound care.

(2) Environmental hygiene in the dialysis unit.

Linens (sheets, pillowcases, and blanket covers) should be changed for each patient. The exterior of the dialysis machine, bed rails, and over tables should be cleaned at the end of each dialysis session. Stethoscopes, thermometers, and blood pressure cuffs should be cleaned after each use. Instruments in the dialysis room should be cleaned and disinfected with either 0.05–0.1% sodium hypochlorite, potassium hydrogen peroxymonosulfate, or alcohol-based disinfectants. Forceps and trays, among others, should be disinfected with hot water (80 °C for 10 min) or thoroughly pre-cleaned with a cleaning agent before each use, immersed in 0.1% sodium hypochlorite for 30 min, and then thoroughly rinsed with water. The above infection control measures are recommended in normal times, and the use of PPE and environmental sanitation are also preventive measures against contact and droplet infection of COVID-19.

A survey of dialysis facilities in Japan [18] revealed that several infection prevention measures were implemented during the COVID-19 pandemic, including health checks of staff and patients, wearing of masks before and after hemodialysis, and disinfection of frequently contacted areas. The implementation rate of these measures was significantly improved compared with that of the pre-pandemic rate, reaching >90%. However, because of the high risk of infectious disease transmission in the hospital setting during a pandemic, alternative end-stage renal failure management methods may need to be considered, such as a temporary switch to peritoneal dialysis or the implementation of a home dialysis program [19].

As noted above, the Japanese government recommended that patients who tested positive be hospitalized because of the high mortality rate associated with COVID-19, particularly patients receiving maintenance dialysis and those with a definite need for regular dialysis. However, after experiencing a delta surge, a strategic shift to outpatient care for mildly ill or asymptomatic patients and increased emergency preparedness was necessary. In response to the rise in the Omicron variant, the Tokyo Metropolitan Government opened a temporary medical facility with a dialysis center in January 2022, providing more beds and access to hemodialysis [20]. The hospital ran a smooth ward operation and reduced the number of complications with new patients with positive COVID-19 test results that required treatment and could not be hospitalized.

5. Current Treatment of COVID-19 in Patients Undergoing Dialysis

As of November 2022, the antivirals approved in Japan for treating COVID-19 include remdesivir, molnupiravir, nirmatrelvir/ritonavir, and the recently approved ensitrelvir (Table 1).

Table 1. Current COVID-19 treatment for patients undergoing dialysis.

Type	Antiviral Drug				Immunity Suppressants/Regulators			Neutralizing Antibody	
Name	Remdesivir	Molnupiravir	Nirmatrelvir/Ritonavir	Ensitrelvir	Dexamethasone	Baricitinib	Tocilizumab	Sotrovimab	Casirivimab–imdevimab
Severity to be administered	Mild, Moderate, Severe	Mild, Moderate	Mild, Moderate	Mild, Moderate	Moderate, Severe	Moderate, Severe	Moderate, Severe	Mild	Mild
Response to Omicron	Yes	Yes	Yes	Yes	Yes	Yes	Yes	No	No
Route of administration	Intravenous	Oral	Oral	Oral	Intravenous, oral	Oral	Intravenous	Intravenous	Intravenous
Length of treatment	3–10 days	5 days	5 days	5 days	10 days	14 days	Single dose	Single dose	Single dose
Dosage in dialysis patients	100 mg 4 h before dialysis initiation. Approximately 6 doses	No adjustment required	No administration to dialysis patients	No clinical trials have been conducted in patients with renal dysfunction	No adjustment required	No administration to dialysis patients	No adjustment required	No adjustment required	No adjustment required

Remdesivir is recommended for mild-to-moderate disease within 7 days of onset. Japanese patients with COVID-19 undergoing hemodialysis enrolled by 19 June 2020, with ($N = 98$) and without ($N = 294$) remdesivir, were studied using propensity matching [16]. Patients receiving remdesivir had a significantly better prognosis than those not receiving it. In addition, the remdesivir-treated group had a shorter hospital stay. In a retrospective study of 486 patients (407 on hemodialysis and 79 on peritoneal dialysis) in the United States, 112 (23%) received remdesivir [21]. The estimated 30-day mortality rate was 0.74 (95% confidence interval, 0.52–1.05) in the remdesivir-treated group compared with the non-treated group. These results suggest that remdesivir is an effective treatment option for patients undergoing maintenance hemodialysis.

Molnupiravir was the first oral antiviral drug approved in Japan to treat COVID-19 [22]. It does not require dosage adjustment according to renal function or volume adjustment in patients undergoing hemodialysis, making it easy to use in outpatient settings [23]. However, the disadvantage is that the capsule formulation is large and challenging to take internally. Nirmatrelvir/ritonavir is another oral antiviral drug approved in Japan [24]. As ritonavir inhibits drug metabolism in CYP3A to maintain drug blood levels, it increases the blood levels of drugs metabolized by CYP3A. Calcium channel blockers and statins are typical examples, but many other drugs, such as tranquilizers, are also affected. Dose adjustment is required in patients with moderately impaired renal function, and administration is not recommended for patients with severe renal dysfunction, including those on maintenance dialysis. Clinical trials have not been conducted on ensitrelvir in patients with renal dysfunction, and its efficacy in those undergoing hemodialysis requires further study.

Omicron strains have been classified into five strains (BA.1, BA.2, BA.3, BA.4, and BA.5). The BA.2 strain has been the primary epidemic strain; however, since July 2022, the BA.2 strain has been rapidly replaced by the BA.5 strain in many countries, including Japan. The inhibitory effects of different antibodies and antiviral drugs on Omicron strains isolated from clinical specimens are being investigated [25]. The neutralizing activity of sotrovimab and casirivimab–imdevimab [26] was significantly lower against all strains after BA.2 than the effect against the conventional stress (from Wuhan). The efficacy of tixagevimab and cilgavimab was similarly reduced. In contrast, bebtelovimab showed a high neutralizing activity against BA.2.12.1, BA.4, and BA.5 strains. Furthermore, the efficacy of the three antiviral drugs (remdesivir, molnupiravir, and nirmatrelvir) was subsequently analyzed, and they were found to effectively inhibit the growth of BA.2.12.1, BA.4, and BA.5 strains.

6. Conclusions

This paper outlines the impact and treatment of COVID-19 on patients undergoing hemodialysis, which has not yet reached a global consensus. Therefore, it is important to continue to elucidate the pathogenesis of severe disease in patients with hemodialysis, leading to expanded vaccination and the establishment of more effective treatment strategies.

Author Contributions: D.K.; writing—original draft preparation, K.K.; writing—review and editing. All authors have read and agreed to the published version of the manuscript.

Funding: This research was funded by Grants-in-Aid for Research from the National Center for Global Health and Medicine, grant number 21A-2002.

Institutional Review Board Statement: The study was conducted in accordance with the Declaration of Helsinki and was approved by the Institutional Review Board of the National Center for Global Health and Medicine (NCGM-G-003616-00, Approval Date: 7 August 2020).

Informed Consent Statement: Not applicable.

Data Availability Statement: Not applicable.

Conflicts of Interest: The authors declare no conflict of interest.

References

1. Matsunaga, N.; Hayakawa, K.; Terada, M.; Ohtsu, H.; Asai, Y.; Tsuzuki, S.; Suzuki, S.; Toyoda, A.; Suzuki, K.; Endo, M.; et al. Clinical Epidemiology of Hospitalized Patients With Coronavirus Disease 2019 (COVID-19) in Japan: Report of the COVID-19 Registry Japan. *Clin. Infect. Dis.* **2021**, *73*, e3677–e3689. [CrossRef]
2. Katagiri, D.; Ishikane, M.; Asai, Y.; Kinoshita, N.; Ota, M.; Moriyama, Y.; Ide, S.; Nakamura, K.; Nakamoto, T.; Nomoto, H.; et al. Evaluation of Coronavirus Disease 2019 Severity Using Urine Biomarkers. *Crit. Care Explor.* **2020**, *2*, e0170. [CrossRef]
3. Mureșan, A.V.; Russu, E.; Arbănași, E.M.; Kaller, R.; Hosu, I.; Arbănași, E.M.; Voidăzan, S.T. Negative Impact of the COVID-19 Pandemic on Kidney Disease Management-A Single-Center Experience in Romania. *J. Clin. Med.* **2022**, *11*, 2452. [CrossRef] [PubMed]
4. Katagiri, D. For safe and adequate blood purification therapy in severe COVID-19—What we have learned so far. *Glob. Health Med.* **2022**, *4*, 94–100. [CrossRef] [PubMed]
5. Katagiri, D.; Ishikane, M.; Asai, Y.; Izumi, S.; Takasaki, J.; Katsuoka, H.; Kondo, I.; Ide, S.; Nakamura, K.; Nakamoto, T.; et al. Direct hemoperfusion using a polymyxin B-immobilized polystyrene column for COVID-19. *J. Clin. Apher.* **2021**, *36*, 313–321. [CrossRef] [PubMed]
6. Kikuchi, K.; Nangaku, M.; Ryuzaki, M.; Yamakawa, T.; Hanafusa, N.; Sakai, K.; Kanno, Y.; Ando, R.; Shinoda, T.; Nakamoto, H.; et al. COVID-19 of dialysis patients in Japan: Current status and guidance on preventive measures. *Ther. Apher. Dial.* **2020**, *24*, 361–365. [CrossRef]
7. Ashby, D.R.; Caplin, B.; Corbett, R.W.; Asgari, E.; Kumar, N.; Sarnowski, A.; Hull, R.; Makanjuola, D.; Cole, N.; Chen, J.; et al. Severity of COVID-19 after Vaccination among Hemodialysis Patients: An Observational Cohort Study. *Clin. J. Am. Soc. Nephrol. CJASN* **2022**, *17*, 843–850. [CrossRef]
8. Brunelli, S.M.; Sibbel, S.; Karpinski, S.; Marlowe, G.; Walker, A.G.; Giullian, J.; Van Wyck, D.; Kelley, T.; Lazar, R.; Zywno, M.L.; et al. Comparative Effectiveness of mRNA-based BNT162b2 Vaccine versus Adenovirus Vector-Based Ad26.COV2.S Vaccine for the Prevention of COVID-19 among Dialysis Patients. *J. Am. Soc. Nephrol.* **2022**, *33*, 688–697. [CrossRef]
9. Frittoli, M.; Cassia, M.; Barassi, A.; Ciceri, P.; Galassi, A.; Conte, F.; Cozzolino, M.G. Efficacy and Safety of COVID-19 Vaccine in Patients on Renal Replacement Therapy. *Vaccines* **2022**, *10*, 1395. [CrossRef]
10. Babel, N.; Hugo, C.; Westhoff, T.H. Vaccination in patients with kidney failure: Lessons from COVID-19. *Nat. Rev. Nephrol.* **2022**, *18*, 708–723. [CrossRef]
11. Blake, P.G.; Hladunewich, M.A.; Oliver, M.J. COVID-19 Vaccination Imperatives in People on Maintenance Dialysis: An International Perspective. *Clin. J. Am. Soc. Nephrol.* **2021**, *16*, 1746–1748. [CrossRef] [PubMed]
12. Moreno, N.F.; McAdams, R.; Goss, J.A.; Galvan, N.T.N. COVID-19 Vaccine Efficacy and Immunogenicity in End-Stage Renal Disease Patients and Kidney Transplant Recipients. *Curr. Transplant. Rep.* **2022**, *9*, 174–184. [CrossRef] [PubMed]

13. Kikuchi, K.; Nangaku, M.; Ryuzaki, M.; Yamakawa, T.; Yoshihiro, O.; Hanafusa, N.; Sakai, K.; Kanno, Y.; Ando, R.; Shinoda, T.; et al. Effectiveness of SARS-CoV-2 vaccines on hemodialysis patients in Japan: A nationwide cohort study. *Ther. Apher. Dial.* **2022**, *27*, 19–23. [CrossRef] [PubMed]
14. Mahalingasivam, V.; Su, G.; Iwagami, M.; Davids, M.R.; Wetmore, J.B.; Nitsch, D. COVID-19 and kidney disease: Insights from epidemiology to inform clinical practice. *Nat. Rev. Nephrol.* **2022**, *18*, 485–498. [CrossRef]
15. Perl, J.; Thomas, D.; Tang, Y.; Yeung, A.; Ip, J.; Oliver, M.J.; Blake, P.G. COVID-19 among Adults Receiving Home versus In-Center Dialysis. *Clin. J. Am. Soc. Nephrol. CJASN* **2021**, *16*, 1410–1412. [CrossRef]
16. Kikuchi, K.; Nangaku, M.; Ryuzaki, M.; Yamakawa, T.; Yoshihiro, O.; Hanafusa, N.; Sakai, K.; Kanno, Y.; Ando, R.; Shinoda, T.; et al. Survival and predictive factors in dialysis patients with COVID-19 in Japan: A nationwide cohort study. *Ren. Replace. Ther.* **2021**, *7*, 59. [CrossRef]
17. The Japanese Associations of Dialysis Physicians. *Guidelines for Standard Hemodialysis Procedure and Prevention of Infection in Maintenance Hemodialysis Facilities*, 5th ed.; The Japanese Associations of Dialysis Physicians: Tokyo, Japan, 2020.
18. Sugawara, Y.; Iwagami, M.; Kikuchi, K.; Yoshida, Y.; Ando, R.; Shinoda, T.; Ryuzaki, M.; Nakamoto, H.; Sakai, K.; Hanafusa, N.; et al. Infection prevention measures for patients undergoing hemodialysis during the COVID-19 pandemic in Japan: A nationwide questionnaire survey. *Ren. Replace. Ther.* **2021**, *7*, 27. [CrossRef]
19. Behlul, S.; Artac Ozdal, M. Risk of COVID-19 and Cost Burden in End-Stage Renal Disease Patients and Policy Implications for Managing Nephrology Services during the COVID-19 Pandemic. *Healthcare* **2022**, *10*, 2351. [CrossRef]
20. Naito, K.; Kikuchi, K.; Watanabe, Y.; Narita, T. Implementation of two novel schemes for patients on dialysis as a response to the COVID-19 surge in Tokyo. *Glob. Health Med.* **2022**, *4*, 253–258. [CrossRef]
21. Zaki, K.E.; Huang, C.W.; Zhou, H.; Chung, J.; Selevan, D.C.; Rutkowski, M.P.; Sim, J.J. Comparison of safety and outcomes related to remdesivir treatment among dialysis patients hospitalized with COVID-19. *Clin. Kidney J.* **2022**, *15*, 2056–2062. [CrossRef]
22. Jayk Bernal, A.; Gomes da Silva, M.M.; Musungaie, D.B.; Kovalchuk, E.; Gonzalez, A.; Delos Reyes, V.; Martín-Quirós, A.; Caraco, Y.; Williams-Diaz, A.; Brown, M.L.; et al. Molnupiravir for Oral Treatment of Covid-19 in Nonhospitalized Patients. *N. Engl. J. Med.* **2022**, *386*, 509–520. [CrossRef] [PubMed]
23. Poznański, P.; Augustyniak-Bartosik, H.; Magiera-Żak, A.; Skalec, K.; Jakuszko, K.; Mazanowska, O.; Janczak, D.; Krajewska, M.; Kamińska, D. Molnupiravir When Used Alone Seems to Be Safe and Effective as Outpatient COVID-19 Therapy for Hemodialyzed Patients and Kidney Transplant Recipients. *Viruses* **2022**, *14*, 2224. [CrossRef]
24. Hammond, J.; Leister-Tebbe, H.; Gardner, A.; Abreu, P.; Bao, W.; Wisemandle, W.; Baniecki, M.; Hendrick, V.M.; Damle, B.; Simón-Campos, A.; et al. Oral Nirmatrelvir for High-Risk, Nonhospitalized Adults with Covid-19. *N. Engl. J. Med.* **2022**, *386*, 1397–1408. [CrossRef] [PubMed]
25. Takashita, E.; Yamayoshi, S.; Simon, V.; van Bakel, H.; Sordillo, E.M.; Pekosz, A.; Fukushi, S.; Suzuki, T.; Maeda, K.; Halfmann, P.; et al. Efficacy of Antibodies and Antiviral Drugs against Omicron BA.2.12.1, BA.4, and BA.5 Subvariants. *N. Engl. J. Med.* **2022**, *387*, 468–470. [CrossRef]
26. Terakawa, K.; Katagiri, D.; Shimada, K.; Sato, L.; Takano, H. Safety of casirivimab/imdevimab administration in a SARS-CoV-2 positive maintenance dialysis patient in Japan. *CEN Case Rep.* **2022**, *11*, 328–332. [CrossRef] [PubMed]

Disclaimer/Publisher's Note: The statements, opinions and data contained in all publications are solely those of the individual author(s) and contributor(s) and not of MDPI and/or the editor(s). MDPI and/or the editor(s) disclaim responsibility for any injury to people or property resulting from any ideas, methods, instructions or products referred to in the content.

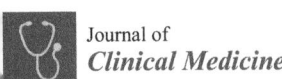

Article

Malnutrition and Insulin Resistance May Interact with Metabolic Syndrome in Prevalent Hemodialysis Patients

Shuzo Kobayashi [1,*], Yasuhiro Mochida [1], Kunihiro Ishioka [1], Machiko Oka [1], Kyoko Maesato [2], Hidekazu Moriya [1], Sumi Hidaka [1] and Takayasu Ohtake [1]

[1] Kidney Disease and Transplant Center, Shonan Kamakura General Hospital, Kamakura 247-8533, Japan
[2] Nephrology, Tokyo Nishi Tokushukai Hospital, Akishima 196-0003, Japan
* Correspondence: shuzo@shonankamakura.or.jp; Tel.: +81-467-46-1717

Abstract: Background: We sought to determine the prevalence of metabolic syndrome (Mets) and whether 100 cm^2 of visceral fatty area (VFA) measured by computed tomography (CT) validates the criteria of waist circumference (WC) in hemodialysis (HD) patients. Methods: The study comprised 141 HD patients. Mets was defined according to the criteria of Adult Treatment Panel III (ATP III) and the modified criteria of National Cholesterol Education Program (NCEP) that defines abdominal obesity as a WC of >=85 cm in men and >=90 cm in women. Results: The prevalence of Mets was 31.9% in men and 13.6% in women. However, the prevalence of patients with a body mass index over 25 in all HD patients was only 11.2%. The visceral fatty area (VFA) measured by CT showed a strong positive correlation with WC. The patients with Mets, comparing with those without Mets, have significantly shorter duration of HD, higher high-sensitive C-reactive protein, and higher Homeostatic Model Assessment for Insulin Resistance (HOMA-IR). In the patients with Mets, there was a significant negative correlation between HOMA-IR and serum albumin levels. Multivariate logistic regression analysis showed that HOMA-IR and short duration of HD were chosen as independent risk factors for Mets. Conclusions: Mets is more prevalent in HD patients. In Japanese HD patients, 100 cm^2 of VFA corresponded to a WC of 85 cm in men and 90 cm in women, thus confirming the validity of the modified criteria. HOMA-IR and serum albumin were significantly correlated in HD patients with Mets.

Keywords: hemodialysis; metabolic syndrome; abdominal obesity; inflammation; atherosclerosis

1. Introduction

In patients on hemodialysis (HD), malnutrition and its related inflammation are known to cause atherosclerosis (malnutrition, inflammation, atherosclerotic syndrome; MIA syndrome) [1], thus leading to cardiovascular disease (CVD). Likewise, metabolic syndrome (Mets), characterized by abdominal obesity, hypertriglyceridemia, low high-density lipoprotein (HDL) cholesterol level, high blood pressure, and high fasting glucose level [2], is also known to be a major leading cause of CVD in the general population [3]. Mets has been associated with an increased risk for diabetes mellitus and CVD, as well as increased CVD and all-cause mortality [3–5]. Chen et al. reported that Mets is prevalent and might be an important factor in the cause of chronic kidney disease (CKD) [6]. In Japan, Mets is a significant determinant of CKD in men under 60 years of age [7].

Besides the fact that Mets is one of the risk factors in CKD, it is important to note that we need to know the prevalence of Mets and its associated factors in maintenance HD patients because malnutrition develops with longer HD duration. In this regard, little information is available, although at the initiation of renal replacement therapy (RRT), there is a report showing that Mets is highly prevalent in incident dialysis patients [8]. Unfortunately, body mass index (BMI) is used instead of the criteria of waist circumferences (WC), and no data on fasting blood are available in that report. Moreover, information on associated factors is not provided.

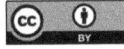

The pathogenesis of Mets and the relationship between Mets and CVD lie in insulin resistance [9]. Insulin resistance is known to develop at an early stage of non-diabetic CKD [10]. We reported a similar result using a hyperinsulinemic euglycemic glucose clamp method and also showed that acidemia and dyslipidemia are independently associated with insulin resistance in CKD [11]. Although RRT improves insulin resistance [12], insulin resistance is still occasionally found in maintenance HD patients [13]. However, it remains unknown concerning the relationship between Mets and insulin resistance in hemodialysis patients.

Therefore, in the present study using fasting blood samples, we first assessed the prevalence of Mets in maintenance HD patients according to the criteria of the Adult Treatment Panel III (ATP III) [2] using modified criteria of WC. We studied the associated factors including insulin resistance expressed by the Homeostasis Model Assessment of Insulin Resistance (HOMA-IR) [14]. Finally, using computer tomography (CT) [15], we confirmed whether or not visceral fat area (VFA) greater than 100 cm^2 corresponds to a WC of 85 cm in men and 90 cm in women, respectively.

2. Materials and Methods

2.1. Study Design and the Subjects

The present study was cross-sectional observational study conducted in our hospital. The protocol was approved by the Tokushukai Group Institutional Review Board (TGE1897-024) and adhered to the tenets of Declaration of Helsinki. The potential subjects comprised 162 patients who were on maintenance HD therapy in dialysis center in our hospital in December 2005. The end date of patient recruitment was 31 December 2005. Patients aged 20 years old or more were enrolled, and there was no upper restriction in age for study entry. Patients with insulin treatment were essentially excluded in this study. Data were collected from maintenance HD patients in December 2005 unless they had acute illness (9 patients) or post-operative conditions (4 patients) within 3 months prior to this study. The patients within 3 months of the initiation of HD (8 patients) were also excluded. The patients visited to our hospital for a 1-day annual check of complications.

The study comprised 141 HD patients (97 men, 44 women). These patients recruited in the present study corresponded to 90% (141/162 patients) of all patients in our hospital and had been treated by regular dialysis for more than 3 months.

2.2. Blood Sampling, WC, and VFA

Blood was drawn in the morning after an overnight fast of at least 12 h on non-dialysis day in the middle of week. EDTA-plasma was used for glucose, insulin, and lipids, and serum for other biochemical assays. Glucose was measured by a glucose oxidase method. Insulin was measured by radioimmunoassay (Insulin RIA-BEAD II: Dinabot Co., Tokyo, Japan). Total cholesterol (TC) and triglycerides (TG) were measured enzymatically. HDL cholesterol was measured after precipitating apolipoprotein B-containing lipoproteins with dextran sulfate and magnesium chloride. High-sensitive C-reactive protein (hsCRP) was measured using a nephelometric immunoassay. WCs of the patients were also measured at a standing position. Finally, 92 patients in men and 20 patients in women who agreed to undergo CT examination received CT examination for measuring VFA, respectively.

2.3. Assessment of Insulin Resistance Using HOMA-IR

Insulin resistance was assessed using HOMA-IR originally described by Mathew et al. [14]. HOMA-IR was calculated using the following formula: HOMA-IR = fasting glucose (mmol/L) × fasting insulin (μU/mL)/22.5.

2.4. BMI and Measurement of VFA Using CT

BMI was calculated as the weight in kilograms divided by the height in meters squared. The amount of abdominal and visceral fat deposition was assessed by CT. The area of the subcutaneous fat and visceral fat was measured in a single cross-sectional scan at the level of the umbilicus. An image histogram was computed for the subcutaneous fat layers in order to determine the range of CT numbers for the fat tissue. The total fat area was then calculated by counting the pixels that had intensities within the selected range of CT numbers. The intraperitoneal space was defined by tracing its contour on the scan image. The total area with the same CT numbers was considered to represent VFA [15].

2.5. Mets Criteria

The ATP III [2] report defines Mets as a constellation of risk factors of metabolic origin including increased abdominal obesity, high triglyceride, low HDL cholesterol, elevated blood pressure, and elevated fasting blood glucose. Elevated blood pressure was defined as systolic or diastolic blood pressure of 130/85 mmHg or higher; low HDL cholesterol level was defined as less than 40 mg/dL; high serum TG levels were defined as 150 mg/dL or more; and elevated fasting glucose level was defined as 110 mg/dL or more. Finally, WC of 85 cm or more in men and 90 cm or more in women was defined as abdominal obesity in Japan as modified NCEP criteria [7].

2.6. Measurement of Blood Pressure

Blood pressure (BP) was measured with a standard mercury sphygmomanometer and cuffs adapted to arm circumferences after the patients had rested in the supine position for at least 5 min prior to HD on the first HD session of a week. Hypertension was also defined as the use of one or more antihypertensive drugs.

2.7. Statistical Analysis

Continuous variables were expressed as mean ± standard deviation (SD) when normally distributed or as median (interquartile range [IQR]) when non-normally distributed. Skewed variables underwent log transformation before statistical analysis. The prevalence of Mets and its individual components (elevated BP level, high plasma glucose level, high triglyceride level, low HDL cholesterol level, and abdominal obesity), as well as the number of Mets components (0, 1, 2, 3, 4, or 5), was determined for the overall study sample. Univariate or multivariate logistic regression analysis was also applied for the determinants of Mets. A *p*-value of less than 0.05 was considered statistically significant. These were analyzed using statistical software (StatView 5; SAS Institute Inc., Carry, NC, USA) for Windows personal computer.

3. Results

The mean age was 67 years, with a range of 34–89 years. Table 1 summarizes the baseline characteristics of the subjects. Body weight, body height, rate of current smoker, rate of diabetes mellitus, TC, and HDL-C were significantly different between men and women, as shown in Table 1.

Table 1. Baseline characteristics of the patients.

	All	Men	Women	P
				(Men vs. Women)
N	141	97	44	
Age (years)	67 ± 11.8	68 ± 10.7	67 ± 12	0.974
HD vintage (months)	83 ± 69	75 ± 62	99 ± 79	0.053
Body height (cm)	161 ± 9.0	165 ± 6.9	153 ± 6.9	<0.001
Body weight (kg)	55.0 ± 10.9	58.2 ± 10.0	48.0 ± 9.4	<0.001
WC (cm)	83.9 ± 9.0	84.7 ± 8.7	82.3 ± 9.7	0.143
BMI (kg/m^2)	21.1 ± 3.4	21.3 ± 3.2	20.5 ± 3.8	0.235
Current smoker, n	35	29	6	0.038
Diabetes mellitus (%)	49.6	55.7	36.4	0.034
TC (mg/dL)	152 ± 34	149 ± 33	162 ± 36	0.043
HDL-C (mg/dL)	47 ± 15	44 ± 14	51 ± 17	0.032
LDL-C (mg/dL)	76 ± 25	75 ± 24	78 ± 25	0.666
TG (mg/dL)	97 ± 69	94 ± 77	101 ± 47	0.585
FBS (mg/dL)	97 ± 33	100 ± 38	89 ± 21	0.072
Insulin (μU/mL)	7.3 ± 11.9	6.3 ± 5.3	9.5 ± 19.3	0.151
HOMA-IR	0.927 (0.593–1.906)	0.921 (0.590–1.991)	0.924 (0.593–1.772)	0.328
Serum albumin (g/dL)	3.67 ± 0.35	3.71 ± 0.33	3.60 ± 0.37	0.251
Systolic BP (mmHg)	143 ± 24	144 ± 25	142 ± 21	0.371
Diastolic BP (mmHg)	77 ± 13	77 ± 13	74 ± 14	0.104

Abbreviations: HD hemodialysis, WC waist circumference, BMI body mass index (kg/m^2), TC total cholesterol, HDL-C high-density lipoprotein cholesterol, LDL-C low-density lipoprotein cholesterol, TG triglyceride, FBS fasting blood glucose, HOMA-IR Homeostasis Model Assessment of Insulin resistance, BP blood pressure.

The prevalence of Mets was 31.9% in men, 13.6% in women, and 26.2% in total according to the modified criteria of NCEP using a definition of a WC of 85 cm or more in men and 90 cm or more in women. The prevalence of HD patients with each Mets component in men and women was shown in Table 2. The prevalence of a WC of 85 cm or more in men and 90 cm or more in women was 53.6% and 25%, respectively. The number of Mets components present in men was 3.8% with no Mets risk factors, 36.5% with one, 44.2% with two, 7.7% with three, and 7.7% with four. The number of Mets components present in women was 0% in no Mets risk factors, 45.4% with one, 54.5% with two, and 0% with three and/or four.

Table 2. Prevalence of Mets component in HD patients.

	Men	Women
Waist ≥ 85 cm, n (%)	52 (53.6)	
Waist ≥ 90 cm, n (%)		11 (25.0)
HDL < 40 mg/dL, n (%)	41 (42.3)	13 (29.5)
TG ≥ 150 mg/dL, n (%)	11 (11.3)	7 (15.9)
FBS ≥ 110 mg/dL, n (%)	23 (23.7)	7 (15.9)
HTN ≥ 130/85 mmHg, n (%)	80 (82.5)	38 (86.4)

Abbreviations: Mets metabolic syndrome, HDL high-density lipoprotein, TG triglyceride, FBS fasting blood glucose, HTN hypertension.

The VFA measured by CT showed a strong positive correlation with WC in both men ($R^2 = 0.390$, $p < 0.0001$) and women ($R^2 = 0.472$, $p < 0.0001$) as shown in Figure 1. In Japanese HD patients, 100 cm^2 of VFA corresponded to a WC of 85 cm in men and 90 cm in women, thus confirming the validity of the modified criteria.

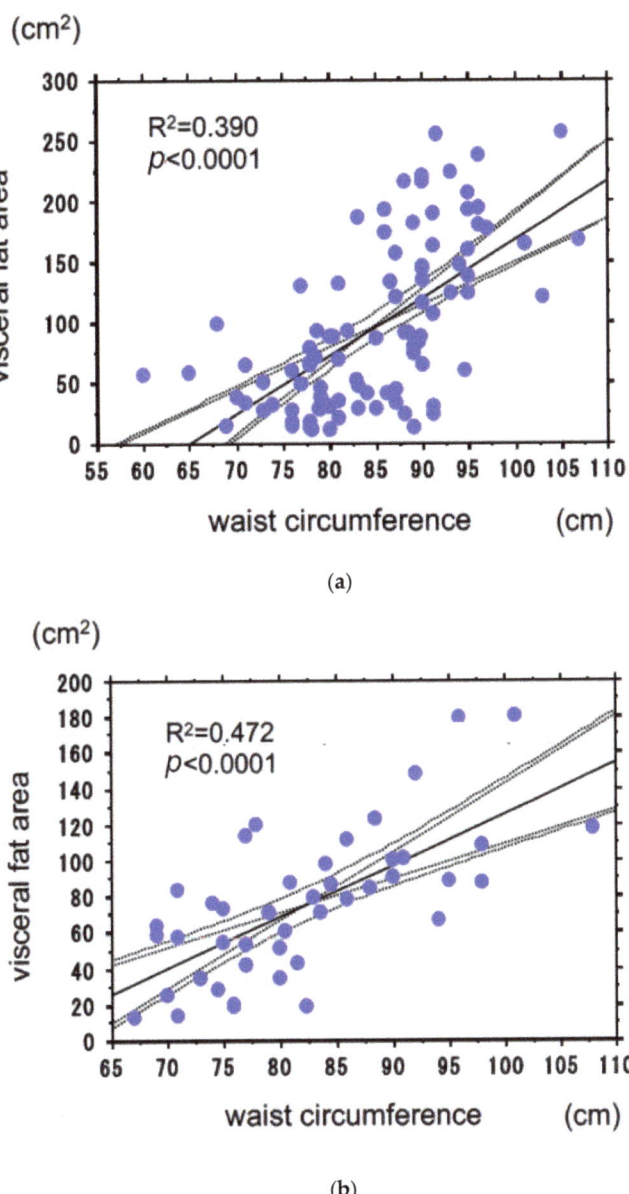

Figure 1. The relationship between visceral fat area and waist circumferences in men (**a**), the relationship between visceral fat area and waist circumferences in women. (**b**). Abbreviations: VFA visceral fat area, WC waist circumference.

HOMA-IR showed a skewed distribution with a median of 0.922, and 20% of the patients had the value greater than 2.0 of HOMA-IR.

The patients with Mets, comparing with those without Mets, had significantly greater WC, shorter duration of HD, greater BMI, higher hsCRP, higher HOMA-IR, higher FBS, and higher TG, as shown in Table 3. In patients undergoing HD for more than 10 years, the prevalence of Mets became 10% (3 patients/30 patients) (data not shown).

Table 3. Characteristics of the patients with or without Mets.

	Mets+	Mets−	p-Value
Number of patients, n (%)	37 (26.2)	104 (73.8)	
Sex (Male/Female)	31:6	66:38	<0.05
Age (years)	67.3 ± 9.2	68.2 ± 11.9	NS
WC (cm)	92.3 ± 5.9	80.9 ± 8.1	<0.0001
HD duration (months)	54.5 ± 39.8	92.5 ± 73.8	<0.005
BMI (kg/m^2)	23.4 ± 3.2	20.2 ± 3.1	<0.0001
Serum albumin (g/dL)	3.65 ± 0.37	3.68 ± 0.34	NS
HOMA-IR	1.818 (0.818–2.818)	0.788 (0.332–1.244)	<0.0001
hsCRP (mg/dL)	0.208 (0.001–0.700)	0.083 (0.001–0.245)	<0.05
TC (mg/dL)	151 ± 37	153 ± 33	NS
HDL-C (mg/dL)	37 ± 10	49 ± 15	NS
LDL-C (mg/dL)	79 ± 27	75 ± 24	NS
TG (mg/dL)	136 ± 109	83 ± 39	0.0001
FBS (mg/dL)	109 ± 14	93 ± 27	0.005
Systolic BP (mmHg)	148 ± 23	143 ± 24	NS
Diastolic BP (mmHg)	75 ± 14	77 ± 13	NS

Abbreviations: WC waist circumference, HD hemodialysis, BMI body mass index, HOMA-IR Homeostasis Model Assessment of Insulin resistance, hsCRP high-sensitive C-reactive protein, TC total cholesterol, HDL-C high-density lipoprotein cholesterol, LDL-C low-density lipoprotein cholesterol, TG triglyceride, FBS fasting blood glucose, BP blood pressure.

In all patients, a significant negative correlation between serum albumin and hsCRP (R^2 = 0.101, $p < 0.001$), and a negative weak correlation between the duration of HD and HOMA-IR (R^2 = 0.032, $p < 0.05$) were found [Figure 2]. On the contrary, the prevalence of serum albumin levels less than 3.7 g/dL was 45.2% in men and 70.5% in women, respectively. The prevalence of the patients with BMI less than 18.5 was 17.5% in men, and 27.3% in women, respectively. The prevalence of patients with a BMI greater than 25 in all HD patients was only 11.2%.

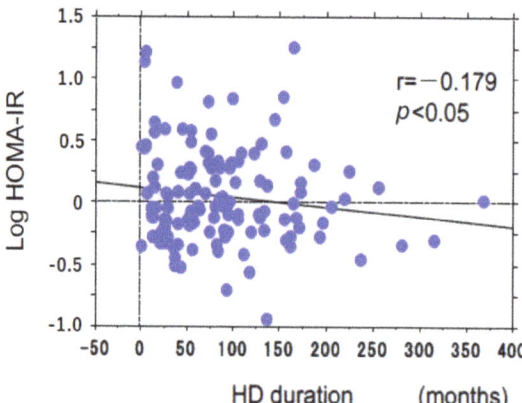

Figure 2. The relationship between HOMA-IR and HD duration (months) ($p < 0.05$, r = −0.179). Abbreviations: HOMA-IR Homeostasis Model Assessment of Insulin resistance, HD hemodialysis.

Regarding the correlation between HOMA-IR and serum albumin levels, there was a significant negative correlation only in patients with Mets (R^2 = 0.349, $p < 0.001$), while in patients without Mets, there was no significant correlation (R^2 < 0.001, p = 0.957) (Figure 3). In a study of univariate regression analysis associated with HOMA-IR, only serum albumin level was chosen as a significant determinant [Table 4] in patients with Mets, while other parameters, including age, HD duration, WC, BMI, hsCRP, TC, TG, and HDL cholesterol, did not show any significant correlation.

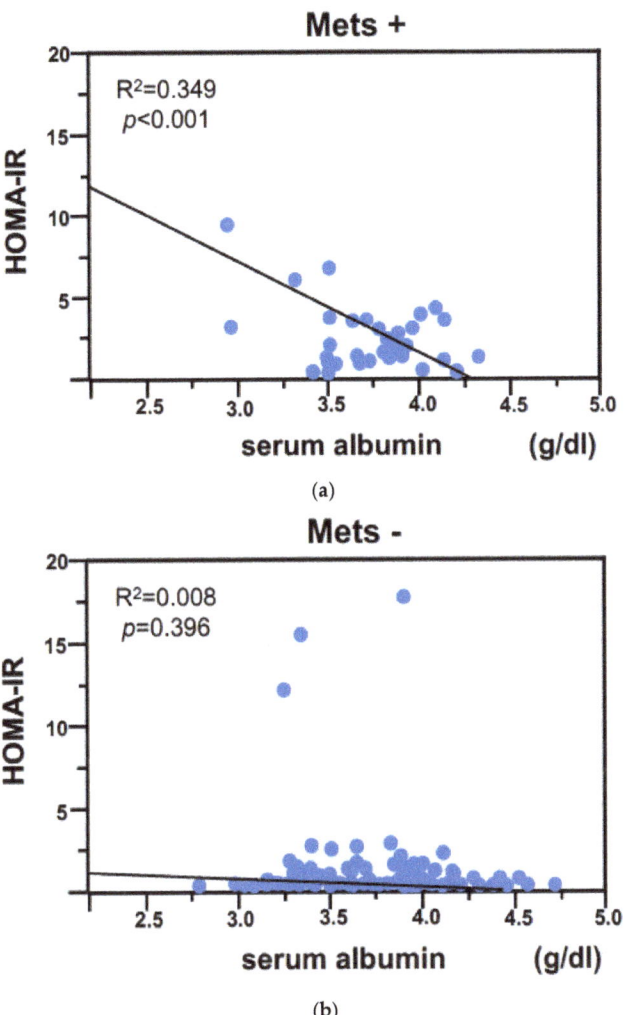

Figure 3. The relationship between HOMA-IR and serum albumin in patients with Mets (**a**) and relationship between HOMA-IR and serum albumin in patients without Mets (**b**).

Table 4. Univariate regression analysis associated with HOMA-IR.

	R	p-Value
Age (years)	0.150	0.414
HD duration (months)	0.120	0.513
Serum albumin (g/dL)	−0.401	0.023
hsCRP (mg/dL)	0.121	0.509
WC (cm)	0.077	0.678
BMI (kg/m^2)	0.046	0.803
TC (mg/dL)	0.158	0.393
LDL-C (mg/dL)	0.208	0.393
TG (mg/dL)	0.056	0.756
Systolic BP (mmHg)	−0.315	0.078
Diastolic BP (mmHg)	−0.333	0.063

Abbreviations: HOMA-IR Homeostasis Model Assessment of Insulin Resistance, HD hemodialysis, hsCRP high-sensitive C-reactive protein, WC waist circumference, BMI body mass index, LDL-C low-density lipoprotein cholesterol, TG triglyceride, BP blood pressure.

The results of multivariate logistic regression analysis on the determinants of Mets, when factors other than the modified NCEP criteria were entered, demonstrated that HOMA-IR, as well as short duration of HD, BMI, and sex (men vs. women), were chosen as independent risk factors [Table 5].

Table 5. Univariate and multivariate logistic regression analysis on the determinants of Mets, when factors other than the modified NCEP criteria were entered.

	Multivariate			Univariate	
	OR (95% CI)	p-Value		OR (95% CI)	p-Value
Sex, vs. women	7.226 (1.618–32.264)	<0.01		2.975 (1.138–7.777)	<0.01
Age (years)	0.980 (0.930–1.033)	NS		0.992 (0.966–1.026)	NS
BMI (kg/m^2)	1.344 (1.130–1.598)	<0.001		1.362 (1.187–1.562)	<0.0001
LDL-C (mg/dL)	1.001 (0.981–1.021)	NS		1.007 (0.992–1.022)	NS
Serum albumin (g/dL)	0.352 (0.042–2.983)	NS		0.806 (0.272–2.384)	NS
HD duration (months)	0.986 (0.976–0.997)	<0.05		0.989 (0.981–0.997)	<0.01
log HOMA-IR	5.230 (1.286–21.280)	<0.05		6.164 (2.025–18.759)	<0.01
log hsCRP	1.250 (0.526–2.970)	NS		2.109 (1.103–4.034)	<0.05

Abbreviations: BMI body mass index, LDL-C low-density lipoprotein cholesterol, HD hemodialysis, HOMA-IR Homeostasis Model Assessment of Insulin Resistance, hsCRP high-sensitive C-reactive protein.

4. Discussions

Mets is known as a cause of end-stage renal disease (ESRD) and CVD. It is reasonable to find high prevalence of Mets in HD patients [16,17]. However, the results are of interest due to the potentially conflicting nature of malnutrition and Mets in dialysis patients. In HD patients, whether Mets-related risk factors depend on visceral adiposity or uremia per se remains unknown. Although the present study does not provide a clear answer for this, we demonstrated that Mets was more prevalent in HD patients as well as in non-dialysis general populations, despite the prevalence of patients with a BMI over than 25 being only 11.2%. Mets tends to become less prevalent with the duration of HD. In patients with Mets, however, the higher the degree of malnutrition developing, the greater the proportion of patients who have insulin resistance with inflammation. Therefore, abdominal obesity may also play an important role in atherosclerosis as well as malnutrition in HD patients. In contrast to the general population, obesity is associated with improved survival [18] and decreased hospitalization rate [18] among patients with ESRD. In addition, the association between obesity and improved prognosis remained significant even after adjustment for serum albumin [18]. It may be hypothesized that a higher level of adiposity may provide a survival advantage for patients with ESRD.

Regarding the report on the prevalence of Mets in HD patients, Young et al. showed that Mets is highly prevalent in incident dialysis [8]. However, the patients were studied at the initiation of dialysis therapy in contrast to our report dealing with maintenance HD patients. Moreover, fasting blood samples were not used for evaluating each metabolic component and BMI was used instead of WC. In this regard, our study is the first report showing the precise prevalence of Mets in maintenance HD patients.

There are accumulating data that (visceral) abdominal obesity and attendant risk factors are associated with increased risk for CVD [16,19]. In a prospective study (Quebec Cardiovascular Study) in which more than 2000 middle-aged men were followed over 5 years, two clinical characteristics associated with visceral obesity were the strongest independent risk factors for ischemic heart disease: fasting hyperinsulinemia and increased apolipoprotein B concentrations [20]. Abdominal obesity is often accompanied by insulin resistance and hyperinsulinemia [9]. This hyperinsulinemia may, in turn, contribute to increased CVD and stroke. Insulin resistance in HD patients has been reported to be an independent predictor of CVD and mortality [13]. In the present study, the distribution of HOMA-IR was similar to that report [13], which means that insulin resistance still remains after the initiation of RRT. However, it appears that the prevalence of insulin resistance becomes less with the duration of HD.

Serum albumin level itself was not a determinant of Mets in HD patients. However, there was a significant correlation between serum albumin levels and insulin resistance in patients with Mets, whereas the association was not seen in patients without Mets. Therefore, the significance of serum albumin is thought not to be a determinant of Mets, but rather an important component in the pathophysiology of Mets in HD patients. In the patients with Mets, hypoalbuminemia is associated with increased HOMA-IR. Comparing patients without Mets, the patients with Mets have significantly higher hsCRP levels. Therefore, in prevalent HD patients, insulin resistance may play an important role for atherosclerosis through the interaction between malnutrition and inflammation. In patients with Mets, the higher the degree of malnutrition developing, the greater the proportion of patients who have insulin resistance with inflammation. In this regard, it is reported that TNF-α could play a role in the development of insulin resistance in humans, both in muscle and in vascular tissue [21]. Sustained low-grade inflammation could be one factor that explains why CKD and CVD often develop simultaneously. It is well known that insulin resistance is associated with endothelial dysfunction [22], which underlies atherosclerotic CVD. HOMA-IR showed a negative correlation with HD duration in our study. However, because it was a weak correlation, the result should be interpreted with caution. Further study might be necessary to confirm the relationship between HOMA-IR and HD duration.

Mets has been exposed to vigorous critique [23], while others are arguing that Mets is of great value [24]. Moreover, a role of Mets remains unclear in maintenance HD patients. Our study may provide a clue to consider Mets as well as malnutrition and its related atherosclerosis through insulin resistance.

There are several limitations to the current study. The present study is a cross-sectional and observational study in a single hospital. However, we do not want to obtain any causality between Mets and cardiovascular events. Second, we evaluated Mets according to the modified NCEP criteria, because in Japan these criteria were authorized by the Japanese Society of Internal Medicine in 2005 by changing the definition of WC. Tanaka and Iseki et al. have already reported the relationship between the Mets and CKD [7] using these modified criteria. The relationship between NCEP criteria and modified criteria is well documented in their report. Indeed, the prevalence of Mets was 12.4% when NCEP criteria was used, while the prevalence increased up to 21.2% when modified criteria was used with a similar rate reported in the USA [6]. The discrepancy might be related to the difference in the prevalence and degree of obesity between the two countries [25]. Evaluation of nutritional status including prealbumin, muscle consumption, upper arm muscle circumference, and comprehensive score was not evaluated in this study. Therefore, full assessment of nutritional status was not performed. However, the objective of the present study was to reveal a relationship between malnutrition and atherosclerosis in terms of metabolic syndrome, which is known to be an independent risk factor for cardiovascular disorders. In order to discuss this issue, we focused on serum albumin levels being an important nutritional factor. It is no doubt that serum albumin, although affected by inflammation, plays an important role as one of many nutritional markers. Future study is necessary to clarify the association between nutritional status by precise nutritional assessment and Mets in patients undergoing HD. Finally, regarding a difference between % of males versus females in the present study, in an overview of regular dialysis treatment in Japan as of 31 December 2009 reported by the Japanese Society for Dialysis Therapy, there are, in Japan, 173,391 men versus 106,722 women in regular dialysis treatment, a ratio (Men/Women) of 1.72, which clearly shows a predominance of men over women, with a similarity to our study (men 97/women 44). Despite the limitations described above, we believe that the data obtained from this study provide evidence of an important issue considering nutritional status and abdominal obesity in maintenance HD patients.

In conclusion, we demonstrate that Mets is more prevalent in HD patients. Mets tends to become less prevalent with the duration of HD and the development of malnutrition. In Japanese HD patients, 100 cm^2 of VFA corresponded to a WC of 85 cm in men and 90 cm in women, thus confirming the validity of the modified criteria. HOMA-IR and serum albumin were significantly correlated in HD patients with Mets, not in those without Mets. Malnutrition and insulin resistance may interact with metabolic syndrome in patients with prevalent HD.

Author Contributions: Conceptualization, S.K.; methodology, S.K.; investigation, S.K., Y.M., K.I., M.O., K.M., H.M., S.H. and T.O.; writing and editing, T.O. and S.K. All authors have read and agreed to the published version of the manuscript.

Funding: This study received no external funding.

Institutional Review Board Statement: This study was reviewed and approved by the Tokushukai Groups Ethics Committee (approval number TGE01897-024).

Informed Consent Statement: This study was a retrospective observational study. Ethical committee approved this study and the method of consent acquisition (TGE01897-024). Consent was obtained by opt out method. There were no patients who expressed to opt out of the study.

Data Availability Statement: The datasets used and/or analyzed during the current study are available from the corresponding author on reasonable request.

Conflicts of Interest: The authors declare no conflict of interest.

References

1. Stenvinkel, P.; Heimburger, O.; Paulter, F.; Diczfalusy, U.; Wang, T.; Berglund, L.; Jogestrand, T. Strong associations between malnutrition, inflammation and atherosclerosis in chronic renal failure. *Kidney Int.* **1999**, *55*, 1899–1911. [CrossRef] [PubMed]
2. National Cholesterol Education Program. Executive Summary of the Third report of National Cholesterol Education Program (NCEP) Expert Panel on Detection, Evaluation, and Treatment of High Blood Cholesterol in Adults (Adults Treatment Panel III). *JAMA* **2001**, *285*, 2486–2497. [CrossRef] [PubMed]
3. Lakka, H.M.; Laaksonen, D.E.; Lakka, T.A.; Niskanen, L.K.; Kumpusualo, E.; Tuomilehto, J.; Salonen, J. The metabolic syndrome and total and cardiovascular disease mortality in middle-aged men. *JAMA* **2002**, *288*, 2709–2716. [CrossRef]
4. Haffner, S.M.; Valdez, R.A.; Hazuda, H.P.; Mitchell, B.D.; Morales, P.A.; Stern, M.P. Prospective analysis of the insulin-resistance syndrome (syndrome X). *Diabetes* **1992**, *41*, 715–722. [CrossRef]
5. Isomaa, B.; Almgren, P.; Tuomi, T.; Forsen, B.; Lahti, K.; Nissen, M.; Taskinen, M.R.; Groop, L. Cardiovascular morbidity and mortality associated with the metabolic syndrome. *Diabetes Care* **2001**, *24*, 683–689. [CrossRef] [PubMed]
6. Chen, J.; Muntner, P.; Hamm, L.L.; Jones, D.W.; Batuman, V.; Fonseca, V.; Whelton, P.K.; He, J. The metabolic syndrome and chronic kidney disease in U.S. adults. *Ann. Intern. Med.* **2004**, *140*, 167–174. [CrossRef]
7. Tanaka, H.; Shiohira, Y.; Uezu, Y.; Higa, A.; Iseki, K. Metabolic syndrome and chronic kidney disease in Okinawa, Japan. *Kidney Int.* **2006**, *69*, 369–374. [CrossRef]
8. Young, D.O.; Lund, R.J.; Haynatzki, G.; Dunlay, R.W. Prevalence of the metabolic syndrome in an incident dialysis population. *Hemodial. Int.* **2007**, *11*, 86–95. [CrossRef]
9. McFarlane, S.I.; Banerji, M.; Sowers, J.R. Insulin resistance and cardiovascular disease. *J. Clin. Endcrinol. Metab.* **2001**, *86*, 713–718. [CrossRef]
10. Chen, J.; Muntner, P.; Hamm, L.L.; Fonseca, V.; Batuman, V.; Whelton, P.K.; He, J. Insulin resistance and risk of chronic kidney disease in nondiabetic US adults. *J. Am. Soc. Nephrol.* **2003**, *14*, 469–477. [CrossRef]
11. Kobayashi, S.; Maesato, K.; Moriya, H.; Ohtake, T.; Ikeda, T. Insulin resistance in patients with chronic kidney disease. *Am. J. Kidney Dis.* **2004**, *45*, 275–280. [CrossRef] [PubMed]
12. Kobayashi, S.; Maejima, S.; Ikeda, T.; Nagase, M. Impact of dialysis therapy on insulin resistance in end-stage renal disease: Comparison of hemodialysis and continuous ambulatory peritoneal dialysis. *Nephrol. Dial. Transpl.* **2000**, *15*, 65–70. [CrossRef] [PubMed]
13. Shinohara, K.; Shoji, T.; Emoto, M.; Tahara, H.; Koyama, H.; Ishimura, E.; Miki, T.; Tabata, T.; Nishizawa, Y. Insulin resistance as an independent predictor of cardiovascular mortality in patients with end-stage renal disease. *J. Am. Soc. Nephrol.* **2002**, *13*, 1894–1900. [CrossRef] [PubMed]
14. Matthews, D.R.; Hosker, J.P.; Rudenski, A.S.; Naylor, B.A.; Treacher, D.F.; Turner, R.C. Homeostasis model assessment: Insulin resistance and beta-cell function from fasting plasma glucose and insulin concentrations in man. *Diabetologia* **1985**, *28*, 412–419. [CrossRef]
15. Tokunaga, K.; Matsuzawa, Y.; Ishikawa, K.; Tarui, S. A novel technique for the determination of body fat by computed tomography. *Int. J. Obes.* **1983**, *7*, 437–445.
16. Delautre, A.; Chantrel, F.; Dimitrov, Y.; Klein, A.; Imhoff, O.; Muller, C.; Schauder, N.; Hannedouche, T.; Krummel, T. Metabolic syndrome in haemodialysis patients: Prevalence, determinants and association to cardiovascular outcomes. *BMC Nephrol.* **2020**, *21*, 343. [CrossRef]

17. Alswat, K.A.; Althobaiti, A.; Alsaadi, K.; Alkhaldi, A.S.; Alharthi, M.M.; Abuharba, W.A.; Alzaidi, A.A. Prevalence of metabolic syndrome among the endo-stage renal disease patients on hemodialysis. *J. Clin. Med. Res.* **2017**, *9*, 687–694. [CrossRef]
18. Johansen, K.L.; Young, B.; Kaysen, G.A.; Chertow, G.M. Association of body size with outcomes among patients beginning dialysis. *Am. J. Clin. Nutr.* **2004**, *80*, 324–332. [CrossRef]
19. Okamoto, T.; Morimoto, S.; Ikenoue, T.; Furumatsu, Y.; Ichihara, A. Visceral fat level is an independent risk factor for cardiovascular mortality in hemodialysis patients. *Am. J. Nephrol.* **2014**, *39*, 122–129. [CrossRef]
20. Tchernof, A.; Lamarchi, B.; Prud'omme, A.; Nadeau, A.; Moorjani, S.; Labrie, F.; Lupien, P.J.; Despres, J.P. The dense LDL phenotype: Association with plasma lipoprotein levels, visceral obesity, and hyperinsulinemia in men. *Diabetes Care* **1996**, *19*, 629–637. [CrossRef]
21. Rask-Madsen, C.; Dominguez, H.; Ihlemann, N.; Hermann, T.; Kober, L.; Trop-Pedersen, C. Tumor necrosis factor-α inhibits insulin's stimulating effect on glucose uptake and endothelium-dependent vasodilation in humans. *Circulation* **2003**, *108*, 1815–1821. [CrossRef]
22. Steinberg, H.O.; Chaker, H.; Leaming, R.; Johnson, A.; Brechtel, G.; Baron, A.D. Obesity/insulin resistance is associated with endothelial dysfunction: Implications for the syndrome of insulin resistance. *J. Clin. Investig.* **1996**, *97*, 2601–2610. [CrossRef]
23. Kahn, R.; Buse, J.; Ferrannini, E.; Stern, M. The metabolic syndrome: Time for a critical appraisal: Joint statement from the American Diabetes Association and the European Association for the Study of Diabetes. *Diabetes Care* **2005**, *28*, 2289–2304. [CrossRef] [PubMed]
24. Gotto, A.M., Jr.; Blackburn, G.L.; Dailey, G.E., III; Garber, A.J.; Grundy, S.M.; Sobel, B.E.; Weir, M.R. The metabolic syndrome: A call to action. *Coron Artery Dis.* **2006**, *17*, 77–80. [CrossRef] [PubMed]
25. Iseki, K.; Ikemiya, Y.; Kinjo, K.; Inoue, T.; Iseki, C.; Takishita, S. Body mass index and the risk of development of end-stage renal disease in a second cohort. *Kidney Int.* **2004**, *65*, 1870–1876. [CrossRef] [PubMed]

Disclaimer/Publisher's Note: The statements, opinions and data contained in all publications are solely those of the individual author(s) and contributor(s) and not of MDPI and/or the editor(s). MDPI and/or the editor(s) disclaim responsibility for any injury to people or property resulting from any ideas, methods, instructions or products referred to in the content.

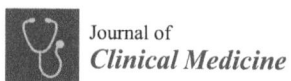

Article

Combined Prognostic Value of Preprocedural Protein–Energy Wasting and Inflammation Status for Amputation and/or Mortality after Lower-Extremity Revascularization in Hemodialysis Patients with Peripheral Arterial Disease

Yoshitaka Kumada [1], Norikazu Kawai [1], Narihiro Ishida [1], Yasuhito Nakamura [1], Hiroshi Takahashi [2], Satoru Ohshima [3], Ryuta Ito [3], Hideo Izawa [2], Toyoaki Murohara [4] and Hideki Ishii [5],*

[1] Department of Cardiovascular Surgery, Matsunami General Hospital, Kasamatsu 501-6062, Japan; ykumada1206@gmail.com (Y.K.); norikazu.kawai@gmail.com (N.K.); alpineskierjp@aol.com (N.I.); o2001070@yahoo.co.jp (Y.N.)
[2] Department of Cardiology, Fujita Health University School of Medicine, Toyoake 470-1192, Japan; hirotaka@fujita-hu.ac.jp (H.T.); izawa@fujita-hu.ac.jp (H.I.)
[3] Department of Cardiology, Nagoya Kyoritsu Hospital, Nagoya 454-0933, Japan; kaku@nagoya-pet.or.jp (S.O.); ryu-i@msi.biglobe.ne.jp (R.I.)
[4] Department of Cardiology, Nagoya University Graduate School of Medicine, Nagoya 466-8550, Japan; murohara@med.nagoya-u.ac.jp
[5] Department of Cardiovascular Medicine, Gunma University Graduate School of Medicine, 3-39-22 Showa-machi, Maebashi 371-8511, Japan
* Correspondence: hkishii@med.nagoya-u.ac.jp; Tel.: +81-27-220-8271; Fax: +81-27-220-8158

Citation: Kumada, Y.; Kawai, N.; Ishida, N.; Nakamura, Y.; Takahashi, H.; Ohshima, S.; Ito, R.; Izawa, H.; Murohara, T.; Ishii, H. Combined Prognostic Value of Preprocedural Protein–Energy Wasting and Inflammation Status for Amputation and/or Mortality after Lower-Extremity Revascularization in Hemodialysis Patients with Peripheral Arterial Disease. *J. Clin. Med.* **2024**, *13*, 126. https://doi.org/10.3390/jcm13010126

Academic Editors: Shuzo Kobayashi, Takayasu Ohtake and Peter Schnuelle

Received: 16 November 2023
Revised: 3 December 2023
Accepted: 20 December 2023
Published: 25 December 2023

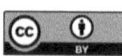

Copyright: © 2023 by the authors. Licensee MDPI, Basel, Switzerland. This article is an open access article distributed under the terms and conditions of the Creative Commons Attribution (CC BY) license (https://creativecommons.org/licenses/by/4.0/).

Abstract: Protein–energy wasting is associated with inflammation and advanced atherosclerosis in hemodialysis patients. We enrolled 800 patients who had undergone successful lower-extremity revascularization, and we investigated the association among the Geriatric Nutritional Risk Index (GNRI) as a surrogate marker of protein–energy wasting, C-reactive protein (CRP), and their joint roles in predicting amputation and mortality. They were divided into lower, middle, and upper tertiles (T1, T2, and T3) according to GNRI and CRP levels, respectively. Regarding the results, the amputation-free survival rates over 8 years were 47.0%, 56.9%, and 69.5% in T1, T2, and T3 of the GNRI and 65.8%, 58.7%, and 33.2% for T1, T2, and T3 of CRP, respectively ($p < 0.0001$ for both). A reduced GNRI [adjusted hazard ratio (aHR) 1.78, 95% confidence interval (CI) 1.24–2.59, $p = 0.0016$ for T1 vs. T3] and elevated CRP (aHR 1.86, 95% CI 1.30–2.70, $p = 0.0007$ for T3 vs. T1) independently predicted amputation and/or mortality. When the two variables were combined, the risk was 3.77-fold higher (95% CI 1.97–7.69, $p < 0.0001$) in patients who occupied both T1 of the GNRI and T3 of CRP than in those who occupied both T3 of the GNRI and T1 of CRP. In conclusion, patients with preprocedurally decreased GNRI and elevated CRP levels frequently experienced amputation and mortality, and a combination of these two variables could more accurately stratify the risk.

Keywords: lower-extremity revascularization; peripheral artery disease; hemodialysis; geriatric nutritional risk index; C-reactive protein

1. Introduction

Recently, the prevalence of chronic kidney disease (CKD) has been significantly increasing [1–3]. Renal impairment is associated with a high incidence of cardiovascular disease [4–6]. Thus, cardio-renal interaction has received attention. In particular, it has been reported that end-stage CKD patients requiring maintenance hemodialysis (HD) therapy are recognized as the highest-risk population for cardiovascular disease, including peripheral artery disease (PAD) [7–9]. Lower-limb revascularization such as bypass surgery or endovascular therapy (EVT) has been commonly performed to treat PAD. However, poorer prognoses, such as higher amputation or mortality rates, remain a major clinical problem in patients with advanced CKD after revascularization, regardless of whether it was bypass surgery [10,11] or EVT [12,13], compared to those without. Unfortunately, the dismal outcomes have not been improved over the last decade despite improvements in the medical management of HD patients over the same period [14–17]. In such a situation, simple risk stratification to predict future outcomes may be clinically important in patients on HD.

On the other hand, nutritional status is one of the key points in patients with CKD. In clinical settings, protein–energy wasting (PEW) [18–20], a state of decreased body protein mass and energy fuel, is commonly seen in patients with CKD [21,22]. PEW can result from a poor diet as well as inflammatory processes [23,24], and inflammatory status itself is associated with higher cardiovascular and all-cause mortality in this population [25,26]. Moreover, we previously reported that the presence of PEW and inflammatory status was independently associated with a reduced ankle–brachial index (ABI) and that patients with these factors had poorer survival rates than those without [27]. Therefore, in this study, we investigated the association of preprocedural Geriatric Nutritional Risk Index (GNRI) values [28,29], which may be a surrogate marker of PEW, and C-reactive protein (CRP) levels with limb amputation and/or mortality after lower-extremity revascularization in patients with CKD undergoing HD.

2. Methods

2.1. Patients

This was a retrospective study. From January 2009 to April 2018, a total of 800 consecutive HD patients who underwent successful lower-extremity revascularization (535 undergoing EVT and 265 undergoing bypass surgery) after the measurement of preprocedural GNRI and CRP levels at Matsunami General Hospital (Kasamatsu, Japan) and Nagoya Kyoritsu Hospital (Nagoya, Japan) were enrolled in this study. Patients with acute limb ischemia were excluded in advance.

Clinical information including patients' characteristics and established risk factors, indications for revascularization, and target lesions for PAD was obtained from medical records. Briefly, in all patients undergoing EVT, iliac and femoropopliteal lesions were expanded with an ordinary balloon at first. A stent was implanted if there was a residual stenosis with a luminal diameter >30% and/or a residual flow-limiting dissection. In contrast, no stent was used in infrapopliteal lesions, even if residual stenosis or dissection was observed after balloon angioplasty. As for bypass surgery, we chose the ipsilateral or contralateral great saphenous vein as the graft. The operation was performed under general anesthesia.

The study was conducted according to the guidelines of the Declaration of Helsinki and approved by the Ethics Committees of Matsunami General Hospital (code: 573) and Nagoya Kyoritsu Hospital (code: K132-02), respectively. The need to obtain written informed consent and provide information regarding how to opt out of this study on the website of each hospital was waived due to the retrospective nature of the study.

2.2. GNRI and CRP Measurements

Blood samples were collected before the day of the procedure to measure serum albumin and CRP levels. We calculated the GNRI from individually obtained serum albumin levels and each patient's height and body weight [30]:

$$\text{GNRI} = [14.89 \times \text{albumin (g/dL)}] + [41.7 \times (\text{body weight/ideal body weight})]$$

The body weight/ideal body weight ratio was set to one when the patient's body weight exceeded the ideal body weight. Ideal body weight was defined as the value calculated from the patient's actual height and a body mass index of 22 [30]. Enrolled patients received HD therapy one day prior to the procedure, and body weight after HD therapy was checked to calculate the GNRI. Serum CRP levels were measured using a latex-enhanced, highly sensitive CRP immunoassay. Then, according to GNRI and CRP levels, enrolled subjects were divided into tertiles, respectively.

2.3. Follow-Up

We routinely followed up the enrolled patients after discharge at 1, 3, and 6 months during the first year. Thereafter, we followed up them at yearly intervals and additionally performed duplex scanning to check for lower-limb ischemia. If we could not conduct a hospital follow-up, the patient was interviewed over the telephone if possible, and the follow-up ended on the day of the last visit if we could not confirm the status of the patient. The follow-up period ended in January 2019. The primary outcome was amputation-free survival (AFS), officially defined as freedom from above-ankle amputation of the index limb or death from any cause [31].

2.4. Statistical Analyses

All statistical analyses were performed using SPSS version 21 (IBM Corp., Armonk, NY, USA).

Normally distributed variables were expressed as the mean ± SD, and asymmetrically distributed data were given as the median and interquartile range. Differences among the groups were evaluated using one-way analysis of variance or the Kruskal–Wallis test for continuous variables and the chi-square test for categorical variables. Using the Kaplan–Meier method, the AFS rates of the groups were expressed. In addition, a log-rank test was used to compare the differences. Hazard ratios (HRs) and 95% confidence intervals (CIs) were calculated for each factor using Cox proportional hazards models. To identify factors independently predicting the outcome, we entered all baseline variables with $p < 0.05$ in a univariable analysis into a multivariate model. To clarify whether the predictability of amputation and/or mortality could improve after the addition of the GNRI alone, CRP alone, and both into a baseline model with established risk factors, the C-index, net reclassification improvement (NRI), and integrated discrimination improvement (IDI) were calculated. The C-index, which is defined as the area under receiver operating characteristic curve between the individual predicted probabilities of the endpoints and the incidence of the endpoints, was compared among all the predictive models [32]. NRI estimates were used to quantify how much better one model predicted the outcome compared to another without the variable of interest [33]. Differences were defined to be statistically significant at a two-sided p value less than 0.05.

3. Results

3.1. Patient Characteristics

Patients were divided into tertiles according to GNRI levels, respectively (tertile 1 (T1): <88.1; T2: 88.1–96.7; T3: >96.7), and CRP levels (T1: <2.0 mg/L; T2: 2.0–12.6 mg/L; T3: >12.6 mg/L) (Figure 1).

The enrolled patients' characteristics are shown in Tables 1 and 2. Those with lower GNRI values had higher CRP levels [11.3 (2.9–44.5) mg/L, 4.0 (1.0–14.0) mg/L, and 3.0 (1.0–12.0) mg/L in T1, T2, and T3, respectively; $p < 0.0001$] and a higher prevalence of ulcer/gangrene (49.6%, 44.6%, and 27.7% in T1, T2, and T3, respectively; $p < 0.0001$). Similarly, those with higher CRP also had lower GNRI values (94.3 ± 9.4, 93.1 ± 9.7, and 89.1 ± 10.1 in T1, T2, and T3, respectively; $p < 0.0001$) and higher prevalence of ulcer/gangrene (23.5%, 34.5%, and 63.9% in T1, T2, and T3, respectively; $p < 0.0001$).

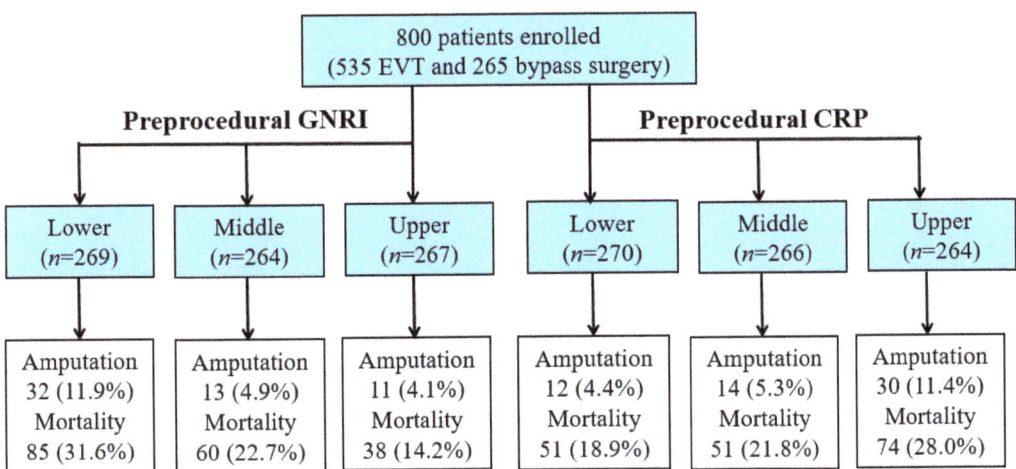

Figure 1. Study design and events.

Table 1. Patient clinical characteristics depending on GNRI levels.

		GNRI			
	All Patients (n = 800)	<88.1 (n = 269)	88.1–96.7 (n = 264)	>96.7 (n = 267)	p Value
Male gender (%)	66.9	62.5	67.4	70.7	0.12
Age (years)	67 ± 10	69 ± 10	67 ± 9	66 ± 10	0.0024
Diabetes (%)	63.3	63.2	64.7	61.8	0.78
Hypertension (%)	62.1	58.0	61.7	66.7	0.12
Dyslipidemia (%)	24.5	18.2	25.8	29.6	0.0076
Smoking (%)	25.7	18.6	31.4	27.2	0.0078
Body mass index (kg/m^2)	21.2 ± 3.3	19.2 ± 2.9	21.0 ± 2.6	23.3 ± 3.0	<0.0001
Coronary artery disease (%)	63.5	58.7	63.9	67.8	0.092
Stroke (%)	16.9	18.6	15.5	16.5	0.63
Indications (%)					<0.0001
Claudication	47.1	36.8	43.9	60.4	
Rest pain	12.3	13.6	11.5	11.9	
Ulcer/gangrene	40.6	49.6	44.6	27.7	
GNRI	92.0 ± 9.8	81.4 ± 5.8	92.3 ± 2.4	102.4 ± 5.3	<0.0001
CRP (mg/L)	5.1 (2.0–20.0)	11.3 (2.9–44.5)	4.0 (1.0–14.0)	3.0 (1.0–12.0)	<0.0001
Preprocedural ABI	0.62 (0.45–0.79)	0.65 (0.41–0.87)	0.57 (0.44–0.79)	0.64 (0.49–0.77)	0.35
Procedure (%)					<0.0001
Bypass surgery	33.1	38.7	39.8	21.0	
Endovascular therapy	66.9	61.3	60.2	79.0	
Number of lesions	825	282	271	272	
Target artery (%)					<0.0001
Iliac	18.1	22.7	17.6	14.3	
Femoropopliteal	62.1	52.8	59.1	72.8	
Below-knee	21.3	24.5	23.3	12.9	

GNRI, Geriatric Nutritional Risk Index; CRP, C-reactive protein; ABI, ankle–brachial index.

Table 2. Patient clinical characteristics depending on serum CRP levels.

	Serum CRP			p Value
	<2.0 mg/L (n = 270)	2.0–12.6 mg/L (n = 266)	>12.6 mg/L (n = 264)	
Male gender (%)	62.6	69.2	68.9	0.19
Age (years)	66 ± 10	67 ± 10	69 ± 10	0.046
Diabetes (%)	60.4	60.9	63.3	0.091
Hypertension (%)	63.7	61.7	61.0	0.80
Dyslipidemia (%)	25.9	24.8	22.7	0.68
Smoking (%)	27.5	24.8	24.9	0.75
Body mass index (kg/m^2)	20.9 ± 3.1	21.2 ± 3.0	21.5 ± 3.7	0.15
Coronary artery disease (%)	63.2	65.0	63.5	0.78
Stroke (%)	18.6	18.4	13.6	0.22
Indications (%)				<0.0001
Claudication	61.9	49.6	29.6	
Rest pain	14.6	15.9	6.5	
Ulcer/gangrene	23.5	34.5	63.9	
GNRI	94.3 ± 9.4	93.1 ± 9.7	89.1 ± 10.1	<0.0001
CRP (mg/L)	1.0 (1.0–2.0)	5.9 (3.9–8.0)	39.5 (20.0–70.0)	<0.0001
Preprocedural ABI	0.65 (0.47–0.79)	0.63 (0.44–0.82)	0.57 (0.43–0.76)	0.23
Procedure (%)				<0.0001
Bypass surgery	22.2	30.5	47.0	
Endovascular therapy	77.8	69.5	53.0	
Number of lesions	274	271	280	
Target artery (%)				<0.0001
Iliac	22.3	18.5	13.6	
Femoropopliteal	69.7	64.6	52.1	
Below-knee	8.0	17.0	34.3	

GNRI, Geriatric Nutritional Risk Index; CRP, C-reactive protein; ABI, ankle–brachial index.

3.2. Predictive Value of the GNRI and CRP

A total of 56 (7.0%) patients required major amputation during the follow-up period (median, 43 months), and 183 (22.9%) patients died. Kaplan-Meier analysis showed that the AFS rates for 8 years were 47.0%, 56.9%, and 69.5% in T1, T2, and T3 of the GNRI and 65.8%, 58.7%, and 33.2% in T1, T2, and T3 of CRP, respectively ($p < 0.0001$ for both) (Figure 2).

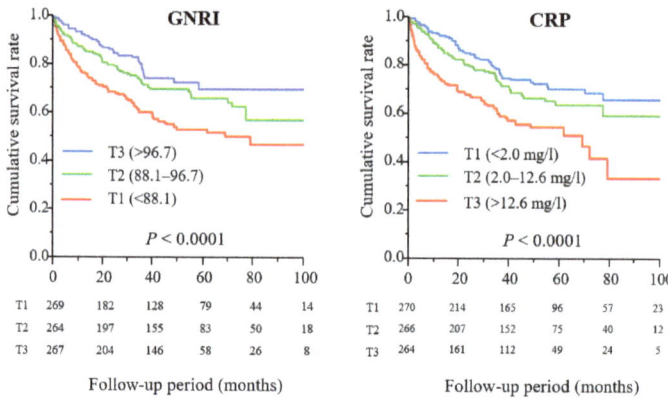

Figure 2. Amputation-free survival rates in tertiles of GNRI (left panel) and CRP (right panel).

After adjustment for male sex, age, previous coronary artery disease, procedure (EVT vs. bypass surgery), below-the-knee artery disease, and ulcer/gangrene as covariates with $p < 0.05$ in a univariate analysis, a decreased GNRI [adjusted HR 1.78, 95% CI 1.24–2.59, $p = 0.0016$ for T1 vs. T3] and elevated CRP (adjusted HR 1.86, 95% CI 1.30–2.70, $p = 0.0007$

for T3 vs. T1) were identified as independent predictors of amputation and/or mortality (Table 3). Similar results were obtained for the amputation and mortality rates.

Table 3. Predictive value of GNRI and CRP for amputation and mortality.

	Non-Adjusted		Adjusted **	
	HR (95% CI)	p Value	HR (95% CI)	p Value
Amputation or death				
GNRI (vs. T3)		<0.0001 *		0.0070 *
T2	1.46 (1.03–2.09)	0.031	1.42 (0.97–2.09)	0.070
T1	2.18 (1.57–3.07)	<0.0001	1.78 (1.24–2.59)	0.0016
CRP (vs. T1)		<0.0001 *		0.0026 *
T2	1.32 (0.93–1.89)	0.11	130 (0.90–1.91)	0.15
T3	2.33 (1.67–3.27)	<0.0001	1.86 (1.30–2.70)	0.0007
Amputation				
GNRI (vs. T3)		<0.0001 *		0.032 *
T2	1.11 (0.78–2.44)	0.79	1.05 (0.46–2.39)	0.89
T1	3.17 (1.70–6.37)	0.0002	2.01 (1.04–4.12)	0.034
CRP (vs. T1)		0.0003 *		0.045 *
T2	1.26 (0.58–2.79)	0.54	1.01 (0.45–2.23)	0.98
T3	3.35 (1.75–6.85)	0.0001	2.02 (1.02–4.25)	0.042
Mortality				
GNRI (vs. T3)		0.0002 *		0.0083 *
T2	1.51 (1.03–2.23)	0.032	1.51 (0.99–2.33)	0.052
T1	2.12 (1.48–3.09)	<0.0001	1.87 (1.25–2.84)	0.0020
CRP (vs. T1)		0.0004 *		0.043 *
T2	1.30 (0.89–1.90)	0.17	1.29 (0.86–1.94)	0.20
T3	2.03 (1.42–2.93)	<0.0001	1.64 (1.11–2.45)	0.012

*: p for trend. **: adjusted for male sex, age, previous coronary artery disease, endovascular therapy (vs. bypass surgery), below-knee artery disease, and ulcer/gangrene as covariates with $p < 0.05$ in a univariate analysis.

3.3. Combined Predictive Value of the GNRI and CRP

The combination of the two variables could stratify the risk of amputation and/or mortality, and the risk was 3.77-fold higher (95% CI 1.97–7.69, $p < 0.0001$) in patients occupying GNRI T1 and CRP T3 than in those occupying GNRI T3 and CRP T1 (Figure 3).

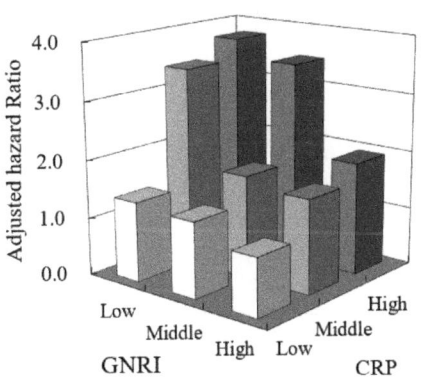

$P < 0.0001$ for trend

The adjusted HR was 3.77 (95% CI 1.97–7.69) for patients with lower GNRI and higher CRP vs. those with higher GNRI and lower CRP.

Figure 3. Adjusted hazard ratio (HR) for amputation and/or mortality in combinations of tertiles of GNRI and CRP.

Similar results were also obtained for amputation and mortality (adjusted HR 3.64, 95% CI 1.32–12.8, $p = 0.0018$ for amputation and adjusted HR 3.68, 95% CI 1.76–8.39, $p < 0.0001$ for mortality for GNRI T1 with CRP T3 vs. GNRI T3 with CRP T1, respectively) (Figure 4).

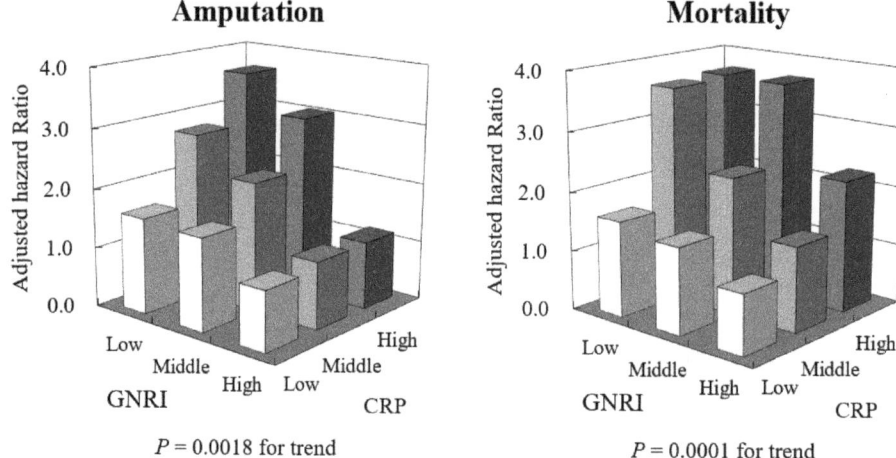

$P = 0.0018$ for trend $P = 0.0001$ for trend

The adjusted HR for patients with lower GNRI and higher CRP vs. those with higher GNRI and lower CRP was 3.64 (95% CI 1.32–12.8) for amputation, and 3.68 (95%CI 1.76–8.39) for mortality.

Figure 4. Adjusted hazard ratio (HR) for amputation (left panel) and mortality (right panel) in combinations of tertiles of GNRI and CRP.

For model discrimination, the addition of both the GNRI and CRP to a predicting model with established risk factors improved the C-index (from 0.661 to 0.716, $p = 0.0021$), NRI (0.508, $p < 0.0001$), and IDI (0.042, $p < 0.0001$). They were even greater than those of either individual variable (NRI 0.145, $p = 0.047$ and IDI 0.006, $p = 0.035$ vs. the GNRI alone and NRI 0.427, $p < 0.0001$ and IDI 0.029, $p < 0.0001$ vs. CRP alone, respectively) (Table 4). The measurement of both PEW and CRP can more accurately stratify risk in hemodialysis patients with PAD who undergo EVT.

Table 4. Discrimination performance of each prediction model for amputation or mortality using the C-index, net reclassification improvement (NRI) and integrated discrimination improvement (IDI).

	C-Index (95% CI)	p Value	NRI	p Value	IDI	p Value
Established risk factors *	0.661	reference		reference		reference
+GNRI	0.710	0.0060	0.456	<0.0001	0.037	<0.0001
+CRP	0.681	0.0034	0.217	0.0063	0.014	0.0001
+GNRI and CRP	0.716	0.0021	0.508	<0.0001	0.042	<0.0001
+GNRI and CRP vs. +GNRI	0.006 **	0.047	0.145	0.047	0.006	0.035
+GNRI and CRP vs. +CRP	0.035 **	0.038	0.427	<0.0001	0.029	<0.0001

*: model includes male sex, age, previous coronary artery disease, endovascular therapy (vs. bypass surgery), below-knee artery disease, and ulcer/gangrene. **: estimated difference.

4. Discussion

Our results clearly demonstrated that a preprocedural decline in the GNRI and an elevated CRP level, which might reflect PEW and chronic inflammation status, resulted in poor AFS after lower-limb revascularization in patients undergoing HD and that the combination of the two variables could more accurately stratify the risk of poor AFS and could provide significantly better predictive performance than either variable alone. Because a simple method for risk stratification in such a high-risk population is attractive, our findings might be of significance in clinical practice.

Numerous studies have reported consistently poorer prognosis after lower-limb revascularization in patients undergoing HD than in the general population in spite of advances in the medical management of HD [10–17]. In previous studies, we reported the following findings: (1) Severe/moderate nutritional risk (GNRI < 92) was higher in patients undergoing HD (53%) than in the elderly general population (21–43%) despite HD patients (average of 64 years) being younger than the elderly general population (80–85 years) [22]. (2) In patients who underwent bypass surgery, preprocedural CRP levels were markedly higher in HD patients than in non-HD patients (median of 11 mg/L vs. 4 mg/L) [34]. (3) Interestingly, preprocedural elevated CRP levels could predict poor AFS only in HD patients and not non-HD patients who underwent infrapopliteal bypass surgery [34]. Thus, our findings in the present study might be reasonably explained, and PEW and chronic inflammation status, a CKD-specific morbidity, might be considered to be one of the causes of poor AFS after lower-limb revascularization in HD population.

In addition, we previously reported that the limb salvage rate after bypass surgery was comparable between HD and non-HD patients when performing propensity score matching with unfavorable factors, including preprocedural CRP levels [35]. This fact suggests the possibility of improved prognosis if inflammation status is adequately managed, even in patients undergoing HD. In this context, the recently developed wound, ischemia, and foot infection (WIfI) scoring system is considered important for assessing the risk of poor AFS [36]. Unfortunately, WIfI scores were not measured in the present study. The association among variables included in WIfI scores and prognosis in such a high-risk population should be clarified in the near future.

The condition of PEW was previously referred to as malnutrition, inflammation, and atherosclerosis (MIA) syndrome before it was officially defined by the International Society of Renal Nutrition and Metabolism (ISRNM) [23,24]. We have previously reported the close association of both a decreased GNRI and elevated CRP with an abnormal ABI [27]. An abnormal ABI also reportedly reflects not only PAD but also systemic atherosclerosis [37,38]; thus, the previous findings might manifest as MIA syndrome. In this context, patients with decreased preprocedural GNRI values and elevated CRP levels were considered to have advanced atherosclerosis and poor prognosis in the present study. Thus, physicians should pay more attention to these unfavorable conditions in those with malnutrition and elevated inflammatory status.

Finally, the addition of both preprocedural GNRI and CRP levels to a predictive model with established risk factors such as age, infrapopliteal disease, and ulcer/gangrene significantly improved the predictability of poor AFS after revascularization to a greater extent than the addition of the GNRI or CRP alone. Thus, measurement of both variables before procedures might be clinically beneficial for predicting prognosis more accurately because these variables are also easily obtained in daily practice.

The present study has several limitations. First, it was a non-randomized, retrospective study. Second, all the study participants were Japanese, a group that reportedly has a lower atherosclerotic risk than patients in the United States and Europe [39]. Third, the study participants were from two centers only. Fourth, once again, we could not assess the WIfI scores. The lack of data regarding wound or infection status in the limbs might be the most important limitation of the study. Last, there were no precise data on medications. These limitations should be considered when interpreting our results.

5. Conclusions

Although lower-extremity revascularization is commonly performed in hemodialysis patients, poor prognosis remains a major problem. In our study, a preprocedural decline in the GNRI and an elevated CRP level, which reflect PEW and chronic inflammation status, are closely associated with poor AFS after lower-limb revascularization in chronic HD patients. Furthermore, the combination of the two variables could not only stratify the risk of amputation and/or mortality but also improve predictive performance when added to established risk factors. Our findings might easily stratify clinical outcomes in HD population at high risk.

Author Contributions: Conceptualization: Y.K., H.T., H.I. (Hideo Izawa), T.M. and H.I. (Hideki Ishii); methodology: Y.K., H.T., H.I. (Hideo Izawa), T.M. and H.I. (Hideki Ishii); software: H.T.; validation: Y.K., H.T., H.I. (Hideo Izawa), T.M. and H.I. (Hideki Ishii); formal analysis: H.T.; investigation: Y.K., N.K., N.I., Y.N., H.T., S.O., R.I., H.I. (Hideo Izawa), T.M. and H.I. (Hideki Ishii); resources: Y.K., N.K., N.I., Y.N., S.O. and R.I.; data curation: Y.K., N.K., N.I., Y.N., S.O. and R.I.; writing—original draft preparation: Y.K., H.T. and H.I. (Hideo Izawa); writing—review and editing: Y.K., N.K., N.I., Y.N., H.T., S.O., R.I., H.I. (Hideo Izawa), T.M. and H.I. (Hideki Ishii); visualization: H.T.; supervision: Y.K., H.T., H.I. (Hideo Izawa), T.M. and H.I. (Hideki Ishii); project administration: Y.K., H.T., H.I. (Hideo Izawa), T.M. and H.I. (Hideki Ishii); funding acquisition: none available. All authors have read and agreed to the published version of the manuscript.

Funding: H. Izawa received grant support through his institution from Bayer, Sumitomo Pharma, PDR Pharma, Biotronik Japan, Abbott Japan, Boston Scientific Japan, Japan Lifeline, and Medtronic Japan and honoraria for lectures from Otsuka, Novartis, Eli Lilly Japan, Bayer, Nippon Boehringer Ingelheim and Daiichi Sankyo. T.M. received lecture fees from Bayer Pharmaceutical Co., Ltd.; Daiichi Sankyo Co., Ltd.; Dainippon Sumitomo Pharma Co., Ltd.; Kowa Co., Ltd.; MSD K.K.; Mitsubishi Tanabe Pharma Co.; Nippon Boehringer Ingelheim Co., Ltd.; Novartis Pharma K.K.; Pfizer Japan Inc.; Sanofi-aventis K.K.; and Takeda Pharmaceutical Co., Ltd. T.M. received unrestricted research grants for the Department of Cardiology, Nagoya University Graduate School of Medicine, from Astellas Pharma Inc.; Daiichi Sankyo Co., Ltd.; Dainippon Sumitomo Pharma Co., Ltd.; Kowa Co., Ltd.; MSD K.K.; Mitsubishi Tanabe Pharma Co.; Nippon Boehringer Ingelheim Co., Ltd.; Novartis Pharma K.K.; Otsuka Pharma Ltd.; Pfizer Japan Inc.; Sanofi-aventis K.K.; Takeda Pharmaceutical Co., Ltd.; and Teijin Pharma Ltd. H. Ishii received lecture fees from Astellas Pharma Inc.; Astrazeneca Inc.; Bayer Pharmaceutical Co., Ltd.; Bristol-Myers Squibb Inc.; Chugai Pharmaceutical Co., Ltd.; Daiichi-Sankyo Pharma Inc.; and MSD K.K.

Institutional Review Board Statement: The study was conducted according to the guidelines of the Declaration of Helsinki and approved by the Ethics Committees of Matsunami General Hospital (code: 573) and Nagoya Kyoritsu Hospital (code: K132-02), respectively.

Informed Consent Statement: The need to obtain written informed consent and provide information regarding how to opt out of this study on the website of each hospital was waived due to the retrospective nature of the study.

Data Availability Statement: The data presented in this study are available on request from the corresponding author.

Acknowledgments: Part of this study was presented at the European Society of Cardiology Congress in 2023.

Conflicts of Interest: The authors declare no conflicts of interest.

References

1. GBD Chronic Kidney Disease Collaboration. Global, regional, and national burden of chronic kidney disease, 1990–2017: A systematic analysis for the Global Burden of Disease Study 2017. *Lancet* **2020**, *395*, 709–733. [CrossRef] [PubMed]
2. GBD 2017 Causes of Death Collaborators. Global, regional, and national age-sex-specific mortality for 282 causes of death in 195 countries and territories, 1980–2017: A systematic analysis for the Global Burden of Disease Study 2017. *Lancet* **2018**, *392*, 1736–1788. [CrossRef] [PubMed]
3. Foreman, K.J.; Marquez, N.; Dolgert, A.; Fukutaki, K.; Fullman, N.; McGaughey, M.; Pletcher, M.A.; Smith, A.E.; Tang, K.; Yuan, C.W.; et al. Forecasting life expectancy, years of life lost, and all-cause and cause-specific mortality for 250 causes of death: Reference and alternative scenarios for 2016—40 for 195 countries and territories. *Lancet* **2018**, *392*, 2052–2090. [CrossRef]
4. Mok, Y.; Ballew, S.H.; Matsushita, K. Prognostic Value of Chronic Kidney Disease Measures in Patients with Cardiac Disease. *Circ. J.* **2017**, *81*, 1075–1084. [CrossRef] [PubMed]
5. Matsushita, K.; Sang, Y.; Chen, J.; Ballew, S.H.; Shlipak, M.; Coresh, J.; Peralta, C.A.; Woodward, M. Novel "Predictor Patch" Method for Adding Predictors Using Estimates from Outside Datasets—A Proof-of-Concept Study Adding Kidney Measures to Cardiovascular Mortality Prediction. *Circ. J.* **2019**, *83*, 1876–1882. [CrossRef] [PubMed]

6. Kai, T.; Oka, S.; Hoshino, K.; Watanabe, K.; Nakamura, J.; Abe, M.; Watanabe, A. Renal Dysfunction as a Predictor of Slow-Flow/No-Reflow Phenomenon and Impaired ST Segment Resolution After Percutaneous Coronary Intervention in ST-Elevation Myocardial Infarction with Initial Thrombolysis in Myocardial Infarction Grade 0. *Circ. J.* **2021**, *85*, 1770–1778. [CrossRef] [PubMed]
7. Sarnak, M.J.; Levey, A.S.; Schoolwerth, A.C.; Coresh, J.; Culleton, B.; Hamm, L.L.; McCullough, P.A.; Kasiske, B.L.; Kelepouris, E.; Klag, M.J.; et al. Kidney disease as a risk factor for development of cardiovascular disease: A statement from the American Heart Association Councils on Kidney in cardiovas-cular Disease, High Blood Pressure Research, Clinical Cardiology, and Epidemiology and Prevention. *Circulation* **2003**, *108*, 2154–2169. [CrossRef] [PubMed]
8. Rajagopalan, S.; Dellegrottaglie, S.; Furniss, A.L.; Gillespie, B.W.; Satayathum, S.; Lameire, N.; Saito, A.; Akiba, T.; Jadoul, M.; Ginsberg, N.; et al. Peripheral arterial disease in patients with end-stage renal disease: Observations from the Dialysis Outcomes and Practice Patterns Study (DOPPS). *Circulation* **2006**, *114*, 1914–1922. [CrossRef]
9. Morooka, H.; Tanaka, A.; Inaguma, D.; Maruyama, S. Peripheral artery disease at the time of dialysis initiation and mortality: A prospective observational multicenter study. *BMJ Open* **2020**, *10*, e042315. [CrossRef]
10. Owens, C.D.; Ho, K.J.; Kim, S.; Schanzer, A.; Lin, J.; Matros, E.; Belkin, M.; Conte, M.S. Refinement of survival prediction in patients undergoing lower extremity bypass surgery: Stratification by chronic kidney disease classification. *J. Vasc. Surg.* **2007**, *45*, 944–952. [CrossRef]
11. Schanzer, A.; Mega, J.; Meadows, J.; Samson, R.H.; Bandyk, D.F.; Conte, M.S. Risk stratification in critical limb ischemia: Derivation and validation of a model to predict amputation-free survival using multicenter surgical outcomes data. *J. Vasc. Surg.* **2008**, *48*, 1464–1471. [CrossRef] [PubMed]
12. Conrad, M.F.; Kang, J.; Cambria, R.P.; Brewster, D.C.; Watkins, M.T.; Kwolek, C.J.; LaMuraglia, G.M. Infrapopliteal balloon angioplasty for the treatment of chronic occlusive disease. *J. Vasc. Surg.* **2009**, *50*, 799–805.e4. [CrossRef] [PubMed]
13. Aulivola, B.; Gargiulo, M.; Bessoni, M.; Rumolo, A.; Stella, A. Infrapopliteal angioplasty for limb salvage in the setting of renal failure: Do results justify its use? *Ann. Vasc. Surg.* **2005**, *19*, 762–768. [CrossRef] [PubMed]
14. Rao, A.; Baldwin, M.; Cornwall, J.; Marin, M.; Faries, P.; Vouyouka, A. Contemporary outcomes of surgical revascularization of the lower extremity in patients on dialysis. *J. Vasc. Surg.* **2017**, *66*, 167–177. [CrossRef] [PubMed]
15. Ambur, V.; Park, P.; Gaughan, J.P.; Golarz, S.; Schmieder, F.; Van Bemmelen, P.; Choi, E.; Dhanisetty, R. The impact of chronic kidney disease on lower extremity bypass outcomes in patients with critical limb ischemia. *J. Vasc. Surg.* **2019**, *69*, 491–496. [CrossRef] [PubMed]
16. Dawson, D.B.; Telles-Garcia, N.A.; Atkins, J.L.; Mina, G.S.; Abreo, A.P.; Virk, C.S.; Dominic, P.S. End-stage renal disease patients un-dergoing angioplasty and bypass for critical limb ischemia have worse outcomes compared to non-ESRD patients: Systematic review and meta-analysis. *Catheter. Cardiovasc. Interv.* **2021**, *98*, 297–307. [CrossRef] [PubMed]
17. Gkremoutis, A.; Bisdas, T.; Torsello, G.; Schmitz-Rixen, T.; Tsilimparis, N.; Stavroulakis, K.; Collaborators, C. Early outcomes of patients with chronic kidney disease after revascularization for critical limb ischemia. *J. Cardiovasc. Surg.* **2021**, *62*, 104–110. [CrossRef]
18. Fouque, D.; Kalantar-Zadeh, K.; Kopple, J.; Cano, N.; Chauveau, P.; Cuppari, L.; Franch, H.; Guarnieri, G.; Ikizler, T.A.; Kaysen, G.; et al. A proposed nomenclature and diagnostic criteria for protein–energy wasting in acute and chronic kidney disease. *Kidney Int.* **2008**, *73*, 391–398. [CrossRef]
19. Ishida, J.; Kato, A. Recent Advances in the Nutritional Screening, Assessment, and Treatment of Japanese Patients on Hemodialysis. *J. Clin. Med.* **2023**, *12*, 2113. [CrossRef]
20. Piccoli, G.B.; Cederholm, T.; Avesani, C.M.; Bakker, S.J.; Bellizzi, V.; Cuerda, C.; Cupisti, A.; Sabatino, A.; Schneider, S.; Torreggiani, M.; et al. Nutritional status and the risk of malnutrition in older adults with chronic kidney disease—implications for low protein intake and nutritional care: A critical review endorsed by ERN-ERA and ESPEN. *Clin. Nutr.* **2023**, *42*, 443–457. [CrossRef]
21. Kopple, J.D. McCollum Award Lecture, 1996, protein-energy malnutrition in maintenance dialysis patients. *Am. J. Clin. Nutr.* **1997**, *65*, 1544–1557. [CrossRef] [PubMed]
22. Takahashi, H.; Ito, Y.; Ishii, H.; Aoyama, T.; Kamoi, D.; Kasuga, H.; Yasuda, K.; Maruyama, S.; Matsuo, S.; Murohara, T.; et al. Geriatric nutritional risk index accurately predicts cardio-vascular mortality in incident hemodialysis patients. *J. Cardiol.* **2014**, *64*, 32–36. [CrossRef] [PubMed]
23. Hanna, R.M.; Ghobry, L.; Wassef, O.; Rhee, C.M.; Kalantar-Zadeh, K. A Practical Approach to Nutrition, Protein-Energy Wasting, Sarcopenia, and Cachexia in Patients with Chronic Kidney Disease. *Blood Purif.* **2020**, *49*, 202–211. [CrossRef] [PubMed]
24. Jankowska, M.; Cobo, G.; Lindholm, B.; Stenvinkel, P. Inflammation and Protein-Energy Wasting in the Uremic Milieu. *Contrib. Nephrol.* **2017**, *191*, 58–71. [PubMed]
25. Cobo, G.; Lindholm, B.; Stenvinkel, P. Chronic inflammation in end-stage renal disease and dialysis. *Nephrol. Dial. Transplant.* **2018**, *33* (Suppl. S3), iii35–iii40. [CrossRef] [PubMed]
26. Takahashi, R.; Ito, Y.; Takahashi, H.; Ishii, H.; Kasuga, H.; Mizuno, M.; Suzuki, Y.; Yuzawa, Y.; Maruyama, S.; Murohara, T.; et al. Combined Values of Serum Albumin, C-Reactive Protein and Body Mass Index at Dialysis Initiation Accurately Predicts Long-Term Mortality. *Am. J. Nephrol.* **2012**, *36*, 136–143. [CrossRef] [PubMed]
27. Ishii, H.; Takahashi, H.; Ito, Y.; Aoyama, T.; Kamoi, D.; Sakakibara, T.; Umemoto, N.; Kumada, Y.; Suzuki, S.; Murohara, T. The Association of Ankle Brachial Index, Protein-Energy Wasting, and Inflammation Status with Cardiovascular Mortality in Patients on Chronic Hemodialysis. *Nutrients* **2017**, *9*, 416. [CrossRef] [PubMed]

28. Bouillanne, O.; Morineau, G.; Dupont, C.; Coulombel, I.; Vincent, J.-P.; Nicolis, I.; Benazeth, S.; Cynober, L.; Aussel, C. Geriatric Nutritional Risk Index: A new index for evaluating at-risk elderly medical patients. *Am. J. Clin. Nutr.* **2005**, *82*, 777–783. [CrossRef]
29. Takahashi, H.; Inoue, K.; Shimizu, K.; Hiraga, K.; Takahashi, E.; Otaki, K.; Yoshikawa, T.; Furuta, K.; Tokunaga, C.; Sakakibara, T.; et al. Comparison of Nutritional Risk Scores for Predicting Mortality in Japanese Chronic Hemodialysis Patients. *J. Ren. Nutr.* **2017**, *27*, 201–206. [CrossRef]
30. Yamada, K.; Furuya, R.; Takita, T.; Maruyama, Y.; Yamaguchi, Y.; Ohkawa, S.; Kumagai, H. Simplified nutritional screening tools for patients on maintenance hemodialysis. *Am. J. Clin. Nutr.* **2008**, *87*, 106–113. [CrossRef]
31. Conte, M.S.; Geraghty, P.J.; Bradbury, A.W.; Hevelone, N.D.; Lipsitz, S.R.; Moneta, G.L.; Nehler, M.R.; Powell, R.J.; Sidawy, A.N. Suggested objective performance goals and clinical trial design for evaluating catheter-based treatment of critical limb ischemia. *J. Vasc. Surg.* **2009**, *50*, 1462–1473. [CrossRef] [PubMed]
32. DeLong, E.R.; DeLong, D.M.; Clarke-Pearson, D.L. Comparing the Areas under Two or More Correlated Receiver Operating Characteristic Curves: A Nonparametric Approach. *Biometrics* **1988**, *44*, 837–845. [CrossRef] [PubMed]
33. Pencina, M.J.; D'Agostino, R.B., Sr.; D'Agostino, R.B., Jr.; Vasan, R.S. Evaluating the added predictive ability of a new marker: From area under the ROC curve to reclassification and beyond. *Stat. Med.* **2008**, *27*, 157–172; discussion 207–212. [CrossRef] [PubMed]
34. Kumada, Y.; Kawai, N.; Ishida, N.; Mori, A.; Ishii, H.; Ohshima, S.; Ito, R.; Umemoto, N.; Takahashi, H.; Murohara, T. Impact of Hemodialysis on Clinical Outcomes in Patients Undergoing Lower Extremity Bypass Surgery for Peripheral Artery Disease—10-year Follow-Up Study. *Angiology* **2022**, *73*, 744–752. [CrossRef] [PubMed]
35. Kumada, Y.; Nogaki, H.; Ishii, H.; Aoyama, T.; Kamoi, D.; Takahashi, H.; Murohara, T. Clinical outcome after infrapopliteal bypass surgery in chronic hemodialysis patients with critical limb ischemia. *J. Vasc. Surg.* **2015**, *61*, 400–404. [CrossRef] [PubMed]
36. Mills, J.L., Sr.; Conte, M.S.; Armstrong, D.G.; Pomposelli, F.B.; Schanzer, A.; Sidawy, A.N.; Andros, G. Society for Vascular Surgery Lower Extremity Guidelines Committee. The Society for Vascular Surgery Lower Extremity Threatened Limb Classification System: Risk stratification based on Wound, Ischemia, and foot Infection (WIfI). *J. Vasc. Surg.* **2014**, *59*, 220–234.e2. [CrossRef] [PubMed]
37. Ono, K.; Tsuchida, A.; Kawai, H.; Matsuo, H.; Wakamatsu, R.; Maezawa, A.; Yano, S.; Kawada, T.; Nojima, Y. Ankle-brachial blood pressure index predicts all-cause and cardiovascular mortality in hemodialysis patients. *J. Am. Soc. Nephrol.* **2003**, *14*, 1591–1598. [CrossRef]
38. Curry, S.J.; Krist, A.H.; Owens, D.K.; Barry, M.J.; Caughey, A.B.; Davidson, K.W.; Doubeni, C.A.; Epling, J.W., Jr.; Kemper, A.R.; Kubik, M.; et al. Screening for Peripheral Artery Disease and Cardiovascular Disease Risk Assessment with the Ankle-Brachial Index: US Preventive Services Task Force Recommendation Statement. US Preventive Services Task Force. *JAMA* **2018**, *320*, 177–183.
39. Sekikawa, A.; Ueshima, H.; Kadowaki, T.; El-Saed, A.; Okamura, T.; Takamiya, T.; Kashiwagi, A.; Edmundowicz, D.; Murata, K.; Sutton-Tyrrell, K.; et al. Less Subclinical Atherosclerosis in Japanese Men in Japan than in White Men in the United States in the Post-World War II Birth Cohort. *Am. J. Epidemiol.* **2007**, *165*, 617–624. [CrossRef]

Disclaimer/Publisher's Note: The statements, opinions and data contained in all publications are solely those of the individual author(s) and contributor(s) and not of MDPI and/or the editor(s). MDPI and/or the editor(s) disclaim responsibility for any injury to people or property resulting from any ideas, methods, instructions or products referred to in the content.

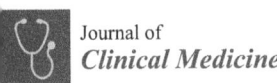

Article

Association of Hyperkalemia and Hypokalemia with Patient Characteristics and Clinical Outcomes in Japanese Hemodialysis (HD) Patients

Masao Iwagami [1,2], Yuka Kanemura [3], Naru Morita [3], Toshitaka Yajima [3,*], Masafumi Fukagawa [4] and Shuzo Kobayashi [5]

1. Department of Health Services Research, Institute of Medicine, University of Tsukuba, Tsukuba 305-8575, Japan
2. Faculty of Epidemiology and Population Health, London School of Hygiene and Tropical Medicine, London WC1E 7HT, UK
3. Cardiovascular, Renal, and Metabolism, Medical Affairs, AstraZeneca K.K., Osaka 530-0011, Japan
4. Division of Nephrology, Endocrinology, and Metabolism, Tokai University School of Medicine, Isehara 259-1193, Japan
5. Kidney Disease and Transplant Center, Shonan Kamakura General Hospital, Kamakura 247-8533, Japan
* Correspondence: toshitaka.yajima@astrazeneca.com; Tel.: +81-6-4802-3600; Fax: +81-3-3457-9301

Abstract: This study aimed to examine the characteristics and clinical outcomes of Japanese hemodialysis patients with dyskalemia. A retrospective study was conducted using a large Japanese hospital group database. Outpatients undergoing thrice-a-week maintenance hemodialysis were stratified into hyperkalemia, hypokalemia, and normokalemia groups based on their pre-dialysis serum potassium (sK) levels during the three-month baseline period. Baseline characteristics of the three groups were described and compared for the following outcomes during follow-up: all-cause mortality, all-cause hospitalization, major adverse cardiovascular events (MACE), cardiac arrest, fatal arrhythmia, and death related to arrhythmia. The study included 2846 eligible patients, of which 67% were men with a mean age of 65.65 (SD: 12.63) years. When compared with the normokalemia group (n = 1624, 57.06%), patients in the hypokalemia group (n = 313, 11.00%) were older and suffered from malnutrition, whereas patients in the hyperkalemia group (n = 909, 31.94%) had longer dialysis vintage. The hazard ratios for all-cause mortality and MACE in the hypokalemia group were 1.47 (95% confidence interval [CI], 1.13–1.92) and 1.48 (95% CI, 1.17–1.86), respectively, whereas that of death related to arrhythmia in the hyperkalemia group was 3.11 (95% CI, 1.03–9.33). Thus, dyskalemia in maintenance hemodialysis patients was associated with adverse outcomes, suggesting the importance of optimized sK levels.

Keywords: dyskalemia; maintenance hemodialysis; hypokalemia; hyperkalemia

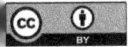

1. Introduction

Despite the rapid progress of dialysis treatments and techniques, patients who are undergoing hemodialysis (HD) still have a poor prognosis. The mortality rate of maintenance dialysis patients in the United States continues to be unacceptably high and was reported at approximately 20% per year in 2020 [1–3]. On the other hand, according to data from the Japanese Society for Dialysis Therapy in 2020, the mortality rate for chronic dialysis patients in Japan is roughly half of that in the US at about 10%. This difference is difficult to explain solely by differences in dialysis methods and techniques, and moreover, even after considering the differences in socioeconomic factors and comorbidities, there are racial/ethnic differences in the mortality of maintenance dialysis patients [4–9].

Recent studies have shown that, compared with serum potassium (sK) levels of 4.6–4.9 mEq/L, sK levels > 5.6 mEq/L involve a higher risk of both all-cause mortality and cardiovascular mortality caused by arrhythmia in end-stage renal disease (ESRD)

patients receiving HD therapy [10–12]. However, prior studies using large HD cohort data revealed that the distribution of sK levels is associated with mortality differently across race/ethnicity in maintenance HD patients [13,14]. According to these reports, higher sK levels at pre-dialysis were associated with higher mortality risk in Caucasian and African-American maintenance HD patients, whereas lower sK levels at pre-dialysis were associated with higher mortality risk in Hispanic patients. Furthermore, the Dialysis Outcomes and Practice Patterns Study (DOPPS) showed that the prevalence and severity of hyperkalemia varied by country [15]. In addition, hyperkalemia excursions over a 4-month period were associated with higher mortality risk in North America and Europe among maintenance HD patients; however, this was not the case in Japan [15]. Therefore, the relationship between the backgrounds and prognosis in patients with dyskalemia on maintenance HD remains to be elucidated in Japan.

To evaluate the impact of dyskalemia on the clinical prognosis of Japanese maintenance HD patients, we designed a comprehensive comparative cohort study, employing a large retrospective multicenter hospital-based database. The aim of this study is to examine the prevalence, incidence, demographics, treatment patterns, comorbidities, nutrition status, and clinical outcomes in Japanese HD patients with hyperkalemia and hypokalemia via comparison to those with normokalemia.

2. Materials and Methods

2.1. Study Design

This is a non-interventional, retrospective, cohort study using electronic health records derived from the Tokushu-kai information system of the Tokushu-kai group hospitals in Japan. Tokushu-kai group is one of the largest medical networks, comprised of 71 hospitals spread across Japan [16–18]. In this study, 63 hospitals among the 71 provided data sets. The overall data set included clinical records of diagnoses, diseases, treatment history, laboratory test results, and all medical procedures including surgery dates and types of examinations.

The study period was from 1 January 2010 to 31 March 2019. The first record of HD was defined as the date of the first HD treatment recorded in the Tokushu-kai information system, as recorded in the data source for each individual patient. The index date was defined as the date three months after the first record of HD for which data were available in the database. The baseline period was defined as the period of three months following the first record of HD for which data were available in the database. For the evaluation of comorbidities, the lookback period was defined as the period of up to 12 months before the first record of HD for which data were available in the database. The follow-up period was from the index date up to the end of the study period or when data from individual patients were no longer available in the claims data set—whichever came first.

2.2. Study Population and Sample Size

All patients with medical records of at least three months and more than one recorded sK level were extracted. The predefined inclusion criteria for the study included male or female patients aged ≥ 18 years at the time of their first HD treatment, patients undergoing maintenance HD three times a week for at least three months, patients with their first HD record, either prevalent or incident HD patients, and patients for whom sK value(s) were available at least once during the baseline period. Patients with less than three dialytic sessions per week were excluded from this study. In addition, we excluded the inpatient group, defined as patients with at least one record of hospitalization during the baseline period because their potassium levels are unlikely to reflect their baseline status due to acute conditions.

The hyperkalemia group (Hyper-K) was defined as patients who had pre-HD sK ≥ 5.1 mmol/L once during the short inter-dialytic interval or pre-HD sK > 5.4 mmol/L once during the long inter-dialytic interval among those who had sK ≥ 5.1 mmol/L twice at any interdialytic interval during the baseline period. Among patients who did not meet the definition of the Hyper-K group, a hypokalemia group (Hypo-K) was defined as patients with sK levels < 3.5 mmol/L at the pre-dialysis stage. A normokalemia group (Normo-K) was defined as patients who met neither the Hyper-K nor the Hypo-K criteria. As shown in Figure 1, patients who met the hyperkalemia criteria were defined as Hyper-K (n = 909). Among the non-Hyper-K group, patients who met the hypokalemia criteria were stratified into Hypo-K (n = 313) and Normo-K (n = 1624). In this study, 20 patients satisfying the criteria of both hyperkalemia and hypokalemia were stratified into the Hyper-K group based on the pre-defined grouping method of this study.

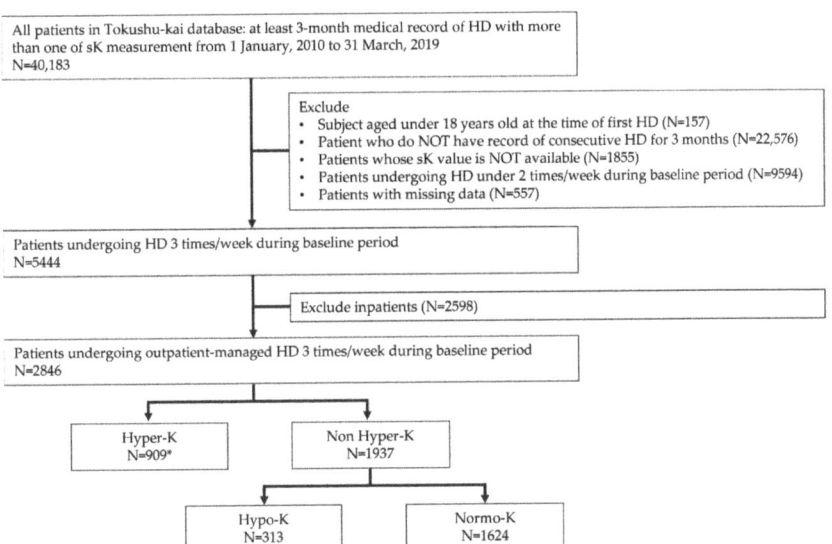

Figure 1. Flow diagram of patient inclusion in the study. Abbreviations: HD—hemodialysis; sK—serum potassium * Hyper-K group includes patients with both hyperkalemia and hypokalemia (n = 20).

2.3. Prevalence of Dyskalemia

The prevalence of hyperkalemia or hypokalemia during the baseline period in patients undergoing maintenance HD was estimated. Hyperkalemia and hypokalemia were collected with the same criteria as the study population definition. For this analysis, patients (n = 20) who had both hyperkalemia and hypokalemia during the baseline period contributed to the calculation of the prevalence of hyperkalemia and hypokalemia, respectively. The prevalence of dyskalemia was stratified into five groups based on dialysis vintage at baseline; the groups were <1 year, $1 \leq$ to <2 years, $2 \leq$ to <5 years, $5 \leq$ to <10 years, and $\geq$10 years.

2.4. Covariate and Outcome Measures

Patient demographics, clinical characteristics, treatment patterns, and laboratory data were measured during the baseline period and comorbidities were evaluated during the lookback period [Table S1].

The clinical outcomes measured during the follow-up period were all-cause mortality, MACE, hospitalization (all-cause), cardiac arrest, fatal arrhythmia defined as ventricular tachycardia, torsade de pointes or ventricular fibrillation, and death related to arrhythmia. Death related to arrhythmia was defined as death within 3 days of a fatal arrhythmia [Table S2].

2.5. Statistical Analyses

The baseline characteristics and treatment of patients were summarized. Differences in the prevalence of dyskalemia among dialysis vintage groups were statistically tested by the chi-square test. The Benjamini–Hochberg Procedure was used to correct for multiple comparisons.

The hazard ratios (HRs) of clinical outcomes were analyzed by the Cox proportional hazard model. Crude and adjusted HRs were calculated. For the adjusted model, the covariates used were age, gender, dialysis vintage, index year, body mass index (BMI), albumin, C-reactive protein (CRP), urea reduction ratio (URR), serum calcium, serum phosphorus (centralized by subtracting the mean), serum phosphorus squared (squared after centralized), hemoglobin, HD treatment time, Charlson Comorbidity Index (CCI), and history of the following comorbidities: heart failure, diabetes, cardiovascular comorbidities, myocardial infarction, other acute ischemic heart diseases, atherosclerotic heart disease of native coronary artery, chronic ischemic heart disease, stroke, unstable angina, and angina pectoris unspecified. For evaluation of clinical events between dyskalemia groups and the Normo-K group, log-rank test was used for all-cause mortality, MACE, and death related to arrhythmia, while the Fina and Gray test was used for hospitalization, cardiac arrest, and fatal arrhythmia. A p-value of <0.05 was considered statistically significant. All data analyses were performed using R version 3.51 (R Foundation, Vienna, Austria).

3. Results

3.1. Prevalence of Dyskalemia

In total, 5444 patient data sets undergoing HD three times a week during the baseline period were extracted from the database; 2846 outpatients were included in the subsequent analysis [Figure 1]. The mean age of the 2846 outpatients was 65.65 (SD:12.63) years, 67% were male, and the median dialysis vintage was 3.07 years (min 0.10, max 37.29) [Table 1].

Table 1. Baseline outpatient characteristics.

Characteristics	Overall	Hyper-K Group	Hypo-K Group	Normo-K Group
	n = 2846	n = 909 (31.94%)	n = 313 (11.00%)	n = 1624 (57.06%)
Age, year (mean ± SD)	65.65 ± 12.63	65.03 ± 11.95	69.37 ± 12.68	65.28 ± 12.87
Male, n (%)	1909 (67.08)	608 (66.89)	194 (61.98)	1107 (68.17)
BMI, kg/m^2 (mean ± SD)	22.4 ± 8.79	22.25 ± 6.68	21.37 ± 3.59	22.65 ± 10.26
Dialysis vintage at baseline, median years (min, max)	3.07 (0.10, 37.29)	4.27 (0.23, 37.29)	1.49 (0.24, 27.09)	2.70 (0.10, 36.94)
2.0 mEq/L potassium dialysate, n (%)	2846 (100.00)	909 (100.00)	313 (100.00)	1624 (100.00)
Kt/V (mean ± SD)	1.37 ± 0.31	1.40 ± 0.30	1.33 ± 0.32	1.36 ± 0.31
Potassium, mEq/L (mean ± SD)	4.75 ± 0.77	5.44 ± 0.58	3.75 ± 0.65	4.55 ± 0.51
Calcium, mg/dL (mean ± SD)	8.73 ± 0.81	8.80 ± 0.81	8.51 ± 0.75	8.73 ± 0.82
Phosphorus, mg/dL (mean ± SD)	5.45 ± 1.48	5.85 ± 1.48	4.70 ± 1.55	5.36 ± 1.40
Hemoglobin, g/dL (mean ± SD)	10.79 ± 1.34	10.82 ± 1.30	10.64 ± 1.55	10.80 ± 1.32
Total protein, g/dL (mean ± SD)	6.48 ± 0.58	6.48 ± 0.57	6.36 ± 0.69	6.49 ± 0.56
Albumin, g/dL (mean ± SD)	3.63 ± 0.43	3.70 ± 0.39	3.41 ± 0.53	3.64 ± 0.42
Creatinine, mg/dL (mean ± SD)	9.77 ± 2.88	10.54 ± 2.73	7.69 ± 2.58	9.74 ± 2.82
URR, % (mean ± SD)	66.12 ± 8.34	66.57 ± 8.00	66.36 ± 8.83	65.81 ± 8.42
nPCR, g/kg/day (mean ± SD)	0.83 ± 0.24	0.84 ± 0.36	0.79 ± 0.07	0.83 ± 0.15
GNRI (mean ± SD)	93.08 ± 7.41	94.15 ± 7.26	90.51 ± 9.16	92.92 ± 7.07

Table 1. Cont.

Characteristics	Overall n = 2846	Hyper-K Group n = 909 (31.94%)	Hypo-K Group n = 313 (11.00%)	Normo-K Group n = 1624 (57.06%)
Ferritin, ng/mL (median; min, max)	77.80 (0.07, 1970.0)	75.20 (0.19, 1900.9)	82.95 (0.07, 1970.0)	77.15 (0.17, 1961.3)
CRP, mg/dL (median; min, max)	0.11 (0.00, 39.47)	0.10 (0.01, 39.47)	0.20 (0.01, 11.03)	0.11 (0.00, 17.94)
Comorbidities, n (%)				
Diabetes	1558 (54.74)	484 (53.25)	191 (61.02)	883 (54.37)
Hypertension	2587 (90.90)	832 (91.53)	281 (89.78)	1474 (90.76)
Heart failure	1163 (40.86)	371 (40.81)	126 (40.26)	666 (41.01)
Cardiac arrest	6 (0.21)	5 (0.55)	1 (0.32)	0 (0.00)
Myocardial infarction	61 (2.41)	23 (2.53)	5 (1.60)	33 (2.03)
Stroke	383 (13.46)	123 (13.53)	34 (10.86)	226 (13.92)
Peripheral vascular diseases	974 (34.22)	331 (36.41)	94 (30.03)	549 (33.81)
Cerebrovascular diseases	797 (28.00)	249 (27.39)	93 (29.71)	455 (28.02)
Dementia	115 (4.04)	18 (1.98)	38 (12.14)	59 (3.63)
Sarcopenia	213 (7.48)	56 (6.16)	40 (12.78)	117 (7.20)
Medications, n (%)				
β-blockers	671 (23.58)	227 (24.97)	67 (21.41)	377 (23.21)
RAASi (ACEi/ARB/MRA)	1474 (51.79)	544 (59.85)	139 (44.41)	791 (48.71)
ACEi	168 (5.90)	69 (7.59)	22 (7.03)	77 (4.74)
ARB	1406 (49.40)	522 (57.43)	128 (40.89)	756 (46.55)
MRA	22 (0.77)	2 (0.22)	3 (0.96)	17 (1.05)
Laxative agent	1082 (38.02)	289 (31.79)	169 (53.99)	624 (38.42)
Potassium adsorbents (SPS/CPS)	384 (13.49)	193 (21.23)	20 (6.39)	171 (10.53)
CPS	311 (10.93)	149 (16.39)	14 (4.47)	148 (9.11)
SPS	91 (3.20)	52 (5.72)	7 (2.24)	32 (1.97)
Potassium supplements	16 (0.56)	1 (0.11)	7 (2.24)	8 (0.49)
Nutritional guidance	1555 (54.64)	489 (53.80)	202 (64.54)	864 (53.20)

Abbreviations: BMI—body mass index; URR—urea reduction ratio; nPCR—normalized protein catabolism rate; GNRI—geriatric nutrition risk index; CRP—C-reactive protein; RAASi—renin-angiotensin-aldosterone system inhibitor; ACEi—angiotensin-converting enzyme inhibitor; ARB—angiotensin receptor blocker; MRA—mineralocorticoid receptor antagonist; SPS—sodium polystyrene sulfonate; CPS—calcium polystyrene sulfonate.

The prevalence of dyskalemia stratified by dialysis vintage at baseline is shown in Figure 2. As described in Section 2.3, twenty patients who met both hyperkalemia and hypokalemia criteria during the baseline period contributed to the calculation of the prevalence of both hyperkalemia and hypokalemia, respectively. Therefore, 909 (31.94%) and 333 (11.70%) patients met criteria for hyperkalemia and hypokalemia, respectively. The prevalence of hyperkalemia significantly increased with increasing dialysis vintage ($p < 0.001$), whereas the prevalence of hypokalemia significantly decreased with increasing duration of dialysis ($p < 0.001$) [Figure 2].

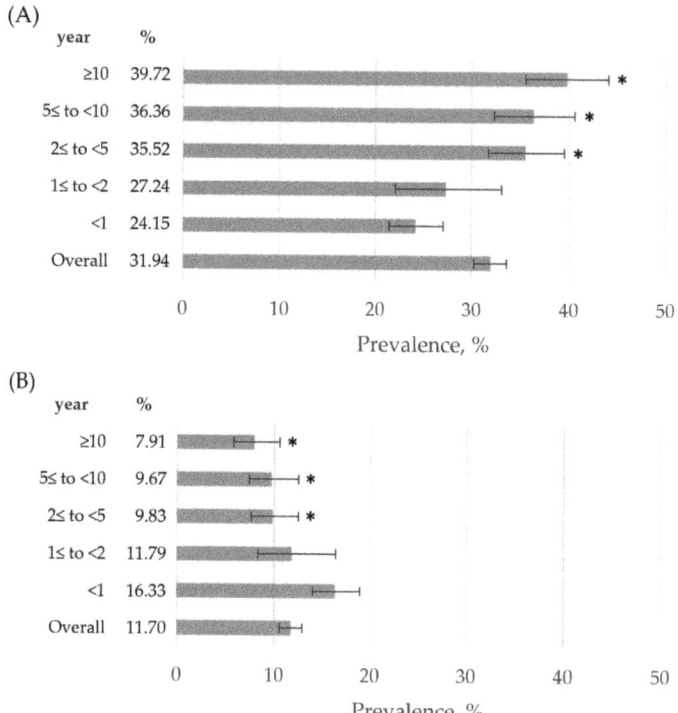

Figure 2. Prevalence of dyskalemia stratified by dialysis vintage at baseline period. (**A**) Prevalence of hyperkalemia (n = 909) during the baseline period by length of dialysis vintage. (**B**) Prevalence of hypokalemia (n = 333) during the baseline period by length of dialysis vintage [Hypo-K group (n = 313) and patients with both hyperkalemia and hypokalemia (n = 20)]. Error bars denote 95% confidence intervals. * $p < 0.01$ versus dialysis vintage of <1 year (the Benjamini–Hochberg Procedure was used to correct for multiple comparisons).

3.2. Baseline Outpatient Characteristics

The baseline characteristics of patients by group are shown in Table 1. Patients in the Hypo-K group (69.37 years, SD: 12.68) tended to be older than in the other groups (approximately 65 years), whereas dialysis vintage in the Hyper-K group (median 4.27 years) tended to be longer than in the other groups (1.49 and 2.70 years in the Hypo-K and Normo-K groups, respectively). All patients in all groups were using dialysate with a potassium concentration of 2.0 mEq/L. As for nutritional status, the Hypo-K group tended to have lower serum total protein, serum albumin, geriatric nutrition risk index (GNRI), and normalized protein catabolic rate (nPCR) than the other groups. These values tended to be in the lower range in all groups when compared with clinical norms [19]. Additionally, the percentage of patients receiving nutritional guidance was higher in the Hypo-K group (64.54%) than in the other groups (approximately 53%). Among inflammatory markers, CRP tended to be higher in the Hypo-K group (median 0.20 mg/dL) than in the other groups (median 0.10 mg/dL and 0.11 mg/dL in the Hyper-K and Normo-K groups, respectively). Among the recorded comorbidities, the prevalence of dementia (12.14%) and sarcopenia (12.78%) in the Hypo-K group were higher than those of the Hyper-K group (1.98% and 6.16%, respectively) and the Normo-K groups (3.63% and 7.20%, respectively). Conversely, arrhythmias tended to be recorded more frequently among the patients in the Hyper-K group compared to the Hypo-K and Normo-K group patients [Table 1].

Among the therapeutic agents used, renin–angiotensin–aldosterone system inhibitors (ACEi/ARB/MRA) were used by 59.85%, 44.41%, and 48.71% of the patients in the Hyper-

K, Hypo-K, and Normo-K groups, respectively. Laxatives were used by 31.79%, 53.99%, and 38.42% of patients in the Hyper-K, Hypo-K, and Normo-K groups, respectively. Potassium adsorbents were used by 21.23% of patients in the Hyper-K group, of which 16.39% was calcium polystyrene sulfonate (CPS) and 5.72% was sodium polystyrene sulfonate (SPS) [Table 1].

3.3. Clinical Outcomes

During the follow-up period, 947 (33.27%) of the 2846 outpatients died, and the mortality rate was 7.78 per 100 person-years [Table S3]. Hypo-K was significantly associated with mortality when compared with Normo-K (HR, 1.47; 95% CI, 1.13 to 1.92) but not when compared with Hyper-K (HR, 0.92; 95% CI, 0.78 to 1.09). The associations of Hypo-K with MACE were also significant when compared with Normo-K (HR, 1.48; 95% CI, 1.17 to 1.86) but not when compared with Hyper-K (HR, 0.97; 95% CI, 0.84 to 1.12) [Figure 3 and Table 2]. On the other hand, Hyper-K was significantly associated with death related to arrhythmia (HR, 3.11; 95% CI, 1.03 to 9.33) [Figure 3 and Table 2].

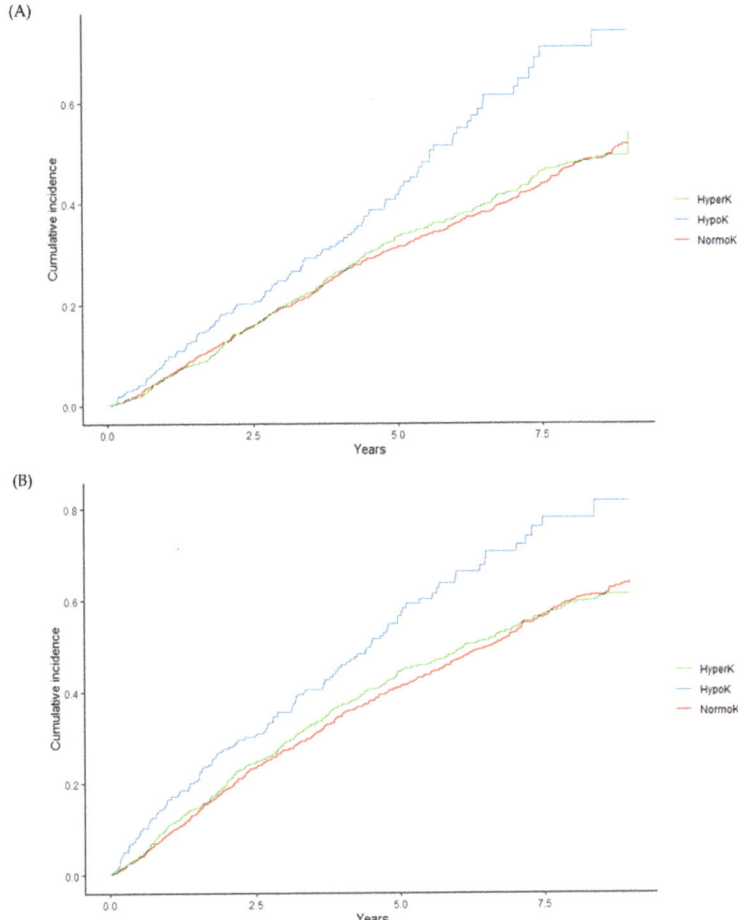

Figure 3. *Cont.*

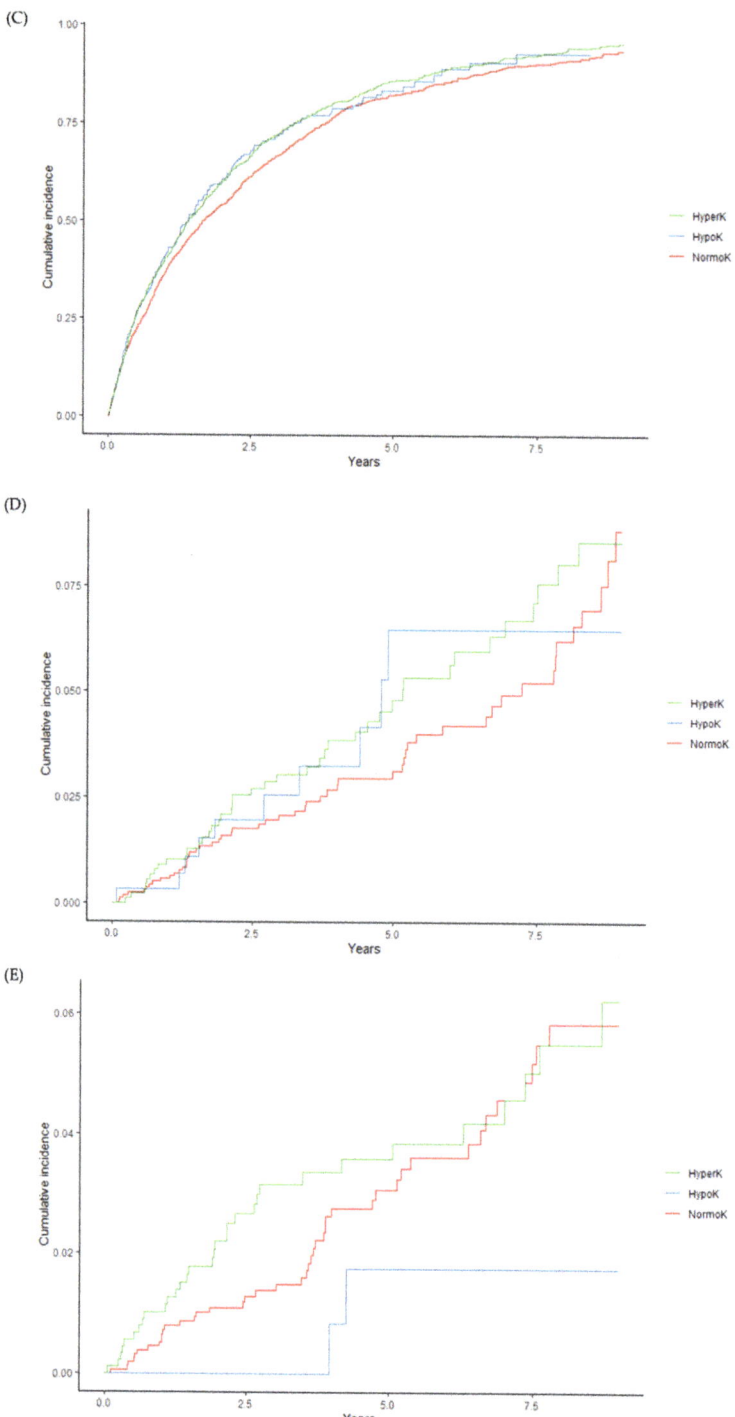

Figure 3. *Cont.*

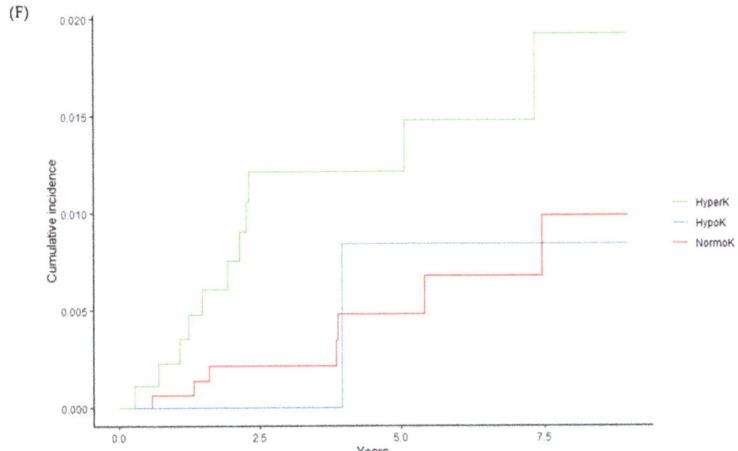

Figure 3. Cumulative incidence of clinical outcomes in Hyper-K, Hypo-K, and Normo-K. (**A**) All-cause mortality in Hyper-K ($p = 0.900$), Hypo-K ($p < 0.001$), and Normo-K; (**B**) MACE in Hyper-K ($p = 0.700$), Hypo-K ($p < 0.001$), and Normo-K; (**C**) hospitalization in Hyper-K ($p = 0.018$), Hypo-K ($p = 0.381$), and Normo-K; (**D**) cardiac arrest in Hyper-K ($p = 0.201$), Hypo-K ($p = 0.364$), and Normo-K; (**E**) fatal arrhythmia in Hyper-K ($p = 0.827$), Hypo-K ($p = 0.214$), and Normo-K; (**F**) death related to arrhythmia in Hyper-K ($p = 0.040$), Hypo-K ($p = 1.000$), and Normo-K. As evaluation of p-values, log-rank testing was used for all-cause mortality, MACE, and death related to arrhythmia, whereas the Fine and Gray test was used for hospitalization, cardiac arrest, and fatal arrhythmia.

Table 2. Association between serum potassium status and clinical outcomes in outpatients.

	N	100 Person-Year	Hazard Ratio (95% C.I.)	
			Crude	Adjusted [a]
All-cause mortality				
Hyper-K ($n = 909$)	314	7.50	1.01 (0.87, 1.16)	0.92 (0.78, 1.09)
Hypo-K ($n = 313$)	120	11.29	1.58 (1.30, 1.94)	1.47 (1.13, 1.92)
Normo-K ($n = 1624$)	513	7.41	1.00 (Reference)	1.00 (Reference)
MACE				
Hyper-K ($n = 909$)	415	10.88	1.02 (0.91, 1.16)	0.97 (0.84, 1.12)
Hypo-K ($n = 313$)	152	16.29	1.57 (1.31, 1.87)	1.48 (1.17, 1.86)
Normo-K ($n = 1624$)	671	10.63	1.00 (Reference)	1.00 (Reference)
Hospitalization				
Hyper-K ($n = 909$)	751	41.97	1.14 (1.04, 1.24)	1.09 (0.98, 1.22)
Hypo-K ($n = 313$)	227	43.54	1.13 (0.98, 1.31)	1.13 (0.94, 1.37)
Normo-K ($n = 1624$)	1216	37.00	1.00 (Reference)	1.00 (Reference)
Cardiac arrest				
Hyper-K ($n = 909$)	41	0.98	1.24 (0.83, 1.86)	1.30 (0.80, 2.12)
Hypo-K ($n = 313$)	10	0.94	1.31 (0.66, 2.60)	1.41 (0.58, 3.38)
Normo-K ($n = 1624$)	54	0.78	1.00 (Reference)	1.00 (Reference)
Fatal arrythmia				
Hyper-K ($n = 909$)	32	0.78	1.25 (0.79, 1.97)	1.44 (0.86, 2.39)
Hypo-K ($n = 313$)	2	0.19	0.31 (0.08, 1.30)	0.28 (0.04, 2.16)
Normo-K ($n = 1624$)	43	0.63	1.00 (Reference)	1.00 (Reference)
Death related to arrythmia				
Hyper-K ($n = 909$)	11	0.26	2.65 (1.03, 6.84)	3.11 (1.03, 9.33)
Hypo-K ($n = 313$)	1	0.09	0.98 (0.12, 8.07)	2.65 (0.31, 22.89)
Normo-K ($n = 1624$)	7	0.10	1.00 (Reference)	1.00 (Reference)

To estimate the hazard ratio, the Normo-K group was used as the reference level. [a] Adjustments: age, gender, dialysis vintage, index year, body mass index (BMI), albumin, C-reactive protein (CRP), urea reduction ratio (URR), serum calcium, serum phosphorus (centralized by subtracting mean), serum phosphorus squared (squared after centralized), hemoglobin, HD treatment time, Charlson Comorbidity Index (CCI), and history of comorbidities: heart failure, diabetes, cardiovascular comorbidities, myocardial infarction, other acute ischemic heart diseases, atherosclerotic heart disease of native coronary artery, chronic ischemic heart disease, stroke, unstable angina, angina pectoris unspecified, heart failure, and diabetes.

4. Discussion

This study sought to understand the characteristics of HD patients with dyskalemia and the association of dyskalemia with clinical outcomes among Japanese patients undergoing maintenance HD.

4.1. Characteristics of Tokushu-kai Hospital Group Database

This study used electronic medical record data between 2010 and 2019 from the Tokushu-kai hospital network. The average age of HD patients in this study population was 68.09 years and 65.65 years before and after excluding the inpatient group, respectively. According to the Current Status of Chronic Dialysis Therapy report by the Japan Society of Dialysis Therapy [20], the average age of chronic dialysis patients showed an upward trend from 66.21 years in 2010 to 69.09 years in 2019. Therefore, the study population was considered almost consistent with the real-world HD patients in Japan.

On the other hand, in terms of mortality, overall mortality in this study through the follow-up period was 947 (33.27%) of 2846 participants, which is 7.78 per 100 person-years. This mortality rate is higher than the data from JDOPPS [21], which found that 562 (14%) of 3967 participants died during the follow-up period, and the overall mortality rate was 6.7 per 100 person-years. This difference may be explained by the characteristics of the database used in this study. The hospital group from which this database is derived actively accepts emergency patients, including those in more severe conditions who have been rejected or have not been able to be treated in other dialysis clinics, and this may have led to the higher mortality rate seen in this study.

4.2. Association of Hypo-K with Baseline Characteristics and Outcomes

In this study, 54% of the hypokalemia group used laxatives, suggesting an association between laxative use and hypokalemia. It has been reported that laxative use was not associated with risk of hypokalemia (K < 3.5 mEq/L) during the preceding 1-year pre-ESKD period. On the other hand, in a group of patients ≥65 years, the use of laxatives contributed to the higher risk of hypokalemia [22]. Despite this previous study, our study demonstrated that over half of the hypokalemia group used laxatives. Therefore, more attention should be paid to the sK trajectory when patients are treated with laxatives, particularly for older patients who may be more prone to laxative-induced hypokalemia than younger patients.

Notably, malnutrition was more prevalent in patients with Hypo-K, in whom nutritional indicators such as serum albumin and total protein were below reference values (3.41 g/L and 6.36 g/dL, respectively, for Hypo-K patients versus reference values of >4.0 g/dL and 6.5 to 8.0 g/dL, respectively). Furthermore, the inflammation marker CRP was higher than the normal values, suggesting a tendency toward malnutrition and inflammation. Many HD patients suffer from protein–energy wasting, also known as uremic malnutrition, as defined by the International Society of Renal Nutrition and Metabolism [23–25]. In contrast to simple malnutrition such as starvation with low nutrient intake, malnutrition in dialysis patients results from increased catabolism due to the effects of inflammatory cytokines, which are more likely to complicate chronic inflammation and atherosclerotic disease and increase the risk of cardiovascular diseases and death [26,27]. The improvement of health-related quality of life (HR-QoL) is a priority issue in HD patients which require more detailed nutritional management, higher ADL, and better nursing care [28–30]. In fact, in the current study, the incidence of death and MACE was significantly higher in Hypo-K patients when compared with Normo-K patients, both with and without adjustment for potential confounding factors.

A strong correlation between malnutrition/low ADL and poor life/health span prognosis in HD patients is also well known [31,32]. This study showed that Hypo-K patients were prone to malnutrition–inflammation status, suggesting that this status may influence clinical outcomes in Hypo-K patients in addition to the direct impact of hypokalemia. Dementia and sarcopenia were more common in the Hypo-K group, despite hypokalemia not necessarily directly affecting cognitive dysfunction; however, it was suggested that hypokalemia is associated with malnutrition, which can lead to sarcopenia and subsequent frailty, which ultimately can result in cognitive decline. Moreover, the consideration of nutritional disorders in maintenance HD patients is particularly important, as such disorders greatly affect vital prognosis and HR-QoL. Thus, nutritional and care-based interventions from nurses and nutritionists as well as the expansion of medical teams and care will be important topics of discussion in the future for better treatment [33]. Despite the fact that sK levels were recorded at pre-dialysis (instead of post-dialysis), about 11% of outpatient HD patients were still categorized in the Hypo-K group in this cohort. This study revealed that hypokalemia reflects a pathological condition with a poor prognosis caused by malnutrition–inflammation. Therefore, optimization of sK levels for the purpose of proper nutritional management and the improvement of ADL may contribute to the improvement of health/lifespan of HD patients. Further research is warranted in this area.

4.3. Association of Hyper-K with Baseline Characteristics and Outcomes

In this study, the prevalence of Hyper-K increased with longer dialysis vintage, culminating at a rate of 39.72% in patients with a dialysis vintage of 10 years or more. According to the United States Renal Data System 2001 report on the number of patients undergoing HD in Japan and the United States by duration of HD, most patients in the United States had a dialysis vintage of two years or less, while many patients had a dialysis vintage of three years or more in Japan. Similarly, the number of patients on dialysis for 10 years or more was 0.17% in the United States and 24.1% in Japan [34]. In addition, according to the statistics of the Japan Society of Dialysis Therapy, 27.8% of patients have been on dialysis for more than 10 years. Furthermore, the proportion of patients with a dialysis vintage of 20 years or more was less than 1% in 1992 but had increased to 8.3% by 2017. These results suggest that the number of patients undergoing dialysis treatment for a longer period will increase in the future in Japan. Taken together with our results, further improvement will be needed for the management of hyperkalemia in Japanese patients on maintenance HD.

In the Hyper-K group, the incidence of mortality and MACE was similar to that of the Normo-K group [15]. According to the data from the DOPPS study, the HR of all-cause mortality in hyperkalemia excursions with sK > 6.0 mEq/L over a 4-month period in Japan was 1.04 (95% CI, 0.78 to 1.39), whereas those in North America and Europe were 1.35 (95% CI, 1.23 to 1.48) and 1.44 (95% CI, 1.23 to 1.68), respectively [15]. Previously, Kim et al. reported racial and ethnic differences in mortality associated with sK levels; however, this study did not include Asian maintenance HD patients [29]. Therefore, it was hypothesized that the Asian HD population, especially the Japanese population, appears to better tolerate higher sK levels than the North American and European HD populations. While the underlying mechanism of racial and ethnic differences in sK levels remains unclear, this may be explained by differences in diet across regions and countries. Further studies are needed to determine the underlying mechanisms for the varying associations between sK level and mortality across race and ethnicity.

On the other hand, the incidence of death related to arrhythmia, defined as death within three days from fatal arrythmia, significantly increased in the Hyper-K group compared with the Normo-K group. According to the Current Status of Chronic Dialysis Therapy report by the Japan Society of Dialysis Therapy [20], potassium-poisoning/sudden death was responsible for 1.7% of the causes of death. It is known that the incidence of sudden cardiac death in Japanese patients is lower than that in the European population [35,36]. This is likely due to the lower complication rate of cardiovascular diseases such as coronary artery disease, congestive heart failure, and left ventricular hypertrophy in the Japanese population [37].

Chronic hyperkalemia not only causes fatal arrhythmia but also restricts the intake of fruits and vegetables, including those that are rich in potassium. Furthermore, fruits and vegetables also offer an abundance of other nutrients such as fiber, minerals, and short-chain fatty acids. These nutrients are associated with a lower risk of cardiovascular disease and mortality [38,39]. It has been reported that potassium intake correlates with the intake of necessary nutrients such as protein, fiber, and energy [40]. Therefore, if excessive nutritional restrictions are imposed as a treatment for hyperkalemia, it may cause malnourishment in HD patients, leading to worse outcomes. Consequently, the importance of properly treating hyperkalemia should be understood and disseminated.

For potassium management, dialysate with a potassium concentration of 2.0 mEq/L is commonly used in Japan, as was the case for all patients in this study and those reported in the DOPPS study [41]. It has been reported that a higher sK gradient is independently associated with a greater risk of all-cause hospitalizations and emergency department visits but not mortality, potentially due to a low number of events [42]. Therefore, to minimize sK fluctuations between pre- and post-dialysis, a personalized management of the sK level and the potassium concentration of the dialysate may be prudent for optimal dialysis treatments. The use of potassium adsorbent was 20% in the Hyper-K group in this study, despite a mean sK level of 5.44 mEq/L. According to data from the DOPPS study in Japan, potassium adsorbent was used in just 1.9% of cases of hyperkalemia, and the frequency was about 6% even when the sK level was >6.0 mEq/L continuing for 4 months or more [15]. In the REVEAL-HK study, which investigated the real-world condition of patients with hyperkalemia in Japan, the frequency of prescribing potassium adsorbent due to hyperkalemia was 37.6% in patients with CKD during the study period, further suggesting that chronic hyperkalemia may persist in many patients without active interventions such as potassium absorbents [43].

4.4. Limitations

This study has limitations, which are inherent due to its retrospective design, and is subject to several biases such as selection bias and confounding factors, despite adjustment. The data used in this study were limited to the Tokushu-kai group of hospitals. Therefore, there may be Tokushu-kai group-specific prescription and treatment patterns. In addition, in hospital-based databases in general, data for patients sent to other hospitals for emergency conditions, as well as those dying at home, cannot be captured. Therefore, absolute risk (differences) of the studied outcomes might be underestimated, whereas the relative risks between the groups (i.e., Hyper-K, Hypo-K, and Normo-K groups) are expected to be estimated correctly. Moreover, since we conducted the study based on the hypothesis that baseline sK impacts the subsequent long-term outcomes, we were unable to examine whether and to what extent change in sK status during the follow-up could affect the outcome. This study was also limited to the Japanese HD population and should be interpreted with caution for other countries, despite the rigorous definition of dyskalemia in the current study.

5. Conclusions

Despite standardized rigorous thrice-weekly dialysis therapy, dyskalemia was prevalent in the patients in this cohort. Hypo-K was characterized by older patients suffering from malnutrition, a higher incidence of all-cause mortality, and MACE. Hyper-K was characterized by a longer history of dialysis and a higher incidence of death related to fatal arrhythmia. Dyskalemia was associated with worse clinical outcomes compared with Normo-K. Therefore, this study emphasized the importance of controlling sK levels in HD patients while also maintaining the nutritional health of each patient. Eliminating patient barriers to better nutritional diets, in combination with the use of potassium binders for hyperkalemia, is expected to improve the worse clinical outcomes and frailty associated with poor nutritional status in maintenance HD patients.

Supplementary Materials: The following supporting information can be downloaded at: https://www.mdpi.com/article/10.3390/jcm12062115/s1, Table S1: List of comorbidities; Table S2: Definition of clinical outcomes; Table S3: Cumulative incidence of clinical outcomes in outpatient managed patients undergoing HD 3 times/week during baseline period.

Author Contributions: Conceptualization: all authors; data curation: Y.K., N.M. and T.Y.; formal analysis: Y.K., N.M. and T.Y.; funding acquisition: T.Y.; investigation: all authors; methodology: M.I., Y.K., N.M. and T.Y.; project administration: N.M. and T.Y.; resources: Y.K., N.M. and T.Y.; supervision: T.Y.; validation: Y.K. and N.M.; visualization: Y.K., N.M. and T.Y.; writing—original draft: M.I., Y.K. and N.M.; writing—review and editing: all authors. All authors have read and agreed to the published version of the manuscript.

Funding: This study and the corresponding analyses were supported and funded by AstraZeneca KK. AstraZeneca also manufactures a drug (sodium zirconium cyclosilicate) that is used to treat hyperkalemia. Authors from AstraZeneca participated in the organization of the study design and interpretation of the results and contributed to the manuscript drafts and revisions and the decision to approve publication of the final manuscript.

Institutional Review Board Statement: This study was reviewed and approved by The Tokushu-kai Group Ethics Committee. The confidentiality of records that could be used to identify patients was not provided to the researchers and is protected by the data provider of the Tokushu-kai Group.

Informed Consent Statement: Informed consent was not required, as patient records were anonymized and deidentified prior to access.

Data Availability Statement: Not applicable.

Acknowledgments: The authors thank Ryo Koto, Hyosung Kim, Kurena Mitsuoka, and Koichi Shirakawa from AstraZeneca for assistance with the statistical analysis, valuable comments, and logistical support, and Masafumi Okada, Seok Won Kim, Shingo Wada, Yuki Kado, Louis Watanabe, and all of the project members from IQVIA Solutions K.K. for providing technical and editorial support, including data analysis, under the guidance of the authors and for providing medical writing support on the initial draft of the paper, which was funded by AstraZeneca K.K., Japan, in accordance with the Good Publication Practice (GPP3) guidelines (http://www.ismpp.org/gpp3; accessed on 1 August 2022).

Conflicts of Interest: M.I., S.K. and M.F. have received a speaker honorarium from AstraZeneca. Y.K., N.M. and T.Y. are employees of AstraZeneca KK.

References

1. Devereaux, P.J.; Schünemann, H.J.; Ravindran, N.; Bhandari, M.; Garg, A.X.; Choi, P.T.; Grant, B.J.; Haines, T.; Lacchetti, C.; Weaver, B.; et al. Comparison of mortality between private for-profit and private not-for-profit hemodialysis centers: A systematic review and meta-analysis. *JAMA* **2002**, *288*, 2449–2457. [CrossRef] [PubMed]
2. Eggers, P.W.; Frankenfield, D.L.; Greer, J.W.; McClellan, W.; Owen, W.F., Jr.; Rocco, M.V. Comparison of mortality and intermediate outcomes between medicare dialysis patients in HMO and fee for service. *Am. J. Kidney Dis.* **2002**, *39*, 796–804. [CrossRef] [PubMed]
3. US Renal Data System 2022 Annul Data Report Figure 6.1a Mortality in Adult ESRD Patients, 2010–2020. Available online: https://usrds-adr.niddk.nih.gov/2022 (accessed on 31 December 2022).
4. Arce, C.M.; Goldstein, B.A.; Mitani, A.A.; Winkelmayer, W.C. Trends in relative mortality between Hispanic and non-Hispanic whites initiating dialysis: A retrospective study of the US Renal Data System. *Am. J. Kidney Dis.* **2013**, *62*, 312–321. [CrossRef] [PubMed]
5. Kucirka, L.M.; Grams, M.E.; Lessler, J.; Hall, E.C.; James, N.; Massie, A.B.; Montgomery, R.A.; Segev, D.L. Association of race and age with survival among patients undergoing dialysis. *JAMA* **2011**, *306*, 620–626. [CrossRef] [PubMed]
6. Yan, G.; Norris, K.C.; Yu, A.J.; Ma, J.Z.; Greene, T.; Yu, W.; Cheung, A.K. The relationship of age, race, and ethnicity with survival in dialysis patients. *Clin. J. Am. Soc. Nephrol.* **2013**, *8*, 953–961. [CrossRef]
7. Murthy, B.V.; Molony, D.A.; Stack, A.G. Survival advantage of Hispanic patients initiating dialysis in the United States is modified by race. *J. Am. Soc. Nephrol.* **2005**, *16*, 782–790. [CrossRef]
8. Frankenfield, D.L.; Rocco, M.V.; Roman, S.H.; McClellan, W.M. Survival advantage for adult Hispanic hemodialysis patients? Findings from the end-stage renal disease clinical performance measures project. *J. Am. Soc. Nephrol.* **2003**, *14*, 180–186. [CrossRef]
9. Saran, R.; Li, Y.; Robinson, B.; Ayanian, J.; Balkrishnan, R.; Bragg-Gresham, J.; Chen, J.T.; Cope, E.; Gipson, D.; He, K.; et al. US Renal Data System 2014 Annual Data Report: Epidemiology of Kidney Disease in the United States. *Am. J. Kidney Dis.* **2015**, *66*, S1–S305. [CrossRef]
10. Kovesdy, C.P.; Regidor, D.L.; Mehrotra, R.; Jing, J.; McAllister, C.J.; Greenland, S.; Kopple, J.D.; Kalantar-Zadeh, K. Serum and dialysate potassium concentrations and survival in hemodialysis patients. *Clin. J. Am. Soc. Nephrol.* **2007**, *2*, 999–1007. [CrossRef]
11. Choi, H.Y.; Ha, S.K. Potassium balances in maintenance hemodialysis. *Electrolytes Blood Press.* **2013**, *11*, 9–16. [CrossRef]

12. Yusuf, A.A.; Hu, Y.; Singh, B.; Menoyo, J.A.; Wetmore, J.B. Serum Potassium Levels and Mortality in Hemodialysis Patients: A Retrospective Cohort Study. *Am. J. Nephrol.* **2016**, *44*, 179–186. [CrossRef]
13. Hayes, J.; Kalantar-Zadeh, K.; Lu, J.L.; Turban, S.; Anderson, J.E.; Kovesdy, C.P. Association of hypo- and hyperkalemia with disease progression and mortality in males with chronic kidney disease: The role of race. *Nephron Clin. Pract.* **2012**, *120*, c8–c16. [CrossRef]
14. Kim, T.; Rhee, C.M.; Streja, E.; Soohoo, M.; Obi, Y.; Chou, J.A.; Tortorici, A.R.; Ravel, V.A.; Kovesdy, C.P.; Kalantar-Zadeh, K. Racial and Ethnic Differences in Mortality Associated with Serum Potassium in a Large Hemodialysis Cohort. *Am. J. Nephrol.* **2017**, *45*, 509–521. [CrossRef]
15. Karaboyas, A.; Robinson, B.M.; James, G.; Hedman, K.; Moreno Quinn, C.P.; De Sequera, P.; Nitta, K.; Pecoits-Filho, R. Hyperkalemia excursions are associated with an increased risk of mortality and hospitalizations in hemodialysis patients. *Clin. Kidney J.* **2021**, *14*, 1760–1769. [CrossRef]
16. Iwagami, M.; Yasunaga, H.; Noiri, E.; Horiguchi, H.; Fushimi, K.; Matsubara, T.; Yahagi, N.; Nangaku, M.; Doi, K. Current state of continuous renal replacement therapy for acute kidney injury in Japanese intensive care units in 2011: Analysis of a national administrative database. *Nephrol. Dial. Transpl.* **2015**, *30*, 988–995. [CrossRef]
17. Miyake, K.; Iwagami, M.; Ohtake, T.; Moriya, H.; Kume, N.; Murata, T.; Nishida, T.; Mochida, Y.; Isogai, N.; Ishioka, K.; et al. Association of pre-operative chronic kidney disease and acute kidney injury with in-hospital outcomes of emergency colorectal surgery: A cohort study. *World J. Emerg. Surg.* **2020**, *15*, 22. [CrossRef]
18. Kubota, K.; Yoshizawa, M.; Takahashi, S.; Fujimura, Y.; Nomura, H.; Kohsaka, H. The validity of the claims-based definition of rheumatoid arthritis evaluated in 64 hospitals in Japan. *BMC Musculoskelet. Disord.* **2021**, *22*, 373. [CrossRef]
19. Ikizler, T.A.; Burrowes, J.D.; Byham-Gray, L.D.; Campbell, K.L.; Carrero, J.J.; Chan, W.; Fouque, D.; Friedman, A.N.; Ghaddar, S.; Goldstein-Fuchs, D.J.; et al. KDOQI clinical practice guidelines for nutrition in CKD: 2020 update. *Am. J. Kidney Dis.* **2019**, *76*, S1–S107. [CrossRef]
20. An Overview of Regular Dialysis Treatment in Japan. Report. 2019. Available online: https://docs.jsdt.or.jp/overview/index2020.html (accessed on 28 October 2022).
21. Ohnishi, T.; Kimachi, M.; Fukuma, S.; Akizawa, T.; Fukuhara, S. Postdialysis Hypokalemia and All-Cause Mortality in Patients Undergoing Maintenance Hemodialysis. *Clin. J. Am. Soc. Nephrol.* **2019**, *14*, 873. [CrossRef]
22. Sumida, K.; Dashputre, A.A.; Potukuchi, P.K.; Thomas, F.; Obi, Y.; Molnar, M.Z.; Gatwood, J.D.; Streja, E.; Kalantar-Zadeh, K.; Kovesdy, C.P. Laxative Use and Risk of Dyskalemia in Patients with Advanced CKD Transitioning to Dialysis. *J. Am. Soc. Nephrol.* **2021**, *32*, 950–959. [CrossRef]
23. Clinical practice guidelines for nutrition in chronic renal failure. K/DOQI, National Kidney Foundation. *Am. J. Kidney Dis.* **2000**, *35*, S17–S104. [CrossRef]
24. Fouque, D.; Kalantar-Zadeh, K.; Kopple, J.; Cano, N.; Chauveau, P.; Cuppari, L.; Franch, H.; Guarnieri, G.; Ikizler, T.A.; Kaysen, G.; et al. A proposed nomenclature and diagnostic criteria for protein-energy wasting in acute and chronic kidney disease. *Kidney Int.* **2008**, *73*, 391–398. [CrossRef] [PubMed]
25. Kalantar-Zadeh, K. Recent advances in understanding the malnutrition-inflammation-cachexia syndrome in chronic kidney disease patients: What is next? *Semin. Dial.* **2005**, *18*, 365–369. [CrossRef] [PubMed]
26. Carracedo, J.; Alique, M.; Vida, C.; Bodega, G.; Ceprián, N.; Morales, E.; Praga, M.; de Sequera, P.; Ramírez, R. Mechanisms of Cardiovascular Disorders in Patients with Chronic Kidney Disease: A Process Related to Accelerated Senescence. *Front. Cell Dev. Biol.* **2020**, *8*, 185. [CrossRef] [PubMed]
27. Sahathevan, S.; Khor, B.-H.; Ng, H.-M.; Gafor, A.H.A.; Mat Daud, Z.A.; Mafra, D.; Karupaiah, T. Understanding Development of Malnutrition in Hemodialysis Patients: A Narrative Review. *Nutrients* **2020**, *12*, 3147. [CrossRef]
28. Cobo, G.; Lindholm, B.; Stenvinkel, P. Chronic inflammation in end-stage renal disease and dialysis. *Nephrol. Dial. Transpl.* **2018**, *33*, iii35–iii40. [CrossRef]
29. Kim, T.; Streja, E.; Soohoo, M.; Rhee, C.M.; Eriguchi, R.; Kim, T.W.; Chang, T.I.; Obi, Y.; Kovesdy, C.P.; Kalantar-Zadeh, K. Serum Ferritin Variations and Mortality in Incident Hemodialysis Patients. *Am. J. Nephrol.* **2017**, *46*, 120–130. [CrossRef]
30. Johansen, K.L.; Chertow, G.M.; Jin, C.; Kutner, N.G. Significance of frailty among dialysis patients. *J. Am. Soc. Nephrol.* **2007**, *18*, 2960–2967. [CrossRef]
31. Jassal, S.V.; Karaboyas, A.; Comment, L.A.; Bieber, B.A.; Morgenstern, H.; Sen, A.; Gillespie, B.W.; De Sequera, P.; Marshall, M.R.; Fukuhara, S.; et al. Functional Dependence and Mortality in the International Dialysis Outcomes and Practice Patterns Study (DOPPS). *Am. J. Kidney Dis.* **2016**, *67*, 283–292. [CrossRef]
32. Kanda, E.; Lopes, M.B.; Tsuruya, K.; Hirakata, H.; Iseki, K.; Karaboyas, A.; Bieber, B.; Jacobson, S.H.; Dasgupta, I.; Robinson, B.M. The combination of malnutrition-inflammation and functional status limitations is associated with mortality in hemodialysis patients. *Sci. Rep.* **2021**, *11*, 1582. [CrossRef]
33. Feroze, U.; Noori, N.; Kovesdy, C.P.; Molnar, M.Z.; Martin, D.J.; Reina-Patton, A.; Benner, D.; Bross, R.; Norris, K.C.; Kopple, J.D.; et al. Quality-of-life and mortality in hemodialysis patients: Roles of race and nutritional status. *Clin. J. Am. Soc. Nephrol.* **2011**, *6*, 1100–1111. [CrossRef]
34. Kalantar-Zadeh, K.; Tortorici, A.R.; Chen, J.L.; Kamgar, M.; Lau, W.L.; Moradi, H.; Rhee, C.M.; Streja, E.; Kovesdy, C.P. Dietary restrictions in dialysis patients: Is there anything left to eat? *Semin. Dial.* **2015**, *28*, 159–168. [CrossRef]

35. Moroi, M.; Tamaki, N.; Nishimura, M.; Haze, K.; Nishimura, T.; Kusano, E.; Akiba, T.; Sugimoto, T.; Hase, H.; Hara, K.; et al. Association between abnormal myocardial fatty acid metabolism and cardiac-derived death among patients undergoing hemodialysis: Results from a cohort study in Japan. *Am. J. Kidney Dis.* **2013**, *61*, 466–475. [CrossRef]
36. Hiyamuta, H.; Tanaka, S.; Taniguchi, M.; Tokumoto, M.; Fujisaki, K.; Nakano, T.; Tsuruya, K.; Kitazono, T. The Incidence and Associated Factors of Sudden Death in Patients on Hemodialysis: 10-Year Outcome of the Q-Cohort Study. *J. Atheroscler. Thromb.* **2020**, *27*, 306–318. [CrossRef]
37. Goodkin, D.; Bragg-Gresham, J.; Koenig, K.; Wolfe, R.; Akiba, T.; Andreucci, V.; Saito, A.; Rayner, H.; Kurokawa, K.; Port, F.; et al. Association of Comorbid Conditions and Mortality in Hemodialysis Patients in Europe, Japan, and the United States: The Dialysis Outcomes and Practice Patterns Study (DOPPS). *J. Am. Soc. Nephrol. JASN* **2003**, *14*, 3270–3277. [CrossRef]
38. Kim, H.; Caulfield, L.E.; Garcia-Larsen, V.; Steffen, L.M.; Coresh, J.; Rebholz, C.M. Plant-Based Diets Are Associated with a Lower Risk of Incident Cardiovascular Disease, Cardiovascular Disease Mortality, and All-Cause Mortality in a General Population of Middle-Aged Adults. *J. Am. Heart Assoc.* **2019**, *8*, e012865. [CrossRef]
39. Chen, X.; Wei, G.; Jalili, T.; Metos, J.; Giri, A.; Cho, M.E.; Boucher, R.; Greene, T.; Beddhu, S. The Associations of Plant Protein Intake with All-Cause Mortality in CKD. *Am. J. Kidney Dis.* **2016**, *67*, 423–430. [CrossRef]
40. Noori, N.; Kalantar-Zadeh, K.; Kovesdy, C.P.; Murali, S.B.; Bross, R.; Nissenson, A.R.; Kopple, J.D. Dietary potassium intake and mortality in long-term hemodialysis patients. *Am. J. Kidney Dis.* **2010**, *56*, 338–347. [CrossRef]
41. Karaboyas, A.; Zee, J.; Brunelli, S.M.; Usvyat, L.A.; Weiner, D.E.; Maddux, F.W.; Nissenson, A.R.; Jadoul, M.; Locatelli, F.; Winkelmayer, W.C.; et al. Dialysate Potassium, Serum Potassium, Mortality, and Arrhythmia Events in Hemodialysis: Results From the Di-alysis Outcomes and Practice Patterns Study (DOPPS). *Am. J. Kidney Dis.* **2017**, *69*, 266–277. [CrossRef]
42. Brunelli, S.M.; Spiegel, D.M.; Du Mond, C.; Oestreicher, N.; Winkelmayer, W.C.; Kovesdy, C.P. Serum-to-dialysate potassium gradient and its association with short-term outcomes in hemodialysis patients. *Nephrol. Dial. Transpl.* **2018**, *33*, 1207–1214. [CrossRef]
43. Kashihara, N.; Kohsaka, S.; Kanda, E.; Okami, S.; Yajima, T. Hyperkalemia in Real-World Patients Under Continuous Medical Care in Japan. *Kidney Int. Rep.* **2019**, *4*, 1248–1260. [CrossRef] [PubMed]

Disclaimer/Publisher's Note: The statements, opinions and data contained in all publications are solely those of the individual author(s) and contributor(s) and not of MDPI and/or the editor(s). MDPI and/or the editor(s) disclaim responsibility for any injury to people or property resulting from any ideas, methods, instructions or products referred to in the content.

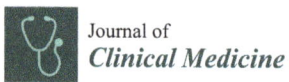 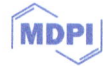

Article

Impact of Vascular Access Flow Suppression Surgery on Cervical Artery Circulation: A Retrospective Observational Study

Koji Hashimoto [1], Makoto Harada [1], Yosuke Yamada [1], Taro Kanno [2], Yutaka Kanno [2] and Yuji Kamijo [1,*]

[1] Department of Nephrology, Shinshu University School of Medicine, 3-1-1 Asahi, Matsumoto 390-8621, Japan; khashi@shinshu-u.ac.jp (K.H.); tokomadaraha724@gmail.com (M.H.); yamada19860603@yahoo.co.jp (Y.Y.)
[2] Kanno Dialysis and Vascular Access Clinic, 2-17-5 Tsukama, Matsumoto 390-0821, Japan; tarosuke0519@yahoo.co.jp (T.K.); kannohd.k-dac@go.tvm.ne.jp (Y.K.)
* Correspondence: yujibeat@shinshu-u.ac.jp; Tel.: +81-263-37-2634

Abstract: Vascular access (VA) flow suppression surgery augments VA flow resistance and can increase other circulation flows hindered by high-flow VA. However, whether VA flow suppression surgery affects cervical circulation has rarely been reported. We aimed to determine the effect of VA flow suppression surgery on the cervical circulation in patients with high-flow VA. This single-center, retrospective, observational study included 85 hemodialysis patients who underwent VA flow suppression surgery at the Kanno Dialysis and Access Clinic between 2009 and 2018. Blood flow in the VA, bilateral vertebral arteries, and common carotid artery was measured before and after VA flow suppression surgery. The VA flow decreased from 1548 mL/min to 693 mL/min postoperatively. The flow of the vertebral artery on the VA side increased from 55 mL/min to 81 mL/min. The flow in the bilateral common carotid arteries also increased. Patients whose symptoms improved postoperatively showed better improvement in the vertebral artery on the VA side. VA flow suppression surgery in patients with high-flow VA increases the flow of the vertebral artery on the VA side and of the bilateral common carotid arteries. High-flow VA can hinder the vertebral and common carotid circulation.

Keywords: hemodialysis; vascular access; high-flow access; cardiovascular events; subclavian steal syndrome

Citation: Hashimoto, K.; Harada, M.; Yamada, Y.; Kanno, T.; Kanno, Y.; Kamijo, Y. Impact of Vascular Access Flow Suppression Surgery on Cervical Artery Circulation: A Retrospective Observational Study. *J. Clin. Med.* **2024**, *13*, 641. https://doi.org/10.3390/jcm13030641

Academic Editor: Maurizio Bossola

Received: 5 January 2024
Revised: 15 January 2024
Accepted: 18 January 2024
Published: 23 January 2024

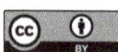

Copyright: © 2024 by the authors. Licensee MDPI, Basel, Switzerland. This article is an open access article distributed under the terms and conditions of the Creative Commons Attribution (CC BY) license (https://creativecommons.org/licenses/by/4.0/).

1. Introduction

Vascular access (VA) is necessary to achieve sufficient dialysis efficiency in patients undergoing hemodialysis (HD). Arteriovenous fistulae (AVF) and arteriovenous grafts (AVG) are widely recognized as being more favorable than central venous catheters in minimizing the risk of infection [1]. AVF and AVG are categorized as vascular access, causing non-physiological blood flow from arteries to veins. Under normal physiological conditions, arterial blood flows into peripheral resistance vessels, and blood passing through the resistance vessels returns to the heart as venous blood. However, once access is created, arterial blood flows directly into the venous circulation without passing through the resistance vessels. Because the flow resistance of the venous circulation is much lower than that of the peripheral resistance vessels, more arterial blood enters the access than the peripheral circulation. Thus, blood flow in the peripheral artery decreases following the creation of an AVF or AVG. Peripheral circulatory disorders caused by VA are known as access-induced distal ischemia [2]. Coldness, numbness, pain, and finger ulceration due to access-induced distal ischemia have been observed. This phenomenon is a severe complication of VA and is reported to occur at a frequency of 1–8% [3].

Considering access-related systemic circulation changes, not only the peripheral arterial circulation but also all the arterial circulation could decrease due to the difference in flow resistance related to shunt access. The vertebral and common carotid arteries arise from the aorta or the subclavian artery. These arterial circulations may also deteriorate due to the access circulation owing to the difference in flow resistance from the limb artery on the AVF side; the effect may increase as the difference in flow resistance increases. The Japanese guidelines for VA state that a VA flow of more than 1500–2000 mL/min is a risk factor for cardiac failure [1]. In addition to the impact on cardiac function, high-flow VA may significantly hinder other systemic circulations due to extremely low flow resistance. A reverse flow phenomenon in the vertebral artery has been observed in some patients with high-flow access [4]. Subclavian steal syndrome (SSS) is caused by insufficient circulation in the vertebral artery. Although classical SSS occurs because of stenosis or the occlusion of the subclavian artery, SSS without arterial stenosis can be caused by a high-flow VA. It has been reported that VA-induced SSS evokes symptoms such as dizziness more often than SSS with stenosis [4]. Another study reported that VA flow suppression surgery improved SSS due to high-flow AVF [5]; however, the number of such case reports is limited, and the clinical influence of the VA on the vertebral circulation is not fully understood. Furthermore, the effect of VA flow suppression surgery on cervical circulation has rarely been reported.

Therefore, we conducted this study to determine the effects of VA flow suppression surgery on cervical circulation in patients with high-flow VA.

2. Materials and Methods

2.1. Patients and Study Design

This was a single-center, retrospective, observational study. The study participants were HD patients who underwent VA flow suppression surgery at the Kanno Dialysis and Access Clinic between September 2009 and November 2018. Patients whose cervical arterial flow was measured before and after blood flow suppression surgery were included in this study. VA flow volume (FV) and the FV of the bilateral vertebral and common carotid arteries were measured before and within 1 week after VA flow suppression surgery. Patients with an occluded vertebral or carotid artery were excluded because the pathogenesis of SSS differs with and without obstruction. Patients with insufficient clinical data were excluded. Other patient information, such as age, sex, dialysis vintage, diabetes, and medical cause for VA flow suppression surgery, were obtained from the medical records. Changes in patient symptoms after surgery were determined by checking the medical records.

We also examined the FV of the bilateral common carotid and vertebral arteries in eight healthy volunteers (HVs) and five patients with end-stage kidney disease (ESKD) before creating the VA for comparison.

The study protocol was approved by the ethics committee of Shinshu University (approval number 4631) and was conducted in accordance with the principles of the Declaration of Helsinki, as revised in 2013. Because of the retrospective nature of the study, informed consent was obtained in the form of an opt-out on the web and a poster announcement.

2.2. Measurement of Blood FV, Resistance Index (RI), and Cardiac Output (CO)

Blood flow was calculated as the FV based on ultrasound findings. The same ultrasonography equipment (Aplio 500; Toshiba, Tokyo, Japan) was used throughout this study. Pre-surgery measurements were performed 1 day before surgery, whereas post-surgery measurements were performed within 1 week after surgery, both at the time of pre-dialysis. The sonographic parameters were measured by the same technician. The estimated VA flow was calculated as the difference between the VA and non-VA sides of the brachial artery blood flow. The FV of the cervical arteries was measured at the straight part of the bilateral common carotid and vertebral arteries without stenosis. The RI of the brachial artery was also measured. In patients with a high origin of the radial artery, the estimated VA flow was calculated as the difference between the sum of the VA-side radial and ulnar artery flows and the non-VA-side brachial artery flow. These patients were excluded from the RI analysis because they could not be compared to other patients with normal branching patterns.

CO was also measured before and after surgery. CO was calculated using the biplane disk summation method based on a previous report [6]. CO pre-surgery measurements were performed 1 day before surgery, while post-surgery measurements were performed within 1 week after surgery, both at the time of pre-dialysis.

2.3. VA Flow Suppression Surgery

VA flow suppression surgery was performed according to the methods described in a previous report [7]. The surgeons selected the appropriate surgical method for each patient. The ligation was performed by ligating and obstructing the target artery using sutures. Banding was performed by narrowing the target artery or runoff vein by wrapping a synthetic graft around the target vessel and suturing the graft. The anastomosis was performed by narrowing the AVF anastomosis site with an exteriorizing anastomosis and suturing. AVG banding was performed by narrowing the synthetic graft via ligation. All VA flow suppression surgical procedures were continued until the VA flow decreased to the target level.

2.4. Statistical Analyses

Continuous variables are presented as medians and ranges, and the Mann–Whitney U test was used to compare the two groups. The Wilcoxon signed-rank test was used to compare two paired groups. Categorical variables are presented as percentages. Logistic regression analysis was used for multivariate analysis. Statistical significance was set at $p < 0.05$. The SPSS software (ver. 27; IBM Japan Corp., Tokyo, Japan) was used for statistical analyses. The datasets generated and/or analyzed in this study are available from the corresponding author upon reasonable request.

3. Results

VA flow suppression surgery was performed in 131 patients during the study period. After applying the exclusion criteria, 85 patients were included in this study (Figure 1). Table 1 presents the patient backgrounds. The median age of the patients was 64 years, and 66% ($n = 56$) were male. Seventy-three percent ($n = 62$) had radiocephalic AVF, and 8% ($n = 7$) had AVG. Eighty-seven percent ($n = 74$) of patients presented with symptoms before the surgery; the most common symptom was exertional breathlessness. The most common reason for VA flow suppression surgery was high-output heart failure. Three patients exhibited high-origin radial artery.

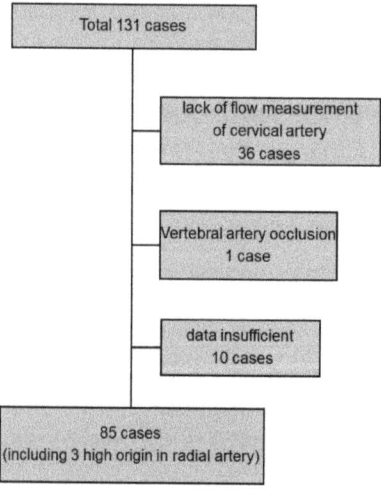

Figure 1. Patient selection.

Table 1. Patient characteristics.

Characteristics	
No. of patients	85
Age (years), n (range)	64 (28–87)
Male, n (%)	56 (66%)
Dialysis vintage (month), m (range)	88 (3–1341)
Diabetes mellitus, n (%)	11 (13%)
Left side access, n (%)	72 (85%)
Access type, n (%)	
Radiocephalic AVF	62 (73%)
Ulnar-basilic AVF	1 (1%)
Brachiocephalic AVF	15 (18%)
AVG	7 (8%)
Symptoms, n (%)	
Exertional breathlessness	51 (60%)
Palpitation	5 (6%)
Distal coldness	10 (12%)
Venous hypertension	12 (14%)
Dizziness	14 (16%)
Tinnitus	9 (11%)
Other neurological symptoms	5 (6%)
Other	4 (5%)
No symptoms	11 (13%)
Reasons for needing blood suppression, n (%)	
High-output heart failure	50 (59%)
Low cardiac function	10 (12%)
Venous hypertension	12 (14%)
Access vessel aneurysm	12 (14%)
Distal steal syndrome	8 (9%)
Subclavian steal syndrome	4 (5%)
Pulmonary hypertension	1 (1%)

Continuous variables are expressed as medians and ranges. Categorical variables were expressed as numbers and percentages. Abbreviation: AVF, arteriovenous fistula; AVG arteriovenous graft.

The median VA flow before VA flow suppression surgery was 1548 mL/min (Table 2). The median VA flow decreased significantly to 693 mL/min after surgery. Anastoplasty, proximal artery banding, and distal artery ligation were the most common surgical methods used to suppress the VA flow. The median preoperative RI was 0.44, which increased to 0.54 postoperatively (Table 3). The median CO was 4.5 L/min before the surgery, which significantly decreased to 4.3 L/min postoperatively.

For flow assessment of the cervical artery, the FV of the vertebral and common carotid arteries are shown in Figures 2 and 3, respectively. The median flow in the vertebral artery in patients with HVs and ESKD was 58 (23–165) mL/min and 90 (27–142) mL/min, respectively (Figure 2). The flows of the VA side vertebral artery in HD patients with high-flow access varied considerably, and four patients (5%) exhibited inverted flow, indicating the subclavian steal phenomenon. The flows of the VA-side vertebral artery were prone to be less than those of the non-VA side; however, the difference was not statistically significant (Table 3). The median flow of the common carotid artery in patients with HVs and ESKD was 440 (244–599) mL/min and 520 (391–677) mL/min, respectively (Figure 3). The median flow in the common carotid artery was identical between the VA and non-VA sides (Table 3). The preoperative flow of the vertebral artery did not differ significantly from that in patients with HVs and ESKD. Meanwhile, the preoperative flows of the common carotid artery were significantly lower than those in patients with ESKD ($p = 0.004$ and

p = 0.006, respectively) and tended to be lower than those in the HVs (p = 0.05, p = 0.06, respectively).

Table 2. Surgical methods for blood flow suppression and changes in the VA flow.

	n (%)	VA Flow (pre) (mL/min)	VA Flow (post) (mL/min)	p	Reduction Rate (%)
All cases	85	1548 (649–2453)	693 (321–1265)	<0.01	53 (18–83)
Surgical methods					
Proximal artery ligation	13 (15%)	1619 (891–2198)	514 (321–995)	<0.01	57 (29–83)
Proximal artery banding	10 (12%)	1396 (1114–2006)	621 (413–1248)	<0.01	57 (18–65)
Proximal artery banding and distal artery ligation	20 (24%)	1561 (1048–2453)	703 (353–1063)	<0.01	56 (29–78)
Anastoplasty	23 (27%)	1584 (649–2447)	723 (357–1248)	<0.01	48 (25–83)
Run-off vein banding	4 (5%)	1354 (904–2143)	666 (353–1265)	<0.01	54 (26–63)
AVG banding	6 (7%)	1252 (1036–1610)	580 (380–801)	<0.01	56 (34–72)
Other	9 (11%)	1633 (1192–2065)	859 (442–1208)	0.03	43 (20–72)

Continuous variables are expressed as medians and ranges. Categorical variables were expressed as numbers and percentages. Preoperative and postoperative differences were compared using the Wilcoxon signed-rank test. Other: Revision using distal inflow (RUDI), 3; distal radial artery ligation, 3; runoff vein ligation, 3. Abbreviations: VA, vascular access; AVG, arteriovenous graft

Table 3. Changes in the VA-related parameters and flow volume of cervical arteries.

Parameters	Pre-Surgery	Post-Surgery	p
Resistance index (RI)	0.44 (0.22~0.64)	0.54 (0.39~0.83)	<0.01
Cardiac output (CO) (L/min)	4.5 (2.4~9.9)	4.3 (2.3~8.6)	<0.01
Vertebral artery			
VA side flow (mL/min)	55 (−70~280)	81 (5~370)	<0.01
Non-VA side flow (mL/min)	70 (10~240)	69 (16~260)	0.20
Common carotid artery			
VA side flow (mL/min)	379 (140~759)	398 (212~850)	0.03
Non-VA side flow (mL/min)	376 (198~910)	397 (141~820)	0.02

Continuous variables are expressed as medians and ranges. Preoperative and postoperative differences were compared using the Wilcoxon signed-rank test.

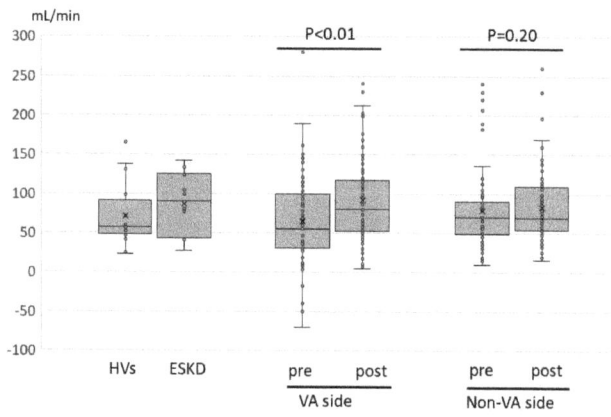

Figure 2. Vertebral artery flow volume of each participant group and changes before and after the surgery. Changes in the vertebral artery flow before and after flow suppression surgery are presented as box-and-whisker plots. Each data is presented as a circle, and the mean value is indicated by x. The p-values for comparison between vertebral artery flow of the HVs and VA side or non-VA side of the study participants were 0.49 and 0.37, respectively. The p-values for comparison between vertebral artery flow of ESKD patients before VA creation and VA side or non-VA side of the study participants were 0.12 and 0.29, respectively. Abbreviations: HVs, healthy volunteers; ESKD, end-stage kidney disease patients before vascular access creation; VA, vascular access.

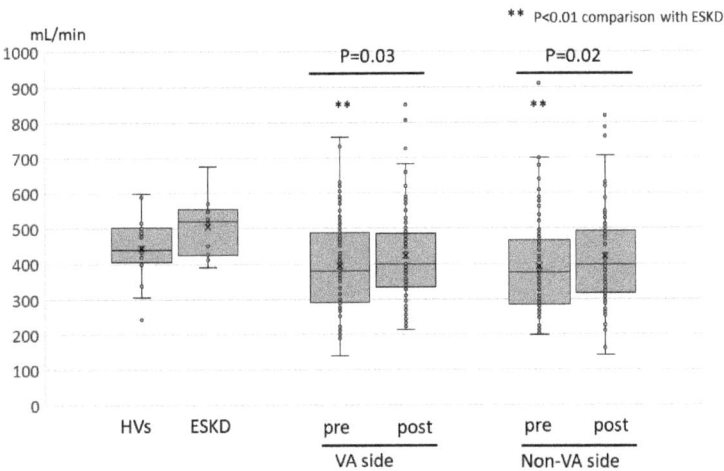

Figure 3. Common carotid artery flow volume of each participant group and changes before and after the surgery. Changes in common carotid artery flow before and after flow suppression surgery are presented as box-and-whisker plots. Each data is presented as a circle, and the mean value is indicated by x. The p-values for comparison between the common carotid artery flow of HVs and the VA side or non-VA side of the study participants were 0.06 and 0.05, respectively. The p-values for comparison between the common carotid artery flow of ESKD patients before VA creation and the VA side or non-VA side of the study participants were 0.005 and 0.004, respectively. Abbreviations: HVs, healthy volunteers; ESKD, end-stage kidney disease patients before vascular access creation; VA, vascular access.

After VA flow suppression surgery, the VA-side vertebral artery flow significantly increased from 55 to 81 mL/min. Four patients with inverted flow patterns returned to normal flow patterns after surgery (Figure S1). The vertebral artery flow on the non-VA side did not significantly change postoperatively (Table 3). VA flow suppression surgery also increased the flow volume of the common carotid arteries on both the VA and non-VA side (379 to 398 mL/min and 376 397 mL/min, respectively) (Table 3).

Symptoms improved in 63 of 74 (85%) patients who presented with symptoms before VA flow suppression surgery. Twenty-five (29%) patients presented with neurological symptoms, such as dizziness and/or tinnitus, which could indicate circulatory insufficiency of the cervical artery, and 18 of these patients had improved symptoms postoperatively. When the improved symptoms (n = 18) were compared with the non-improved symptoms (n = 7), the improved symptom group presented a significant increase in flow change in the VA-side vertebral artery (Table 4). The changes in vertebral artery flow in each patient group according to symptoms are presented in Figure S2. The other arterial flows did not differ between the groups (Table 4).

We conducted a multivariate analysis to investigate the factors related to a larger increasing effect on the vertebral artery after surgery. Age, sex, pre-surgical vertebral artery flow, and CO were selected as basic patient characteristics. The VA flow suppression rate was selected as the effect of VA flow suppression surgery. Multivariate analysis revealed that a lower preoperative CO was associated with a larger flow-increasing effect on the vertebral artery (Table 5).

Table 4. Comparison between the neurological symptom improved group and non-improved group.

	Symptoms Improved	Non-Improved	p
n (%)	17 (68%)	8 (32%)	
Flow reduction rate, n (%)	58.5 (34~78)	61.0 (25~77)	1.00
Vertebral artery			
VA side flow change (mL/min)	48 (−53~160)	2 (−81~90)	0.02
Non-VA side flow change (mL/min)	5 (−48~90)	6 (−30~46)	0.84
Common carotid artery			
VA side flow change (mL/min)	20 (−88~210)	−6 (−100~360)	0.75
Non-VA side flow change (mL/min)	11 (−83~250)	119 (−203~261)	0.37

Continuous variables are expressed as medians and ranges. Categorical variables are expressed as numbers and percentages. Differences between groups were compared using the Mann–Whitney U test. Abbreviations: VA; vascular access.

Table 5. Univariate and multivariate analyses for the flow-increasing effect in the vertebral artery after flow suppression surgery.

Parameters	Univariate			Multivariate		
	Odds Ratio	CI	p	Odds Ratio	CI	p
Age	1.01	0.97–1.04	0.75	1.00	0.96–1.05	0.86
Male	1.15	0.47–2.82	0.76	1.46	0.54–3.89	0.46
Flow reduction rate	1.02	0.99–1.05	0.30	1.02	0.99–1.01	0.99
Pre-Vertebral A flow	1.00	0.99–1.01	0.56	1.00	0.99–1.01	0.49
Pre-CO	0.74	0.54–1.03	0.07	0.70	0.49–0.99	0.04

Factors related to a larger flow-increasing effect in the vertebral artery were analyzed using logistic regression analysis. Abbreviations: Pre-CO, presurgical cardiac output; CI, confidence interval.

Similarly, we investigated factors related to a larger increase in the common carotid artery after surgery. Multivariate analysis revealed that a lower presurgical FV of the common carotid artery was associated with a larger increase in the flow of the common carotid artery (Table 6).

Table 6. Univariate and multivariate analyses for the flow-increasing effect in the common carotid artery after flow suppression surgery.

Parameters	Univariate			Multivariate		
	Odds Ratio	CI	p	Odds Ratio	CI	p
Age	1.00	0.97–1.03	0.98	0.99	0.95–1.03	0.56
Male	0.61	0.25–1.51	0.29	0.86	0.31–2.37	0.77
Flow reduction rate	1.01	0.98–1.04	0.49	1.02	0.99–1.05	0.24
Pre-CCA flow	0.99	0.99–1.00	<0.01	0.99	0.98–0.99	0.01
Pre-CO	0.80	0.58–1.09	0.15	0.90	0.63–1.29	0.57

Factors related to a larger flow-increasing effect in the common carotid artery were analyzed using logistic regression. Pre-CCA, pre-surgical common carotid artery; pre-CO, pre-surgical cardiac output; CI, confidence interval.

4. Discussion

The current study revealed that VA flow suppression surgery for high-flow access increases the FV of the vertebral and common carotid arteries. Previous studies have reported that high-flow VA can invoke SSS [5,8,9]. Although no obstructions or stenoses existed in the subclavian artery, reversed blood flow of the VA-side vertebral artery was observed in patients with high-flow VA due to the pressure gradient via extremely low VA-side flow resistance. This was a high-flow VA-associated subclavian steal phenomenon.

Previous reports have indicated that stopping VA flow via manual compression or closure of the VA normalized the flow pattern of the vertebral artery in cases of high-flow VA-associated subclavian steal phenomenon [4,8]. In this study, the reversed flow patterns of the vertebral artery were all normalized postoperatively. We observed that patients without reversed flow patterns in the vertebral artery also showed improved FV of the vertebral artery postoperatively. This phenomenon may be due to a decrease in the pressure gradient caused by an increase in the VA flow resistance. Patients in this study did not have a significant decrease in the FV of the VA-side vertebral artery compared with the small number of HVs and ESKD patients. However, blood flow in the vertebral artery varies physiologically among individuals, and the FV of the vertebral artery in patients with HVs and ESKD in this study was widely distributed. The small sample size and wide variation in patients with HVs and ESKD in this study may have prevented the detection of such differences. A previous study measuring the FV of the vertebral artery using sonography in 96 healthy people reported that the mean FV of the vertebral artery was 85 ± 37 mL/min [10], which was larger than the data in this study population. Thus, the blood flow of the vertebral artery in patients with high-flow VA might be lower than that in the healthy population.

Reduced blood flow in the vertebral artery may induce circulatory insufficiency in the vertebrobasilar arterial system. Patients with SSS are prone to dizziness due to vertebrobasilar insufficiency [11]. Symptoms, such as dizziness and tinnitus, were frequently observed in this study population next to heart failure symptoms. When we performed a subgroup analysis of patients with these neurological symptoms before surgery, patients with improved postoperative symptoms exhibited a larger increase in vertebral artery flow than patients with non-improved symptoms. Therefore, reduced blood flow in the vertebral artery could induce neurological symptoms, and VA flow suppression surgery for high-flow VA could improve neurological symptoms via augmentation of vertebral artery flow.

It is known that the cerebral blood flow of HD patients is reduced during HD sessions and is affected by the ultrafiltration volume, filtration rate, and the acid–base balance changes [12]. HD patients with insufficient vertebral artery blood flow due to high-flow VA may exhibit symptoms, such as dizziness due to vertebrobasilar insufficiency, during HD sessions. A previous study reported that patients with symptoms had a high risk of stroke [11]. Thus, HD patients with vertebrobasilar insufficiency symptoms should undergo evaluation of their vertebral artery blood flow and VA flow to prevent future stroke.

Our study also revealed that VA flow suppression surgery could improve vertebral artery blood flow in patients with reduced CO. As the proportion of VA flow to the total circulation was large in patients with high-flow VA, the proportion of other systemic circulations was limited, especially in patients with reduced CO. Thus, patients with reduced CO may have markedly increased systemic circulation, including that of the vertebral artery, after surgery. Patients with a high-flow VA and reduced CO may benefit more from surgery.

This study also revealed that blood flow in the common carotid artery improved postoperatively. To the best of our knowledge, this is the first report describing the impact of VA flow suppression surgery on the common carotid artery. When the flow resistance of the VA is significantly lower than that of the systemic circulation, various parts of the circulatory system with flow resistance higher than that of the VA may be affected. The common carotid artery is thicker than the vertebral artery, its flow resistance is lower than that of the vertebral artery, and its blood flow is higher. Thus, because the vertebral arteries inherently have less blood flow than the common carotid arteries, attention tends to focus on the effects on the vertebral arteries, which are more prone to malperfusion symptoms when blood flow is reduced. However, the current results showed that the FV of the common carotid artery was also affected by high-flow VA, which was less than that in patients with ESKD, and was improved by VA flow suppression surgery. Further research is required to verify whether the impact of high-flow VA on the flow of the common carotid artery causes any clinically relevant problems.

This study has several limitations. First, this was a single-center retrospective study, and we could not examine parameters that were not recorded. Therefore, we cannot exclude the effects of uncoordinated confounders. Second, all patients included in this study underwent blood flow suppression surgery for the treatment of high-flow VA; therefore, a selection bias may have been present when deciding on VA flow suppression surgery. Additional studies are required to demonstrate the impact of normal-flow VA on cervical circulation. Third, because the flow volumes of the VA, vertebral artery, and common carotid artery before and after VA flow suppression surgery were measured at one point, it is unclear how long this effect lasts for cervical circulation. A prospective observational study with a longer observation period is required to confirm this finding. Fourth, this was an observational study with no control group, and changes in the symptoms of the patients were examined through interviews with medical staff related to the VA flow suppression surgery. Therefore, the results of this study relating to symptom changes after surgery may have contained information bias.

5. Conclusions

In conclusion, VA flow suppression surgery in patients with high-flow VA increased blood flow to the VA-side vertebral artery and bilateral common carotid arteries along with improving various symptoms caused by high flow volume. High-flow VA can decrease the vertebral and common carotid circulation. Medical staff involved in HD should measure VA flow not only in patients with VA troubles but also in patients who present with neurological symptoms such as dizziness or reduced CO. When the measured VA flow is large, medical staff should consider performing VA flow suppression surgery.

Supplementary Materials: The following supporting information can be downloaded at: https://www.mdpi.com/article/10.3390/jcm13030641/s1, Figure S1: Flow pattern change in the vertebral artery before and after VA flow suppression surgery; Figure S2: (A) Changes in VA side vertebral artery flow volume of each patient group according to the symptoms; (B) Changes in non-VA side vertebral artery flow volume of each patient group according to the symptoms.

Author Contributions: Conceptualization, K.H.; methodology, K.H.; formal analysis, K.H., M.H. and Y.Y.; investigation, K.H., T.K., Y.K. (Yutaka Kanno) and Y.K. (Yuji Kamijo); writing—original draft preparation, K.H.; writing—review and editing, Y.K. (Yuji Kamijo), M.H. and Y.Y. All authors have read and agreed to the published version of the manuscript.

Funding: This research received no external funding.

Institutional Review Board Statement: The study protocol was approved by the ethics committee of Shinshu University (approval number 4631) and was conducted in accordance with the principles of the Declaration of Helsinki, as revised in 2013.

Informed Consent Statement: Because of the retrospective nature of the study, informed consent was obtained in the form of an opt-out on the web and a poster announcement.

Data Availability Statement: Data are contained within the article and supplementary materials.

Acknowledgments: The authors thank Kazunari Shiroi for contributing to accurate sonographic measurements.

Conflicts of Interest: Author Taro Kanno and Yutaka Kanno were employed by the Kanno Dialysis and Vascular Access Clinic. The remaining authors declare that the research was conducted in the absence of any commercial or financial relationships that could be construed as a potential conflict of interest.

References

1. Kukita, K.; Ohira, S.; Amano, I.; Naito, H.; Azuma, N.; Ikeda, K.; Kanno, Y.; Satou, T.; Sakai, S.; Sugimoto, T.; et al. 2011 update Japanese Society for Dialysis Therapy guidelines of vascular access construction and repair for chronic hemodialysis. *Ther. Apher. Dial.* **2015**, *19* (Suppl. S1), 1–39. [CrossRef] [PubMed]
2. Beathard, G.A.; Jennings, W.C.; Wasse, H.; Shenoy, S.; Hentschel, D.M.; Abreo, K.; Urbanes, A.; Nassar, G.; Dolmatch, B.; Davidson, I.; et al. ASDIN white paper: Assessment and management of hemodialysis access-induced distal ischemia by interventional nephrologists. *J. Vasc. Access* **2020**, *21*, 543–553. [CrossRef]

3. Beathard, G.A.; Spergel, L.M. Hand ischemia associated with dialysis vascular access: An individualized access flow-based approach to therapy. *Semin. Dial.* **2013**, *26*, 287–314. [CrossRef] [PubMed]
4. Kargiotis, O.; Siahos, S.; Safouris, A.; Feleskouras, A.; Magoufis, G.; Tsivgoulis, G. Subclavian steal syndrome with or without arterial stenosis: A review. *J. Neuroimaging* **2016**, *26*, 473–480. [CrossRef] [PubMed]
5. Kaneko, Y.; Yanagawa, T.; Taru, Y.; Hayashi, S.; Zhang, H.; Tsukahara, T.; Matsunaga, T.; Ishizu, T. Subclavian steal syndrome in a hemodialysis patient after percutaneous transluminal angioplasty of arteriovenous access. *J. Vasc. Access* **2018**, *19*, 404–408. [CrossRef]
6. Lang, R.M.; Badano, L.P.; Mor-Avi, V.; Afilalo, J.; Armstrong, A.; Ernande, L.; Flachskampf, F.A.; Foster, E.; Goldstein, S.A.; Kuznetsova, T.; et al. Recommendations for cardiac chamber quantification by echocardiography in adults: An update from the American Society of Echocardiography and the European Association of Cardiovascular Imaging. *J. Am. Soc. Echocardiogr.* **2015**, *28*, 1–39. [CrossRef] [PubMed]
7. Kanno, T.; Kamijo, Y.; Hashimoto, K.; Kanno, Y. Outcomes of blood flow suppression methods of treating high flow access in hemodialysis patients with arteriovenous fistula. *J. Vasc. Access* **2015**, *16* (Suppl. S10), S28–S33. [CrossRef] [PubMed]
8. Naidich, J.B.; Weiss, A.; Molmenti, E.P.; Naidich, J.J.; Pellerito, J.S. An interesting observation regarding retrograde vertebral artery flow in patients with dialysis access fistulas. *J. Ultrasound Med.* **2019**, *38*, 2703–2707. [CrossRef]
9. Miyawaki, D.; Nomura, T.; Kubota, H.; Wada, N.; Keira, N.; Tatsumi, T. Angiographic visualization of high-flow arteriovenous fistula-induced subclavian steal syndrome. *Cardiovasc. Interv. Ther.* **2021**, *36*, 544–546. [CrossRef] [PubMed]
10. Yazici, B.; Erdoğmuş, B.; Tugay, A. Cerebral blood flow measurements of the extracranial carotid and vertebral arteries with Doppler ultrasonography in healthy adults. *Diagn. Interv. Radiol.* **2005**, *11*, 195–198. [PubMed]
11. Tan, X.; Bai, H.X.; Wang, Z.; Yang, L. Risk of stroke in imaging-proven subclavian steal syndrome. *J. Clin. Neurosci.* **2017**, *41*, 168–169. [CrossRef]
12. Polinder-Bos, H.A.; García, D.V.; Kuipers, J.; Elting, J.W.J.; Aries, M.J.H.; Krijnen, W.P.; Groen, H.; Willemsen, A.T.M.; van Laar, P.J.; Strijkert, F.; et al. Hemodialysis induces an acute decline in cerebral blood flow in elderly patients. *J. Am. Soc. Nephrol.* **2018**, *29*, 1317–1325. [CrossRef]

Disclaimer/Publisher's Note: The statements, opinions and data contained in all publications are solely those of the individual author(s) and contributor(s) and not of MDPI and/or the editor(s). MDPI and/or the editor(s) disclaim responsibility for any injury to people or property resulting from any ideas, methods, instructions or products referred to in the content.

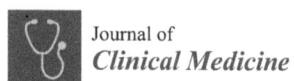

Brief Report

The Influence of Healthy Habits on Cognitive Functions in a Group of Hemodialysis Patients

Piotr Olczyk, Patryk Jerzak, Krzysztof Letachowicz, Tomasz Gołębiowski, Magdalena Krajewska and Mariusz Kusztal *

Department of Nephrology and Transplantation Medicine, Wroclaw Medical University, 50-367 Wroclaw, Poland
* Correspondence: mariusz.kusztal@umw.edu.pl

Abstract: (1) Background: Cognitive impairment (CI) is more prevalent in hemodialysis (HD) patients than in the general population. The purpose of this study was to examine if behavioral, clinical, and vascular variables are linked with CI in individuals with HD. (2) Methods: Initially, 47 individuals with chronic HD volunteered to participate in the trial, but only 27 patients ultimately completed the Montreal Cognitive Assessment (MoCA) and the Computerized Cognitive Assessment Tool (CompBased-CAT). We collected information on smoking, mental activities, physical activity (Rapid Assessment of Physical Activity, RAPA), and comorbidity. The oxygen saturation (rSO2) and pulse wave velocity (PWV; IEM Mobil-O-Graph) of the frontal lobes were measured. (3) Results: Significant associations were discovered between MoCA and rSO2 ($r = 0.44$, $p = 0.02$ and $r = 0.62$, $p = 0.001$, right/left, respectively), PWV ($r = -0.69$, $p = 0.0001$), CCI ($r = 0.59$, $p = 0.001$), and RAPA ($r = 0.72$, $p = 0.0001$). Those who actively occupied their time during dialysis and non-smokers achieved higher cognitive exam results. A multivariate regression study demonstrated that physical activity (RAPA) and PWV had separate effects on cognitive performance. (4) Conclusions: Cognitive skills are related to inter-dialysis healthy habits (physical activity, smoking) and intra-dialysis activities (tasks and mind games). Arterial stiffness, oxygenation of the frontal lobes, and CCI were linked with CI.

Keywords: hemodialysis; cognitive functions; risk factors

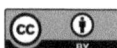

1. Introduction

The prevalence of treated end-stage kidney disease (ESKD) has increased worldwide, likely due to improving ESKD survival, population demographic shifts and increasing access to dialysis programs in countries with growing economies. The unadjusted 5-year survival of ESKD patients on kidney replacement therapy was 41% in the USA, 48% in Europe, and 60% in Japan [1]. Hemodialysis is the most common modality of kidney replacement therapy. In 2020, approximately 786,000 people in the United States had ESKD, 71% of whom were dialysed [2]. Reduced quality of life, especially in the area of mental health, is still the subject of research in this group of patients.

Mild cognitive impairment (MCI) is found in 30% to 60% of the overall population of dialysis patients, and it involves persistent cognitive impairment and behavioural disturbances. One of the hypotheses regarding how chronic kidney disease (CKD) affects cognitive impairment is vascular damage in conjunction with malnutrition or inflammation. Moreover, compelling evidence demonstrates a decline in cerebral mean flow velocity and white matter hyperintensities with hemodialysis.

In connection with the above hypothesis, the factors that may potentially affect the cognitive abilities of hemodialysis patients are the condition of their blood vessels, as well as blood flow and oxygenation of their brain tissue. Arterial stiffness determined by pulse wave velocity (PWV) is one of the validated parameters that shows the overall condition of blood vessels in the body. Studies reveal that hemodialysis patients show increased vascular stiffness compared to patients with CKD stage 4 and patients after kidney transplantation [3]. Brain oxygenation can be non-invasively assessed using near-infrared spectroscopy (NIRS). It has been proven that hemodialysis patients show a significantly reduced rSO2 compared with the general population [4]. On the other hand, the most plausible hypothesis is that the damage may be caused by uremic (neuro) toxins produced in the course of CKD. It is also speculated that kidney failure prevents the production of neuroprotective factors, resulting in the suffering of the brain in CKD [5,6].

The association of a greater frequency of MCI beyond the age of 60 with the age-dominant group of dialysis patients—likewise 60 and older—is also reflected in the increased mortality, therefore, acquires therapeutic importance [7].

Cognitive impairment in hemodialysis patients is common and refers to many domains, such as cognitive-motor function, language, executive function, learning and memory, and complex attention. According to a study conducted, executive function and memory are the cognitive functions most closely linked to mortality [7,8].

Among cognitive function tests, the Montreal cognitive assessment test (MoCA) is characterised by the highest precision [9] with great sensitivity in the group of hemodialysis patients [10]. A recent Cochrane library review of the evidence also underlined the accuracy of the MoCA test for detecting dementia [11]. Computer-Based Cognitive Assessment Tool (CompBased-CAT)—CogniFit—is an advanced assessment made via a web browser or mobile app. It allows the assessment of specific cognitive abilities, such as concentration/attention, memory, reasoning, planning, or coordination. CompBased-CAT has already been validated in other groups of patients [12] and can be efficiently combined with an intervention tailored to the patient's needs (training module).

The purpose of the study was to determine whether vascular stiffness, brain oxidation, comorbidities, and certain healthy behaviours impact cognitive impairment assessed by MoCA and CompBased-CAT in a cohort of hemodialysis patients.

2. Materials and Methods

Seventy-five hemodialysis maintenance patients were considered for the study at the academic dialysis centre. Study exclusion criteria included manual disability of the upper limbs, severe vision problems, being previously diagnosed and treated by a psychiatrist due to dementia or Alzheimer's disease, post-stroke condition, lack of sign of informed consent, less than 3 months on renal replacement therapy, and the patient's refusal to participate in the study. Patients have been adequately dialysed a minimum of 3 times a week and achieved a target $Kt/V > 1.4$. Each patient had the results of basic laboratory tests (urea, potassium, sodium, calcium, phosphates, parathyroid hormone, and haemoglobin level) taken before the dialysis session (Table 1). None of the patients was taking drugs influencing the central nervous system.

Finally, 20 men and 7 women completed all tests and measures in this pilot study (Figure 1). The average age is 51 years (21–80 years), and the average dialysis vintage is 2 years (Table 1). Patients were examined by trained personnel and completed a battery of cognitive tests: The MOCA test and, additionally, the multi-domain cognitive assessment battery by CogniFit™, which is a commercial online application and an example of Comp-Based-CAT. A cognitive function assessment was performed before the hemodialysis session. The Cognifit contains visual, auditory, and cross-modal tasks, including puzzles, problem-solving, and reaction time games. The CogniFit test was completed using a mobile application installed on the tablet (Galaxy Tab A6, Samsung electronics, Korea). All patients had been able to operate mobile devices (tablets, smartphones) before being tested. Due to the need to use both hands for some tasks, it would be impossible for patients with a dialysis fistula to complete the test during a dialysis session. Oxygen saturation (rSO2) of frontal cerebral lobes (INVOS 5100c system) and PWV (IEM Mo-bil-O-Graph) were measured. The INVOS 5100c system uses near-infrared spectroscopy to assess brain oxygenation non-invasively. The IEM Mo-bil-O-Graph uses oscillometric methods by detecting data from the cuff during inflation and converting it using patented algorithms to estimate PWV. Clinical and laboratory data were also recorded. Patient regular passive or active (reading, crossword solving, electronic games) behaviour during sessions was noted. For each patient, the Charlson Comorbidity Index (CCI) was calculated, which is a validated tool for assessing 10-year mortality from patient morbidity data. [13,14]. Physical activity levels were measured using the Physical Activity Rapid Assessment (RAPA), a self-administered questionnaire consisting of nine binary questions (answer yes or no) presented textually and graphically. The questionnaire had already been used in a group of elderly and hemodialysis patients [15,16].

Table 1. Patients' characteristics and results.

	Mean	Median (IQR)/%
Age	51.3	53 (34; 68)
BMI	25.5	24.5 (21.5; 32)
Dialysis vintage	2.37	2 (0.5; 3)
Smoking	13	48%
Diabetes	6	22.20%
Hypertension	16	59.20%
Hemoglobin g/dL	10.7	10.2 (9.6; 11.1)
Urea mg/dL	130	134 (78; 175)
Potassium mmol/L	5.5	5.69 (3.6; 6.1)
Sodium mmol/L	138	140 (131; 145)
Calcium mg/dL	8.9	8.7 (7.3; 12.1)
Phosphorus mg/L	6.3	5.9 (3.1; 10.8)
Parathyroid hormone pg/mL	829	857 (30; 1547)
Residual diuresis (>500 mL)	12	44.40%
Charlson Comorbidity Index (CCI)	4.6	5 (2; 7)
rSO2 front R **	57%	59 (49; 56)
rSO2 front L	54%	53 (49; 66)
MoCA	25.7	28 (23; 29)
RAPA	2.8	3 (0; 6)
Cognifit total score	312.7	321 (212; 371)
Processing speed	269	232 (117; 382)
Shifting of attention	261	214 (58; 384)
Visual short-term memory	254	199 (27; 350)
Auditory short-term memory	315	337 (200; 403)
Working memory	285	256 (188; 423)
Naming	327	373 (98; 528)

BMI—body mass index. ** rSO2 front—oxygen saturation of frontal lobe. R—right. L—left. MoCA—Montreal Cognitive Assessment. RAPA—Physical Activity Rapid Assessment.

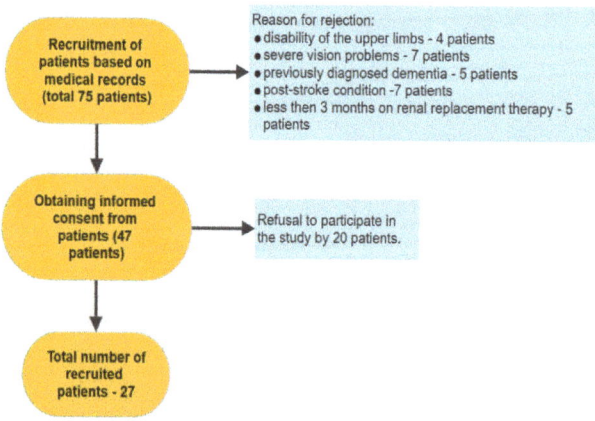

Figure 1. Recruitment process diagram.

With the potential intradialytic hypotension and feeling of exhaustion at the end of the HD session taken into account, all cognitive tests, as well as RAPA and behavioural anamnesis, were taken in the first hour of the session.

Statistical power (sample size estimation) analysis was conducted, determining the minimum r = 0.51, at which the test power was 0.8 (assumptions n = 27, α = 0.05). Multivariate regression analysis was performed among parameters showing significance in univariate analysis (no more than 3 parameters in each model tested).

All procedures performed in this study were in accordance with the ethical standards of our institutional research committee and with the 1964 Helsinki declaration and its later amendments. Informed consent was obtained from all individual participants included in the study.

3. Results

Patients' characteristics, as well as measured results, are displayed in Table 1. The median MoCA score is 28 (IQR 23;29). The CompBased-CAT total score is 321 (IQR 212; 371). Median saturation (rSO2) is more profoundly reduced in the left frontal lobe when compared with the right (53% vs. 59%).

3.1. Univariate Analysis

The MoCA results in univariate analysis correlate with rSO2 front R (r = 0.44, p = 0.02), rSO2 front L (r = 0.62, p = 0.001), PWV (r = −0.69, p = 0.0001), CCI (r = −0.59, p = 0.001), RAPA (r = 0.72, p = 0.0001) (Figure 2). Statistically significant correlations were found between the CompBased-CAT result and rSO2 front R (r = 0.49, p = 0.009), rSO2 front L (r = 0.65, p = 0.0001), PWV (r = −0.64, p = 0.0001), CCI (r = −0.58, p = 0.002), RAPA (r = 0.56, p = 0.002) (Figure 3). Both in the case of correlation with MoCA and Cognifit rSO2, the R front did not reach the required test power. Additionally, the CompBased-CAT score correlates with MoCA (r = 0.85, p = 0.0001). The interrelationships between the parameters are presented in the correlation matrix (Figure 4).

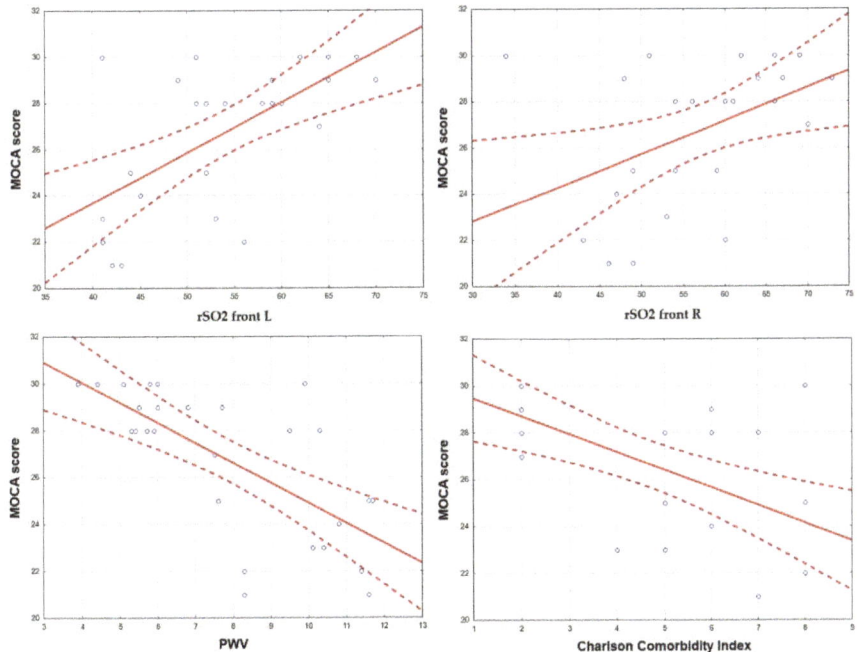

Figure 2. Correlation of the MOCA score with rSO2 front R, rSO2 front L, PWV, and CCI.

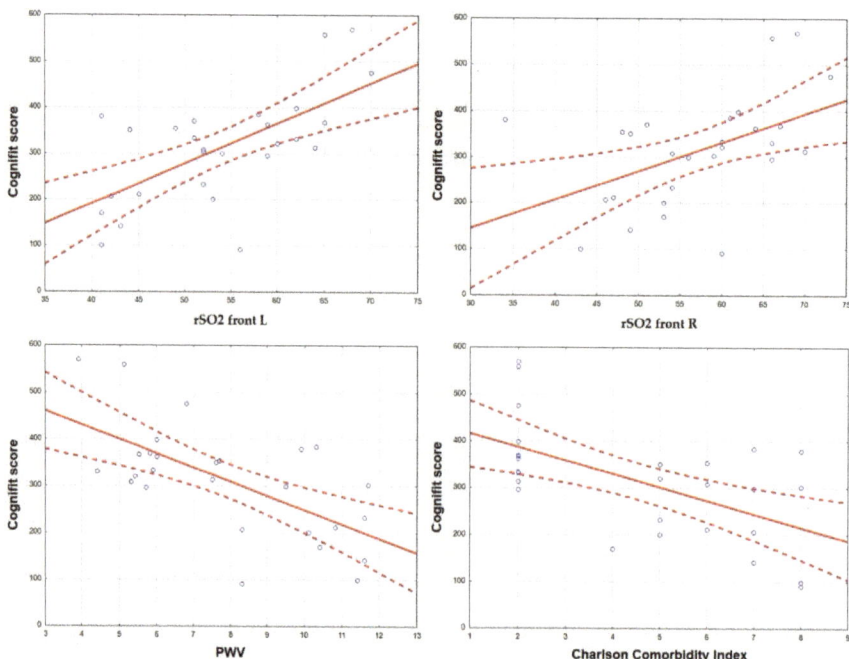

Figure 3. Correlation of the CompBased-CAT (Cognifit score) with rSO2 front R, rSO2 front L, PWV, and CCI.

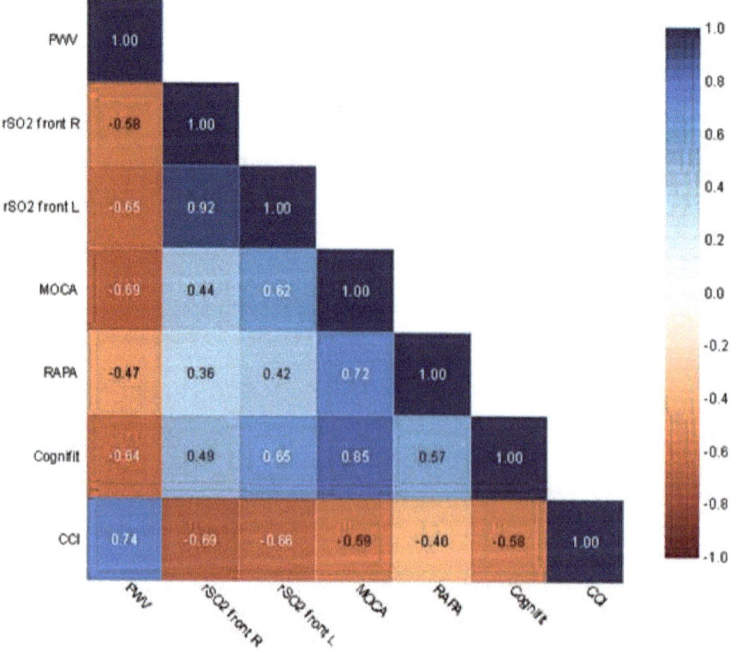

Figure 4. Correlation Matrix.

In addition, patients who actively spend time on dialysis score higher in the CompBased-CAT and MOCA tests (CompBased-CAT: 386 vs. 233, $p = 0.0002$; MOCA: 28.6 vs. 24.7, $p = 0.0002$; and active vs. non-active, respectively) (Figure 5) and use social media (CompBased-CAT: 352 vs. 255, $p = 0.03$; MOCA: 27.8 vs. 25.2, $p = 0.026$; and users vs. non-media users, respectively) (Figure 6). Markedly higher scores in the CompBased-CAT test are obtained by non-smokers (370 vs. 250, $p = 0.006$, non-smokers vs. smokers, respectively); however, in the case of the MoCA test, the difference was not statistically significant (27.7 vs. 25.7, $p = 0.09$) (Figure 7). There was no correlation between the results of cognitive tests and the concentration of urea, potassium, sodium, phosphates, calcium, and haemoglobin before dialysis. In addition, smokers also showed increased vascular stiffness (mean PWV 8.9 vs. 6.9, $p = 0.04$) and less physical activity correlated with increased PWV ($r = -0.47$, $p = 0.014$).

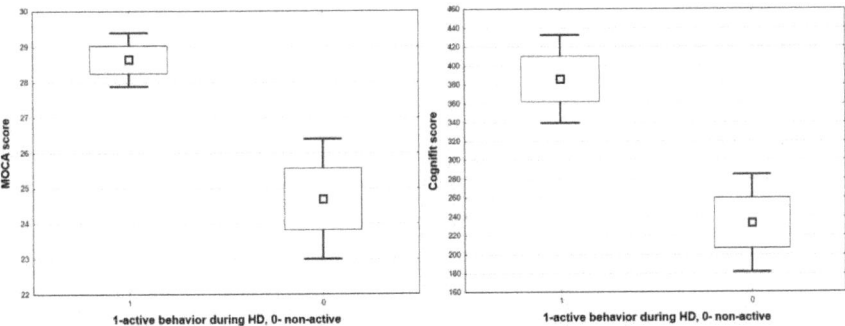

Figure 5. Box-whisker graph of CompBased-CAT (Cognifit score) and MOCA vs. HD session activity.

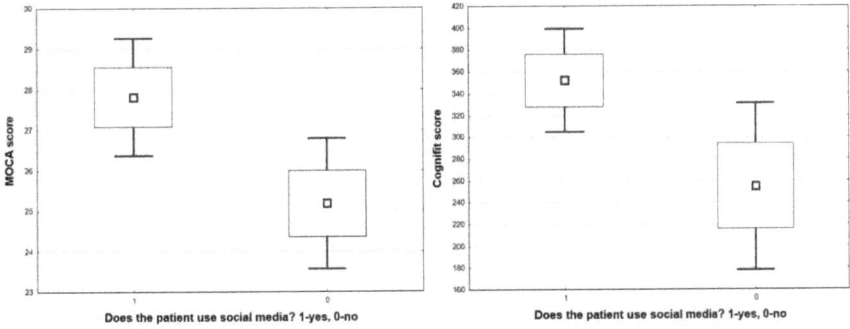

Figure 6. Box-whisker graph of CompBased-CAT (Cognifit score) and MOCA vs. using social media.

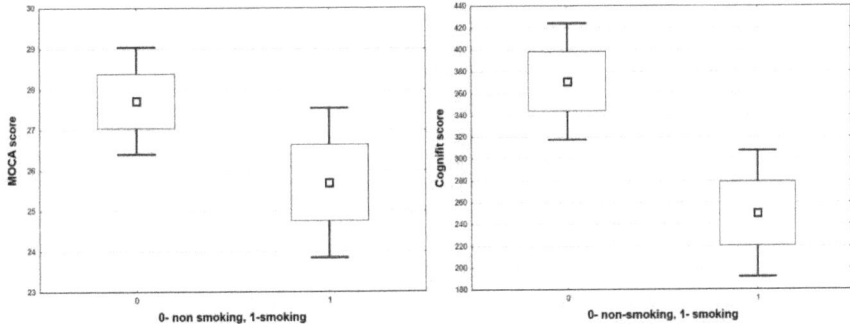

Figure 7. Box-whisker graph of CompBased-CAT (Cognifit score) and MOCA vs. smoking.

3.2. Multivariate Analysis

Results of the multiple linear regression indicate that there is a very strong collective significant effect between the PWV, RAPA, and MOCA (F = 25.76, $p < 0.001$, $R^2 = 0.68$, R^2adj = 0.66) (Table 2). Multivariate analysis of the same parameters with the CompBased-CAT confirms their correlation with cognitive functions (F = 12.03, $p < 0.001$, $R^2 = 0.5$, R^2adj = 0.46). (Table 3). In addition, the correlation between rSO2 front L, RAPA and cognitive function is demonstrated—MOCA (F = 21.63, $p < 0.001$, $R^2 = 0.64$, R^2adj = 0.61) and CompBased-CAT (F = 13.15, $p < 0.001$, $R^2 = 0.52$, R^2adj = 0.48) (Tables 4 and 5). In the multiple linear regression models, the power of the test was above 0.8. No other correlations were found using the multivariate model.

Table 2. MOCA/PWV/RAPA multiple linear regression (adjusted $R^2 = 0.66$; MOCA = 28.892 − 0.563 PWV + 0.810 RAPA).

	Coeff.	SE	t-Stat	Stand Coeff.	p-Value
PWV	−0.56	0.16	−3.5	−0.46	0.002
RAPA	0.81	0.21	3.91	0.51	0.001

Table 3. CompBased-CAT/PWV/RAPA multiple linear regression (adjusted $R^2 = 0.46$; Cognifit = 433.605623 + 20.873369 RAPA − 22.85519 PWV).

	Coeff.	SE	t-Stat	Stand Coeff.	p-Value
PWV	−22.86	7.75	−2.95	−0.48	0.007
RAPA	20.87	9.99	2.09	0.34	0.047

Table 4. MOCA/rSO2 front L/RAPA multiple linear regression (adjusted $R^2 = 0.61$; MOCA = 16.918 + 0.889 RAPA + 0.135 rSO2 front L).

	Coeff.	SE	t-Stat	Stand Coeff.	p-Value
rSO2 L	0.14	0.05	2.88	0.39	0.008
RAPA	0.89	0.21	4.15	0.56	0.0003

Table 5. CompBased-CAT/rSO2 front L/RAPA multiple linear regression (adjusted $R^2 = 0.48$; Cognifit = −109.901 + 21.790 RAPA + 6.681 rSO2 front L).

	Coeff.	SE	t-Stat	Stand Coeff.	p-Value
rSO2 L	6.68	2.09	3.2	0.5	0.004
RAPA	21.79	9.52	2.29	0.36	0.031

4. Discussion

In the current study, cognitive function (executive functions, in particular) measured by the MoCA test and Computer-Based Cognitive Assessment Tool was analysed. Moreover, their relationship to arterial stiffness (a surrogate for vessel damages), frontal lobes oxygen saturation, and healthy habits were analysed in a cohort of hemodialysis patients.

Cognitive impairment in hemodialysis patients, called since the 1960s "dialysis dementia", is still a serious problem influencing patient compliance and, what is more relevant, also survival. In the COGNITIVE-HD study, CI occurred in 474/676 patients. It also occurs significantly more often in dialysis (36%) than in non-dialysed (25%) patients in Japan [17]. Additionally, hemodialysis is associated with a higher risk of CI than peritoneal dialysis, and renal transplantation significantly reduces CI symptoms [18,19]. In the last decades, many risk factors for the loss of cognitive abilities have been identified in hemodialysis patients. There are traditional factors, such as the level of education or the presence of depression and factors related to dialysis, e.g., dialysis vintage and the presence of specific inflammatory factors [20]. Awareness of these factors can help identify the patients most at risk of developing cognitive deficits. To assess cognitive function in hemodialysis patients, both the standardised Montreal cognitive assessment (MoCA) [21] and the novel CompBased-CAT are also good options for those above 60 years of age [12,22]. Such an approach seems to be a feasible assessment strategy for multimorbid older adults with or without cognitive impairment.

In this study, various risk factors of cognitive decline have been assessed. Parameters such as rSO2 of the frontal lobes, PWV, CCI score, physical activity, and the way of spending time during dialysis were examined. The first negative correlation was found between the result of cognitive tests and CCI (CompBased-CAT $r = -0.57$, MoCA $r = -0.59$). CCI has not yet been associated with cognitive impairment in the group of hemodialysis patients. Such a relationship has already been found among patients with mild-to-moderate Alzheimer's disease [23]. Such a relationship has not been confirmed in a group of elderly people with dementia [24]. CCI may be another useful indicator of the risk of cognitive impairment in hemodialysis patients.

We measured the frontal lobe oxygen saturation (rSO2) to confirm the metabolic risk factor of dementia, which is more prominent in dialysis patients. It is mainly due to repeated brain hypoperfusion during hemodialysis sessions, namely, intradialytic blood pressure changes cause declines in cerebral oxygenation saturation during HD. It was recently confirmed in a cerebrovascular reactivity study using a combination of functional MRI and cerebral oxygenation saturation [25]. Studies show that cerebral flow measured using transcranial Doppler ultrasound to measure cerebral arterial mean flow velocity (MFV) is reduced in hemodialysis patients. [26]. The right frontal lobe is related to the formation of new cognitive processes, while the left frontal lobe is crucial "for the cognitive selection driven by the content of working memory and for context-dependent behaviour" [27]. The relationship between the frontal lobes and the results of cognitive tests (MoCA), mainly of executive function, has already been described [28]. In our study, the results of cognitive tests (MoCA, CompBased-CAT) also positively correlated with the saturation of both the left and right frontal lobes. The study clearly shows a stronger relationship between the left frontal lobe saturation and the result of cognitive tests. Further analysis using multifactorial models showed a correlation between RAPA, rSO2 front L, and cognitive functions. This may indicate that physical activity has a positive effect on blood flow through the left frontal lobe, which leads to better results in cognitive functions.

Multivariate regression analysis in our study indicated an independent impact of physical activity score (RAPA), as well as arterial stiffness (PWV), on cognitive function (MoCa and CompBased-CAT). The relationship between cognitive functions and vascular stiffness in a group of hemodialysis patients has already been described [29]. The relationship between physical exercise and cognitive ability is well-known among the general population. Increasing physical exercise may prevent cognitive impairment from developing [30], even in the elderly [31]. It also refers to chronic hemodialysis patients. Authors of a recent systematic review found that physical exercise might improve or at least not worsen cognitive performance in HD patients, whereas the effect of cognitive training has not yet been adequately studied [32]. There is a general feeling that we need more sensitive and specific cognitive tests to measure the effects of interventions in the HD population adequately. This is why we supplemented MoCA with CompBased-CAT, keeping the generational change in mind, which is also taking place among dialysis centre patients—more and more people will be willing to use mobile solutions. A strong correlation with the standardised MoCA questionnaire was obtained.

The next lifestyle habit negatively affecting cognitive function is smoking cigarettes [33]. In a study looking at brain perfusion in patients with ESRD on HD maintenance who also had cognitive impairment, a high number of cortical defects (frontal and temporal lobes) consistent with the multiple-infarct type of dementia were reported. The majority of the patients in the study were current or former smokers [34]. Both smoking and physical activity are modifiable risk factors. This opens the field for conducting interventional studies and for the patient's work to reduce the risk of cognitive dysfunction.

This study also indicates that not only physical but also mental activity is very important in the context of cognitive decline. Patients who use social media and actively spend time during dialysis (computer games, crosswords vs. sleeping, watching TV) also obtained statistically significantly higher results in tests of cognitive functions. This hypothesis is made more likely by the fact that the longest-treated dialysis patients in the world show high mental activity, for example, Helena Garvao, who lived with 44 years of hemodialysis. The patient earned her PhD in linguistics and, at the age of 47, additionally completed studies in Portuguese literature. Furthermore, she worked as a lecturer for 30 years [35].

The cross-sectional design, the low recruitment rate and the relatively small sample size are the main limitations of the study. The potential selection bias of the study was that all patients must have used electronic tablets (some elderly persons might have refused to do it).

In summary, we confirmed that cognitive impairment in hemodialysis patients is multifactorial and healthy habits from the pre-dialysis time play a significant role. We urgently need diagnostic and preventive/therapeutic means in the cognitive field for this population. One must remember that, besides intradialytic interventions (reducing hypoperfusion by limiting ultrafiltration, modifying time, HD to HDF switch, etc.), also promoting physical/mental activity may change the risk of dementia progression. Further studies in this field are expedient.

5. Conclusions

Healthy habits, such as being physically active, not smoking, and inter-dialysis sessions (tasks and mind games, use of social media) are associated with better cognitive functions. Cognitive functions in hemodialysis patients are related to vascular stiffness (PWV), physical activity (RAPA), the blood supply to the frontal lobes (rSO2), and comorbidity (CCI).

Author Contributions: Conceptualisation, P.O. and M.K. (Mariusz Kusztal); methodology, P.O., P.J. and M.K. (Mariusz Kusztal); writing—original draft preparation, P.O. and M.K. (Mariusz Kusztal); writing—review and editing, K.L., T.G., M.K. (Mariusz Kusztal), P.J. and M.K. (Magdalena Krajewska); supervision, M.K. (Magdalena Krajewska). All authors have read and agreed to the published version of the manuscript.

Funding: This study was supported by the Wroclaw Medical University statutory funds (SUBZ.C160.22.051). This was investigator-initiated research. The funding body had no role in the study design, data collection, analyses and interpretation, or in writing the manuscript.

Institutional Review Board Statement: This study was conducted according to the guidelines of the Declaration of Helsinki and approved by the ethics committee of Wroclaw Medical University (protocol code KB-645/2018, date of approval 16 November 2018).

Informed Consent Statement: Informed consent was obtained from all subjects involved in the study.

Data Availability Statement: Not applicable.

Conflicts of Interest: The authors declare no conflict of interest.

References

1. Thurlow, J.S.; Joshi, M.; Yan, G.; Norris, K.C.; Agodoa, L.Y.; Yuan, C.M.; Nee, R. Global Epidemiology of End-Stage Kidney Disease and Disparities in Kidney Replacement Therapy. *Am. J. Nephrol.* **2021**, *52*, 98–107. [CrossRef]
2. Johansen, K.L.; Chertow, G.M.; Foley, R.N.; Gilbertson, D.T.; Herzog, C.A.; Ishani, A.; Israni, A.K.; Ku, E.; Tamura, M.K.; Li, S.; et al. US Renal Data System 2020 Annual Data Report: Epidemiology of Kidney Disease in the United States. *Am. J. Kidney Dis.* **2021**, *77*, A7–A8. [CrossRef]
3. Olczyk, P.; Małyszczak, A.; Gołębiowska, T.; Letachowicza, K.; Szymczaka, A.; Mazanowskaa, O.; Krajewskaa, M.; Kusztala, M. Arterial Stiffness Assessed by Oscillometric Method in Kidney Transplant, Predialysis, and Dialysis Patients. *Transplant. Proc.* **2020**, *52*, 2337–2340. [CrossRef]

4. Hoshino, T.; Ookawara, S.; Goto, S.; Miyazawa, H.; Ito, K.; Ueda, Y.; Kaku, Y.; Hirai, K.; Nabata, A.; Mori, H.; et al. Evaluation of Cerebral Oxygenation in Patients Undergoing Long-Term Hemodialysis. *Nephron Clin. Pract.* **2014**, *126*, 57–61. [CrossRef]
5. Viggiano, D.; Wagner, C.A.; Martino, G.; Nedergaard, M.; Zoccali, C.; Unwin, R.; Capasso, G. Mechanisms of cognitive dysfunction in CKD. *Nat. Rev. Nephrol.* **2020**, *16*, 452–469. [CrossRef]
6. McAdams-DeMarco, M.A.; Daubresse, M.; Bae, S.; Gross, A.L.; Carlson, M.C.; Segev, D.L. Dementia, Alzheimer's Disease, and Mortality after Hemodialysis Initiation. *Clin. J. Am. Soc. Nephrol.* **2018**, *13*, 1339–1347. [CrossRef]
7. Raphael, K.L.; Wei, G.; Greene, T.; Baird, B.C.; Beddhu, S. Cognitive Function and the Risk of Death in Chronic Kidney Disease. *Am. J. Nephrol.* **2011**, *35*, 49–57. [CrossRef] [PubMed]
8. Drew, D.A.; Weiner, D.E.; Tighiouart, H.; Scott, T.; Lou, K.; Kantor, A.; Fan, L.; Strom, J.A.; Singh, A.K.; Sarnak, M.J. Cognitive Function and All-Cause Mortality in Maintenance Hemodialysis Patients. *Am. J. Kidney Dis.* **2015**, *65*, 303–311. [CrossRef] [PubMed]
9. Dautzenberg, G.; Lijmer, J.; Beekman, A. Diagnostic accuracy of the Montreal Cognitive Assessment (MoCA) for cognitive screening in old age psychiatry: Determining cutoff scores in clinical practice. Avoiding spectrum bias caused by healthy controls. *Int. J. Geriatr. Psychiatry* **2020**, *35*, 261–269. [CrossRef]
10. Lee, S.H.; Cho, A.; Min, Y.-K.; Lee, Y.-K.; Jung, S. Comparison of the montreal cognitive assessment and the mini-mental state examination as screening tests in hemodialysis patients without symptoms. *Ren. Fail.* **2018**, *40*, 323–330. [CrossRef] [PubMed]
11. Davis, D.H.; Creavin, S.T.; Yip, J.L.; Noel-Storr, A.H.; Brayne, C.; Cullum, S. Montreal Cognitive Assessment for the detection of dementia. *Cochrane Database Syst. Rev.* **2021**, *13*, CD010775.
12. Yaneva, A.; Massaldjieva, R.; Mateva, N. Initial Adaptation of the General Cognitive Assessment Battery by CompBased-CAT TM for Bulgarian Older Adults. *Exp. Aging Res.* **2022**, *48*, 336–350. [CrossRef]
13. Chan, F.H.-W.; Chan, T.-C.; Luk, J.K.-H.; Chu, L.-W. Validation study of Charlson Comorbidity Index in predicting mortality in Chinese older adults. *Geriatr. Gerontol. Int.* **2014**, *14*, 452–457. [CrossRef]
14. Oliveros, H.; Buitrago, G. Validation and adaptation of the Charlson Comorbidity Index using administrative data from the Colombian health system: Retrospective cohort study. *BMJ Open* **2022**, *12*, e054058. [CrossRef]
15. Topolski, T.D.; LoGerfo, J.; Patrick, D.L.; Williams, B.; Walwick, J.; Patrick, M.M. The Rapid Assessment of Physical Activity (RAPA) Among Older Adults. *Prev. Chronic Dis.* **2006**, *3*, A118.
16. Lopes, A.A.; Lantz, B.; Morgenstern, H.; Wang, M.; Bieber, B.A.; Gillespie, B.W.; Li, Y.; Painter, P.; Jacobson, S.H.; Rayner, H.C.; et al. Associations of Self-Reported Physical Activity Types and Levels with Quality of Life, Depression Symptoms, and Mortality in Hemodialysis Patients. *Clin. J. Am. Soc. Nephrol.* **2014**, *9*, 1702–1712. [CrossRef]
17. van Zwieten, A.; Wong, G.; Ruospo, M.; Palmer, S.C.; Teixeira-Pinto, A.; Barulli, M.R.; Iurillo, A.; Saglimbene, V.; Natale, P.; Gargano, L.; et al. Associations of Cognitive Function and Education Level With All-Cause Mortality in Adults on Hemodialysis: Findings From the COGNITIVE-HD Study. *Am. J. Kidney Dis.* **2019**, *74*, 452–462. [CrossRef] [PubMed]
18. Neumann, D.; Mau, W.; Wienke, A.; Girndt, M. Peritoneal dialysis is associated with better cognitive function than hemodialysis over a one-year course. *Kidney Int.* **2018**, *93*, 430–438. [CrossRef]
19. Dixon, B.S.; the FHN study; VanBuren, J.M.; Rodrigue, J.R.; Lockridge, R.S.; Lindsay, R.; Chan, C.; Rocco, M.V.; Oleson, J.J.; Beglinger, L.; et al. Cognitive changes associated with switching to frequent nocturnal hemodialysis or renal transplantation. *BMC Nephrol.* **2016**, *17*, 1–11. [CrossRef] [PubMed]
20. Olczyk, P.; Kusztal, M.; Gołębiowski, T.; Letachowicz, K.; Krajewska, M. Cognitive Impairment in End Stage Renal Disease Patients Undergoing Hemodialysis: Markers and Risk Factors. *Int. J. Environ. Res. Public Health* **2022**, *19*, 2389. [CrossRef]
21. Tiffin-Richards, F.E.; Costa, A.S.; Holschbach, B.; Frank, R.D.; Vassiliadou, A.; Krüger, T.; Kuckuck, K.; Gross, T.; Eitner, F.; Floege, J.; et al. The Montreal Cognitive Assessment (MoCA)—A Sensitive Screening Instrument for Detecting Cognitive Impairment in Chronic Hemodialysis Patients. *PLoS ONE* **2014**, *9*, e106700. [CrossRef]
22. Wiloth, S.; Lemke, N.; Werner, C.; Hauer, K.; Szturm, T.; Patterson, M.D. Validation of a Computerized, Game-based Assessment Strategy to Measure Training Effects on Motor-Cognitive Functions in People with Dementia. *JMIR Serious Games* **2016**, *4*, e12. [CrossRef]
23. Aubert, L.; Pichierri, S.; Hommet, C.; Camus, V.; Berrut, G.; De Decker, L. Association Between Comorbidity Burden and Rapid Cognitive Decline in Individuals with Mild to Moderate Alzheimer's Disease. *J. Am. Geriatr. Soc.* **2015**, *63*, 543–547. [CrossRef] [PubMed]
24. Kao, S.-L.; Wang, J.-H.; Chen, S.-C.; Li, Y.-Y.; Yang, Y.-L.; Lo, R.Y. Impact of Comorbidity Burden on Cognitive Decline: A Prospective Cohort Study of Older Adults with Dementia. *Dement. Geriatr. Cogn. Disord.* **2021**, *50*, 43–50. [CrossRef] [PubMed]
25. Richerson, W.T.; Schmit, B.D.; Wolfgram, D.F. The Relationship between Cerebrovascular Reactivity and Cerebral Oxygenation during Hemodialysis. *J. Am. Soc. Nephrol.* **2022**, *33*, 1602–1612. [CrossRef] [PubMed]
26. Findlay, M.D.; Dawson, J.; Dickie, D.A.; Forbes, K.P.; McGlynn, D.; Quinn, T.; Mark, P.B. Investigating the Relationship between Cerebral Blood Flow and Cognitive Function in Hemodialysis Patients. *J. Am. Soc. Nephrol.* **2019**, *30*, 147–158. [CrossRef] [PubMed]
27. Goldberg, E.; Podell, K.; Lovell, M. Lateralization of frontal lobe functions and cognitive novelty. *J. Neuropsychiatry Clin. Neurosci.* **1994**, *6*, 371–378. [CrossRef]

28. Gao, Y.; Nie, K.; Huang, B.; Mei, M.; Guo, M.; Xie, S.; Huang, Z.; Wang, L.; Zhao, J.; Zhang, Y.; et al. Changes of brain structure in Parkinson's disease patients with mild cognitive impairment analyzed via VBM technology. *Neurosci. Lett.* **2017**, *658*, 121–132. [CrossRef]
29. Kim, E.D.; Meoni, L.A.; Jaar, B.G.; Shafi, T.; Kao, W.H.L.; Estrella, M.M.; Parekh, R.; Sozio, S.M. Association of Arterial Stiffness and Central Pressure With Cognitive Function in Incident Hemodialysis Patients: The PACE Study. *Kidney Int. Rep.* **2017**, *2*, 1149–1159. [CrossRef] [PubMed]
30. Erickson, K.I.; Hillman, C.; Stillman, C.M.; Ballard, R.M.; Bloodgood, B.; Conroy, D.E.; Macko, R.; Marquez, D.X.; Petruzzello, S.J.; Powell, K.E.; et al. Physical Activity, Cognition, and Brain Outcomes: A Review of the 2018 Physical Activity Guidelines. *Med. Sci. Sports Exerc.* **2019**, *51*, 1242–1251. [CrossRef]
31. Kumar, M.; Srivastava, S.; Muhammad, T. Relationship between physical activity and cognitive functioning among older Indian adults. *Sci. Rep.* **2022**, *12*, 1–13. [CrossRef]
32. Bogataj, Š.; Mesarič, K.K.; Pajek, M.; Petrušič, T.; Pajek, J. Physical exercise and cognitive training interventions to improve cognition in hemodialysis patients: A systematic review. *Front. Public Health* **2022**, *10*. [CrossRef] [PubMed]
33. Amini, R.; Sahli, M.; Ganai, S. Cigarette smoking and cognitive function among older adults living in the community. *Aging Neuropsychol. Cogn.* **2021**, *28*, 616–631. [CrossRef] [PubMed]
34. Lass, P.; Buscombe, J.R.; Harber, M.; Davenport, A.; Hilson, A.J.W. Cognitive Impairment in Patients With Renal Failure Is Associated With Multiple-Infarct Dementia. *Clin. Nucl. Med.* **1999**, *24*, 561–565. [CrossRef] [PubMed]
35. One of the Longest Living Dialysis Patients Shares How She Lives Life on Her Own Terms. Available online: https://www.kidneybuzz.com/one-of-the-longest-living-dialysis-patients-shares-how-she-lives-on-her-terms/2018/2/22/one-of-the-longest-living-dialysis-patients-shares-how-she-lives-on-her-terms (accessed on 5 January 2023).

Disclaimer/Publisher's Note: The statements, opinions and data contained in all publications are solely those of the individual author(s) and contributor(s) and not of MDPI and/or the editor(s). MDPI and/or the editor(s) disclaim responsibility for any injury to people or property resulting from any ideas, methods, instructions or products referred to in the content.

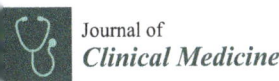

Article

Intradialytic Tolerance and Recovery Time in Different High-Efficiency Hemodialysis Modalities

Agnieszka Zakrzewska [1,†], Jan Biedunkiewicz [2,†], Michał Komorniczak [1], Magdalena Jankowska [1], Katarzyna Jasiulewicz [1], Natalia Płonka [1], Bogdan Biedunkiewicz [1], Sylwia Małgorzewicz [3], Agnieszka Tarasewicz [1], Ewelina Puchalska-Reglińska [4], Janusz Siebert [5], Alicja Dębska-Ślizień [1] and Leszek Tylicki [1,*]

1. Department of Nephrology, Transplantology and Internal Diseases, Medical University of Gdańsk, Smoluchowskiego 17, 80-214 Gdańsk, Poland; michal.komorniczak@gumed.edu.pl (M.K.); magdalena.jankowska@gumed.edu.pl (M.J.); kateolivia@gumed.edu.pl (K.J.); bogdan.biedunkiewicz@gumed.edu.pl (B.B.)
2. Department of Anesthesiology and Intensive Therapy, Faculty of Medicine, Medical University of Gdańsk, 80-214 Gdańsk, Poland; jan.biedunkiewicz@gumed.edu.pl
3. Department of Clinical Nutrition, Medical University of Gdańsk, Dębinki 7, 80-211 Gdańsk, Poland
4. Dialysis Unit, 7th Naval Hospital in Gdańsk, 80-305 Gdańsk, Poland
5. Department of Family Medicine, University Center for Cardiology, Medical University of Gdansk, 80-211 Gdansk, Poland
* Correspondence: leszek.tylicki@gumed.edu.pl
† These authors contributed equally to this work.

Abstract: There are several forms of maintenance high-efficiency hemodialysis (HD), including hemodiafiltrations (HDF) in different technical modes and expanded HD, using dialyzers with medium cut-off membranes. The aim of the study was to assess the intradialytic tolerance and length of dialysis recovery time (DRT) in these modalities. This is an exploratory, crossover study in maintenance HD patients with low comorbidity and no clinical indications for the use of high-efficiency HD, who were exposed to five intermittent dialyses in random order: high-flux hemodialysis (S-HD), expanded HD (HDx), pre-dilution HDF (PRE-HDF), mix-dilution HDF (MIX-HDF) and post-dilution HDF (POST-HDF). Twenty-four dialysis sessions of each method were included in the analysis. Dialysis parameters, including blood flow rate, dialysis fluid flow rate and temperature, and pharmacological treatment were constant. Average total convection volume for post-HDF, pre-HDF and mix-HDF were 25.6 (3.8), 61.5 (7.2) and 47.1 (11.4) L, respectively. During all therapies, patients were monitored for the similarity of their hydration statuses using bioimpedance spectroscopy, and for similar variability over time in systemic blood pressure and cardiac output, while peripheral resistance was monitored using impedance cardiography. The lowest frequency of all intradialytic adverse events were observed during HDx. Delayed DRT was the shortest during PRE-HDF. Patients were also more likely to report immediate recovery while receiving PRE-HDF. These differences did not reach statistical significance; however, the study results suggest that intradialytic tolerance and DRT may depend on the dialysis method used. This supports the need of taking into account patient preferences and quality of life while individualizing high-efficiency therapy in HD patients.

Keywords: hemodialysis; hemodiafiltration; expanded hemodialysis; quality of life

1. Introduction

For some time now, hemodialysis (HD) using high-flux membranes is the standard of chronic dialysis treatment (S-HD) replacing dialysis based on low-flux membranes. Technological advances over the past few decades have contributed to further developments in HD therapy and the introduction of high-efficiency dialysis therapies into clinical practice. Significant technological changes in dialyzer membrane permeability and ultrafiltration-controlled delivery systems permitted the more efficient removal of larger–medium-sized water-soluble toxins. There are several forms of high-efficiency dialysis treatment, which include, among others: hemodiafiltration (HDF) in pre-dilution (PRE-HDF), post-dilution (POST-HDF) and mixed dilution (MIX-HDF) mode and the so-called expanded HD (HDx) using dialyzers with medium cut-of membranes (MCO) [1–3]. The observational studies and some secondary analyses of randomized trials have indicated that high-volume on-line HDF may improve patient survival in comparison to S-HD, regardless of whether pre-dilution or post-dilution mode is used [4,5]. Quite recently, the CONVINCE (Comparison of high-dose HDF with high-flux HD) trial confirmed that the use of high-volume POST-HDF resulted in a lower risk of death from any cause than conventional S-HD [6]. Pending the results of other controlled studies in this area, this method is being used increasingly, especially in patients with high comorbidity, long duration of dialysis therapy and contraindications to kidney transplantation [7]. Some experts recommended the use of high-volume online POST-HDF in patients whose Age-Adjusted Charlson Comorbidity Index (AACCI) is ≥ 8 [8]. Particularly, clinical benefits have been demonstrated in patients with hemodynamic instability, poorly controlled blood pressure (BP), polyneuropathy, calcium–phosphate disorders, pruritus or erythropoietin resistance, among others [3,9]. There is little clinical experience in the use of high-efficiency HD methods in patients with low comorbidity for a chance for a kidney transplant and a potentially short period of dialysis—the vast majority of whom are still dialyzed by classic high-flux HD.

2. Materials and Methods

2.1. Study Design

This is an exploratory, open, crossover (one-center) study in maintenance HD patients who were exposed to (i) high-flux S-HD and four high-efficiency intermittent dialysis modalities in random order: (ii) HDx, (iii) PRE-HDF, (iv) MIX-HDF, (v) POST-HDF. Each patient underwent three sessions in each of these modalities during one week. The second and third sessions of the week entered the final analysis. Patients and dialysis unit staff were not blinded to treatment allocation. The aim of the study was to compare patients' tolerance of dialysis methods in a group of patients with low comorbidity who have no clinical indications for the use of high-efficiency dialysis. The study was conducted according to the guidelines of the Declaration of Helsinki, and approved by the Ethical Committee at the Medical University of Gdansk (no. NKBBN/479-759/2022; 18 November 2022).

2.2. Patients

The inclusion criteria were as follows: adult patients, eligible for kidney transplantation, treated chronically with HD 3 × per week for at least 6 months; dialysis single-pool Kt/V for urea (spKt/Vurea) > 1.2; patient's weight in the range of 60–85 kg; AACCI < 8; achievement of a blood flow of >350 mL/min through a fistula or arteriovenous catheter. Exclusion criteria include life expectancy <6 months, severe incompliance to the HD procedures and accompanying prescriptions, emergency hospitalization within 30 days before entering the study, diabetes, active inflammation, active cancer, hemodynamic instability during HD sessions, poorly controlled BP, uremic polyneuropathy, uremic pruritus, dialysis amyloidosis and erythropoietin resistance. Also, patients needed to have no contraindication for bioimpedance measurement and be able to record dialysis recovery time (DRT).

2.3. Dialysis Prescription and Equipment

All dialysis therapies were performed on Fresenius 5008 dialysis machine with AutoSub Plus system (Fresenius Medical Care, Bad Homburg, Germany). SHD and HDF treatments were performed with high-flux FX 100 dialyzers (effective surface area: 2.2; UF coefficient 73 mL/h × mmHg; Fresenius Medical Care; Bad Homburg, Germany). HDx sessions were performed using Terranova 400 MCO dialyzer (effective surface area: 1.7 m^2, UF coefficient 48 mL/h × mmHg; Baxter, Alliston, ON, Canada). Dialysis session time was set at 4 h for all modalities. Temperature of dialysate was set at 36.5 C degree. Blood flow rate and dialysate flow rate were set to 350 and 500 mL/min, respectively. The dry weight of the patients was confirmed before the start of the study using bioimpedance spectroscopy. The fluid removal of each session (ultrafiltration) was set according to individual patient's interdialytic weight gain plus fluid intake during the procedure and bloodline priming volume. Ultrafiltration profiling and sodium profiling were not used. The electrolyte composition of dialysis fluid was: Na 138–140 mmol/L; K 2.0–3.0 mol/L; HCO_3 32 mmol/L; Ca 1.25–1.5 mmol/L; Mg 0.5 mmol/L; Cl 110 mmol/L; glucose 1.0 g/L (10 patients—83.3%: K—2.0 mmol/L; 11 patients—91.7%: Ca—1.25 mmol/L). All patients received standard heparin as a bolus and continuous infusion in accordance with current practice. Sterile and nonpyrogenic substitution fluid for HDF was produced online by ultrafiltration of the ultrapure dialysate. Substitution fluid rate and convection rate during HDF modalities were optimized automatically using the AutoSub Plus system based on pressure pulse attenuation and cross-membrane pressure assessment (Fresenius Medical Care; St. Wendel, Germany). The basic principle of AutoSub Plus is to avoid excessive hemoconcentration in the dialyzer and maximization of the ultrafiltration flow [10]. For a given patient, dialysis settings were kept unchanged during all treatment modalities, e.g., post-dialysis weight, dialysis session length, composition of the dialysis fluid, blood and dialysis fluid flow, dialysis fluid temperature and anticoagulation dose. The patient's concomitant medications were continued in an unchanged manner.

2.4. Outcomes

During all sessions, adverse events (AEs), DRT, hemodynamic parameters and hydration state were recorded. The results from the middle and the last dialysis sessions in weeks were used in the analysis.

2.4.1. Adverse Events

The frequency of symptomatic hypotension, AEs potentially related to BP/fluid shifts, AEs not classically related to BP/fluids shifts and intradialytic clotting events were recorded. Symptomatic hypotension was defined as a decrease in systolic BP $\geq$ 20 mm Hg, requiring reduction in or cessation of ultrafiltration and/or need for intravenous fluid bolus or head-down tilt of dialysis chair. AEs potentially related to BP/fluid shifts were defined as experiencing breathlessness, cramps (normal BP), dizzy/lightheaded, falling, headache, erratic venous pressures, clotted needle or restless legs. AEs not classically related to BP/fluids shifts were defined as aches in bones, arm pain, back pain, bleeding, constipation, diarrhea, feeling cold, feeling down, feeling hot, generally unwell, heavy legs, increased lethargy, infection (given antibiotics), itch, leg pain, nausea, stomach pains, sweating, swollen abdomen and vomiting. Intradialytic clotting events were defined as either an increase in venous pressures requiring additional anticoagulant dosing or clotting of the extracorporeal circuit [11].

2.4.2. Dialysis Recovery Time

At each dialysis session, the patient was asked the duration of DRT to baseline function, following their antecedent dialysis session. The patients' responses were converted to a number of minutes, as follows [12]:

i. Answers given in minutes were recorded directly.
ii. Answers in hours were multiplied by 60.
iii. Variants of "half a day", including the "next day", were given a value of 720 min.
iv. Variants of "one day" were given a value of 1440 min.
v. Variants of "more than a day" were given a value of 2160 min (36 h).

Given that the distribution of DRT was bimodal with a peak at zero, it was analyzed via separate crossover analysis: percentage of immediate DRT (equal 0 min) and delayed DRT in minutes.

2.4.3. Hemodynamic Monitoring

For real-time hemodynamic measurements, the CardioScreen 2000 (Medis. Medizinische Messtechnik GmbH, Ilmenau, Germany) device was used. CardioScreen 2000 is a feasible and accurate method for non-invasive hemodynamic measurements using methods of impedance cardiography, which utilizes a physiological adaptive signal analysis (PASA) algorithm. Hemodynamic measurements obtained using a PASA algorithm were correlated highly significantly to measurements obtained via the thermodilution method [13]. The following parameters were measured or calculated: systolic BP (SBP), diastolic BP (DBP), mean arterial pressure (MAP), cardiac index (CI), systemic vascular resistance index (SVRI). Hemodynamic parameters were measured in resting position 10 min prior to dialysis, during dialysis (at the following time points: 15, 30, 60, 120, 180, 240 min) and 10 min after dialysis. In order to aggregate the changes in time during the entire dialysis session, the area under the curve (AUC) of BP, CI and SVRI were calculated using the trapezoid method.

2.4.4. Hydration State

Body composition and hydration state had been assessed using a portable whole body bioimpedance spectroscopy device (BCM; Fresenius Medical Care, Bad Homburg, Germany). The measurements were obtained before and after dialysis session in resting position. The extracellular water (ECW), intracellular water (ICW) and total body water (TBW) were calculated from a fluid model [14].

2.5. Statistics

Continuous data are reported as means (±standard deviation, SD) or medians (interquartile ranges, IQR). The Shapiro–Wilk test was used to determine the distribution of continuous variables. Categorical data are reported as percentages of the total. The Wilcoxon signed-rank test or ANOVA was used in the analysis comparing the results of the variables repeatable more than twice. Two-sided $p < 0.05$ was considered to be statistically significant. The statistical analysis was performed using the program Statistica 13.3 (TIBCO Software Inc.; Palo Alto, CA, USA). Given that the distribution of DRT was bimodal with a peak at zero, it was analyzed via separate analysis with 2 models (immediate DRT as categorical variable and delayed DRT as continuous variable).

3. Results

3.1. Characteristics of Patients

Twelve patients met the inclusion criteria and were enrolled to the study, eleven of whom were men (91.67%) and one woman (8.33%), with a mean age of 52.5 ± 15.47 years. Hypertension was diagnosed in 10 (83.3%) patients. A description of the study group is presented in Table 1.

Table 1. Characteristics of the study group.

Gender (men/women)	11/1
Causes of ESRD (*n*/%)	
Autosomal dominant polycystic kidney disease	4/33.4
Glomerulonephritis (primary or secondary)	3/25.0
Hypertensive nephropathy	2/16.7
Renal malformation	1/8.3
Interstitial nephropathy	1/8.3
Other	1/8.3
Age (years)	52.5 (15.5)
AACI (points)	4.5 (2.2)
Dialysis vintage (months)	42.5 (31.04)

Table 1. Cont.

Body mass index (kg/m^2)	23.8 (3.6)
Weight (kg)	73.7 (14.2)
spKt/V$_{urea}$	1.5 (0.3)
Hemoglobin (g/dL)	10.9 (0.9)
Albumin (g/L)	33.1 (4.9)

ESRD: end-stage renal disease; AACI: Age-Adjusted Charlson Comorbidity Index.

3.2. Dialysis Parameters

Dialysis session time, blood flow rate and dialysate flow rate were constant during all modalities. All patients achieved the minimum level of convection for high-volume post-HDF with a substitution volume >21 L. Mean (standard deviation) total convection for post-HDF, pre-HDF and mix-HDF were 25.6 (3.8), 61.5 (7.2) and 47.1 (11.4) L, respectively. The target body weight was achieved during all studied dialysis sessions. The fluid removal, SBP, DBP, TBW, ECW and ICW did not differ between tested treatments. Detailed dialysis parameters and patients' hydration status results are presented in Table 2.

Table 2. Delivered dialysis parameters, systemic blood pressure and hydration status parameters.

	S-HD	HDX	PRE-HDF	MIX-HDF	POST-HDF	p
Time min	240	240	240	240	240	NA
Blood flow mL/min	350	350	350	350	350	NA
Dialysate flow mL/min	500	500	500	500	500	NA
Ultrafiltration mL	2.12 (0.74)	2.33 (0.62)	2.45 (0.8)	2.29 (0.74)	2.19 (0.52)	$p = 0.6$
Ultrafiltration/dry weight %	0.028	0.032	0.034	0.031	0.029	$p = 0.56$
Total convection L	NA	NA	61.5 (7.2)	47.1 (11.4)	25.6 (3.8)	NA
SBP $_{predialysis}$ mmHg	147.7 (27.5)	144.1 (20.3)	147.7 (26.6)	147.3 (20.3)	144.3 (22.4)	$p = 0.95$
DBP $_{predialysis}$ mmHg	88.5 (18.8)	88.3 (16.9)	89.9 (20.4)	89.9 (16.4)	86.1 (18.0)	$p = 0.93$
TBW $_{predialysis}$ l	39.76 (8.04)	41.64 (11.65)	39.05 (6.84)	40.15 (7.32)	39.7 (8.4)	$p = 0.93$
TBW $_{postdialysis}$ l	38.17 (8.03)	40.46 (12.51)	37.5 (6.97)	38.56 (7.29)	37.44 (8.24)	$p = 0.85$
ECW $_{predialysis}$ l	19.1 (3.2)	19.9 (3.3)	20.1 (3.5)	19.3 (3.5)	18.9 (3.2)	$p = 0.74$
ECW $_{postdialysis}$ l	17.2 (3.1)	17.43 (3.1)	17.38 (2.9)	18.2 (5.7)	16.7 (2.9)	$p = 0.77$
ICW $_{predialysis}$ l	21.31 (5.6)	23.3 (7.5)	22.2 (5.1)	20.7 (4.2)	20.8 (5.4)	$p = 0.62$
ICW $_{postdialysis}$ l	21.33 (5.7)	24.5 (8.8)	24.2 (6.5)	21.2 (4.7)	20.7 (5.5)	$p = 0.17$

Note: Ultrafiltration: the fluid removal during the session; total convection: the total volume of convection during the session, which is the sum of the patient's dehydration volume and the volume of the replacement fluid administered; SBP: systolic blood pressure; DBP: diastolic blood pressure; TBW: total body water; ECW: extracellular water; ICW: intracellular water.

3.3. Hemodynamic Parameters

SBP and DBP at the beginning (first minute) and at the end of dialysis (240 min) sessions did not differ between treatments. AUC of SBP, DBP and MAP measurements obtained during dialysis over time did not differ between treatments as well. CI was decreasing ($p < 0.001$ for all methods) while SVRI was increasing ($p < 0.001$ for all methods) during all methods used. The AUC of CI and SVRI measurements obtained during dialysis over time did not differ between the treatments. Detailed results are presented in Table 3 and Figures 1 and 2.

Table 3. Systemic blood pressure and area under the curve (AUC) of hemodynamic parameters.

	S-HD	HDX	PRE-HDF	MIX-HDF	POST-HDF	p
SBP 1st min mmHg	145.8 (24.6)	139.1 (17.2)	143.4 (22.6)	141.2 (18.0)	137.9 (21.9)	$p = 0.75$
SBP 240 min mmHg	142.5 (35.5)	142.2 (28.3)	138.7 (35.7)	140.6 (35.5)	138.8 (29.2)	$p = 0.98$
DBP 1st min mmHg	87.0 (17.5)	86.3 (14.3)	86.1 (16.7)	87.9 (16.6)	83.4 (15.8)	$p = 0.85$
DBP 240 min mmHg	85.7 (17.1)	89.1 (21.3)	84.9 (17.3)	85.3 (20.5)	87.3 (18.7)	$p = 0.91$
AUC SBP	323 816.6 (72,781.6)	318 930.3 (61,252.4)	316 602.0 (68,292.8)	305 190.3 (76,556.9)	313 049.4 (80,028.1)	$p = 0.8$
AUC DPB	194,716.4 (37,664.1)	192,651.0 (53,530.6)	194,253.7 (33,794.1)	190,661.9 (44,971.5)	191,900.7 (44,991.7)	$p = 0.88$
AUC MAP	237,748.1 (46,888.6)	230,184.4 (59,405.4)	235,096.4 (42,932.1)	231,486.3 (53 996.6)	234,209.5 (47,871.5)	$p = 0.23$
AUC CI	6559.2 (1439.5)	6770.9 (1271.3)	6512.5 (1256.4)	6093.9 (1282.4)	6680.9 (1652.9)	$p = 0.65$
AUC SVRI	6,176,119.3 (1,325,662.8)	6,456,193.4 (1,473,702.1)	6,256,567.9 (999,108.8)	7,075,464.9 (1,930,210.7)	6,301,942.5 (1,337,688.1)	$p = 0.34$

SBP: systolic blood pressure; DBP: diastolic blood pressure; MAP: mean arterial pressure; CI: cardiac index; SVRI: systemic vascular resistance index.

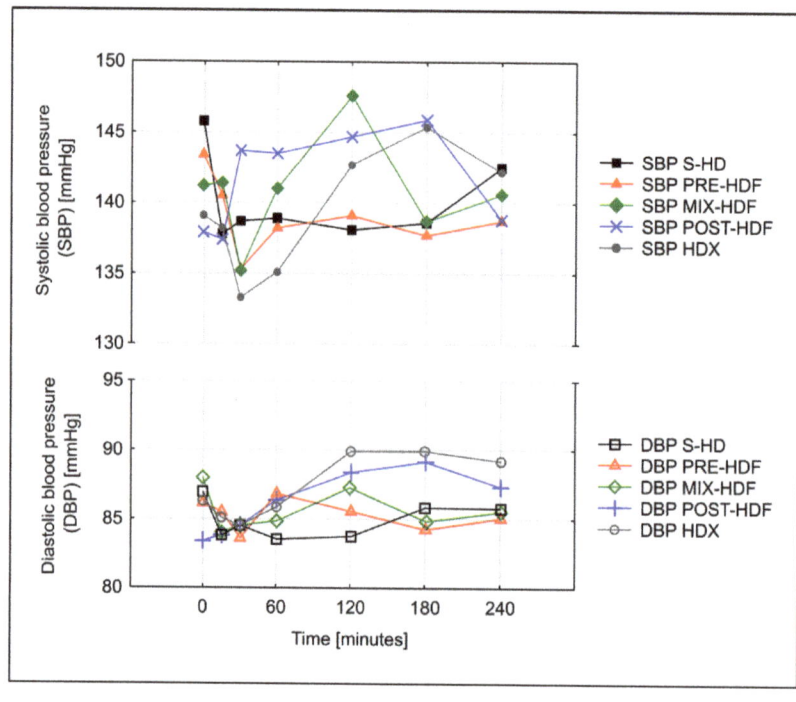

Figure 1. Changes over time in mean systolic (SBP) and diastolic blood (DBP) pressure during various dialysis treatments.

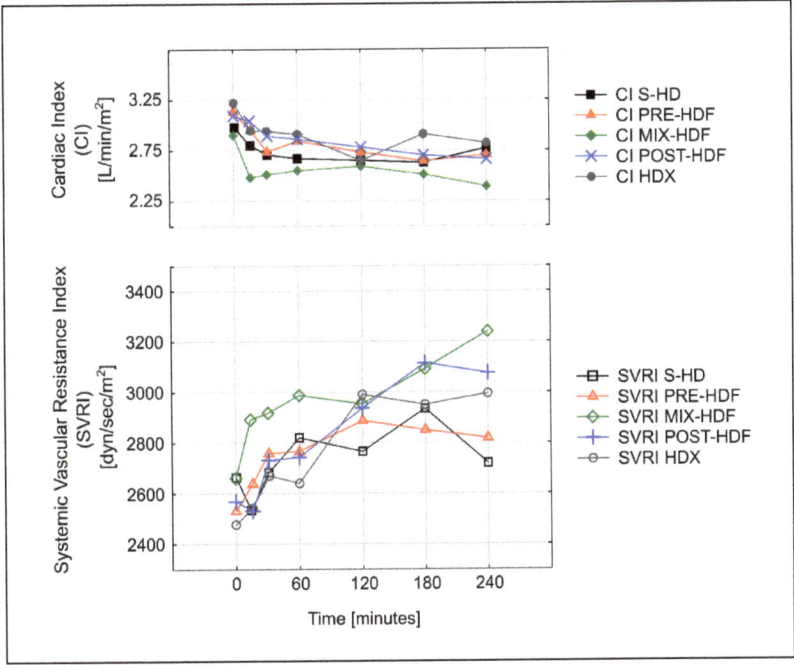

Figure 2. Mean area under the curve (AUC) of changes over time in cardiac index (CI) and systemic vascular resistance index (SVRI) during various treatments.

3.4. Adverse Events and Dialysis Recovery Time

AEs were grouped to those that may or may not have been related to BP changes or fluid shifts and those related to clotting events. There were no incidents of symptomatic intradialytic hypotension during any treatment. The lowest frequency of all AEs was observed with HDx (25%), although the differences did not prove to be statistically significant. Delayed DRT was the shortest during PRE-HDF. Patients were also more likely to report immediate recovery while receiving PRE-HDF (62.5%). However, the differences did not reach statistical significance. Detailed results are presented in Table 4.

Table 4. Adverse events (% events per sessions) and dialysis recovery time (DRT).

	S-HD	HDX	PRE-HDF	MIX-HDF	POST-HDF	p
Symptomatic hypotension n	0	0	0	0	0	$p = 1.0$
AEs potentially related to BP/fluid shifts n	0	1	1	2	4	$p = 0.39$
AEs potentially not related to BP/fluid shifts n	7	4	5	5	2	$p = 0.47$
Intradialytic clotting events n	1	1	2	2	4	$p = 0.51$
All AEs n (%)	8 (33.3%)	6 (25%)	7 (29.2%)	9 (37.5%)	10 (41.7%)	$p = 0.76$
Immediate DRT n (%)	11 (45.8%)	12 (50%)	15 (62.5%)	9 (37.5%)	10 (41.7%)	$p = 0.10$
Delayed DRT min	360.0 (180–720)	180 (120–390)	60 (30–600)	360 (180–360)	390 (60–720)	$p = 0.37$

Note: AEs: adverse events; values are given as number of events (percentage). Multiples of the same episodes within 1 session were treated as a single event. All AEs: all AEs reported by patients and reported in the table, including clotting events; DRT: dialysis recovery time.

4. Discussion

The CONVINCE trail provides the first convincing evidence that patients receiving high-volume POST-HDF have improved survival compared with those receiving high-flux HD [6]. It appears to be a milestone that indicates the therapy of choice for patients treated with long-term dialysis [15]. However, the question of what therapy to offer patients with low comorbidity and a potentially better prognosis or the prospect of transplantation remains unanswered. This may affect even a quarter of the entire population. Typically, such patients are treated with standard hemodialysis using high-flux membranes. The question arises whether it is worth using high-efficiency therapies and which of them is best tolerated by them. Apart from the obvious importance of survival outcome, the quality of life of patients and their tolerance of dialysis treatments should be taken into account [16–18]. Evidence-based medicine did not provide accurate recommendations about the best strategy to provide patients with a greater comfort of dialysis treatment. Therefore, therapy needs to be formulated and personalized, according to the heterogeneity of patients, based on their dominant co-morbidities, clinical characteristics and existing biochemical disorders. The individualization of treatment is based on the choice of dialysis techniques, dialysis membrane, the possibility of automatic regulation and profiling of ultrafiltration, sodium and potassium concentration and temperature in the dialysis bath, which is discussed in detail elsewhere [19].

Maintenance HD patients have a high burden of symptoms that negatively affect their quality of life [20]. Post-dialysis fatigue, intra-dialytic hypotension, cramps and dizziness are the most common symptoms reported by patients [21]. Post-dialysis fatigue and a lack of energy interfere with daily life and are also predictors of mortality [22]. Patients treated with standard HD report average DRT in the range of 2–4 h, with approximately 25% reporting DRT greater than 6 h [23,24]. In the FRENCHIE (French Convective versus Hemodialysis in Elderly) study, 25.9% of patients reported at least one AE during a dialysis session and 20.6% of patients had asymptomatic hypotension [25]. Moreover, patients may prioritize outcomes differently than those set by medical professionals. Focusing on the tolerance of the dialysis procedure and the comfort of life, we compared in the study various high-efficiency dialysis techniques used in the group of patients in whom these therapies are not commonly used. For an objective assessment of intradialytic stability, we used the method of impedance cardiography for real-time hemodynamic measurements.

Convective-based high-efficiency dialytic modalities, including online HDF, have been proposed as an alternative capable of relieving most intradialytic AEs and improving patient outcomes. HDF, used in various modes, including POST-HDF, PRE-HDF and MIX-HDF, provides a more effective removal of soluble middle molecular weight toxins and protein-bound compounds than conventional S-HD [1]. Other potential mechanisms underlying these effects are: (i) better biocompatibility due to the combined use of biocompatible membranes and ultrapure/sterile fluids, which results in a reduction in systemic inflammatory response; and (ii) a favorable impact of HDF on intradialytic hypotensive episodes due to a higher sodium mass transfer and mode-specific thermal effects [26]. Several previous studies investigating the influence of convection-based methods on intradialytic tolerance have yielded conflicting results. The FRENCHIE study compared high-flux HD and POST-HDF in terms of intradialytic tolerance in elderly chronic HD patients (over age 65) and reported significant differences between treatments with fewer episodes of intradialytic symptomatic hypotension and muscle cramps in POST-HDF [25]. Similar conclusions can be drawn from the results of the ESHOL trial [27]. However, in some studies, no improvement was observed in terms of intradialytic tolerance when switching therapy from S-HD to HDF [21,28,29] and some even indicate deterioration. For instance, in the crossover study by Smith J. et al., POST- HDF was associated with an increased rate of symptomatic hypotension compared to S-HD (8.0% vs. 5.3%) and intradialytic tendency to clotting (1.8% vs. 0.7%) [11]. The inclusion criteria we used are probably responsible for the fact that no episodes of intradialytic hypotension were recorded during any procedure in our study. We did not note any significant differences in dialysis tolerance between individual treatments, although some differences were clearly visible. POST-HD was the worst tolerated procedure. At least one AE was observed in almost 42% of POST-HDF sessions. The largest number of clotting events is noteworthy, which is fully understandable considering the highest degree of hemoconcentration during POST-HDF in the dialyzer, increasing the viscosity of the blood before fluid substitution, which results in the deposition of plasma proteins on the membrane surface, the clogging of membrane pores, an increased transmembrane pressure and an occlusion of dialyzer blood channels [30]. PRE-HDF resolves this problem but requires about three times more replacement fluid than POST-HDF. This reduces the risks of clotting and protein deposition and allows much higher ultrafiltration rates of up to 100% of the blood flow rate which can be far lower than in POST-HDF. The cooling effect of replacement solution in large volumes during PRE-HDF may help maintain hemodynamic stability as well [31]. During the PRE-HDF conducted in our study group, we observed fewer adverse symptoms than during POST-HDF. Locatelli et al. demonstrated 54% less intradialytic hypotension events in patients who were treated with PRE-HDF in comparison with a low-flux HD [32]. MIX-HDF is the least frequently used in clinical practice; hence, there is less tolerance studies on this method. In one of the few studies, symptomatic intradialytic hypotension episodes and other AEs occurred similarly in the MIX-HDF and PRE-HDF [33].

Small observational studies indicate that HDx may result in better treatment tolerance than standard HD with less dialysis hypotension and a reduction in DRT [34,35]. Other studies indicate that HDx use may be effective in reducing symptoms of restless leg syndrome, dialysis pruritus and improve quality of life [36,37]. It may be that removing a wider range of toxins, including large middle toxins, accounts for some of these benefits [38]. Compared to HDF, HDx does not increase transmembrane pressure, thus providing minimal stress to the filter [3]. Importantly, the HDX treatment is technically the simplest to perform among the high-efficiency methods, similar to standard hemodialysis, which may also affect the course of the procedure, with fewer complications and AEs. What is noteworthy in our study is that the number of observed and reported AEs was the lowest during HDx.

To the best of our knowledge, there are no studies comparing all high-efficiency dialysis modalities in the context of intradialytic tolerance, only individual small studies comparing PRE-HDF, only in relation to POST-HDF and HDx, and did not show any differences [39–41]. Our study seems to be pioneering in this respect, especially if we take into account the population in which the study was conducted. The lowest frequency of all AEs was observed with HDx (25%) and PRE-HDF (29%), although the differences did not prove to be statistically significant. There were no incidents of symptomatic intradialytic hypotension during any treatment modality. Our patients were characterized by strong cardiovascular stability. The use of impedance cardiography provided us with an indirect insight into cardiac output, blood viscosity and autonomic activity, as sympathetic stimulation constricts peripheral arteries and increases vascular resistance. In line with previous observations, CI decreased while SVRI increased during all methods used [42]. Of note, the CI AUC and SVRI AUC were not statistically different between all modalities, which indicates similar hemodynamic stability during the tested treatments.

Yet, another interesting patient outcome measure that we tracked in our study was the length of DRT. The length of DRT is a recent and reliable method of post-dialysis fatigue assessment, an important patient-reported complaint that affects their quality of life and restricts the ability to perform their daily activities [43]. Davenport et al. found that the DRT ≥ 1 h may be present in more than 75% of HD patients [44]. Most importantly, evidence from the DOPPS study has suggested an association between longer DRT and increased mortality [24]. Thus far, no convincing evidence has been obtained that dialysis methods based on convection, i.e., HDF, shortens the length of DRT [44,45]. There were also no differences in DRT and self-reported intradialytic symptoms with differing convection volumes during HDF [46]. Despite the lack of statistical significance, our results suggest that PRE-HDF may contribute to shortening post-dialysis fatigue more effectively than other compared therapies in the population that was the subject of our study. This improvement concerned both an increase in the percentage of patients who reported a return to well-being immediately after the dialysis, as well as a shortening of DRT in those for whom it required a longer time (Table 4). The analysis of the potential factors responsible for this phenomenon was beyond the scope of our study, but cooling effect of replacement solution in large volumes during PRE-HDF may be at least partially involved [31].

Our study has several strengths: (i) the choice of crossover design was made in order to abrogate the influence of interpatient variability; (ii) a detailed analysis of the variability of hemodynamic parameters over time was performed; (iii) the patients' hydration status was measured and did not differ during individual treatments; (iv) basic dialysis parameters have been unified for all treatment modalities; (v) the high-volume nature of HDF, known to provide the best long-term prognosis, was assured during study. On the other hand, we are aware of the limitations of our study. We had only one woman in our study group, which may raise questions about its homogeneity, given the differences in body composition. However, the exclusion of female participants is a recognized problem in many nephrological studies and we decided against it [47]. The study included only relatively young patients with low comorbidities, who constitute the vast minority in dialysis centers. This means that the study results cannot be generalized to the entire dialysis population. On the other hand, such an approach allowed for the exclusion of most factors that might influence AEs except for the treatment modality (for example, diabetic neuropathy, atherosclerosis, heart failure or malnutrition). Another limitation is the single-center study design. The "center effect" is a well-known problem in studies about dialysis, secondarily to an endless list of aspects related to the clinical and nursing management of the dialysis session. We are convinced that the crossover design of the study should mitigate such a bias to a certain extent. The important limitation is also the small size of the study group. This is the cost that should be paid when eligibility criteria are set to control for many confounders. Taking all these limitations into account, one should be aware that only exploratory conclusions should be drawn.

In conclusion, the study did not find any significant differences in intradialytic AEs and DRT between standard high-flux HD and four high-efficacy HD modalities, including PRE-HDF, MIX-HDF, POST-HDF and HDx. However, the study results may suggest that tolerance of dialysis session and post-dialysis fatigue may vary in some patients when using different high-efficacy modalities. This indicates the necessity of individualizing HD therapy also in relatively young patients with low comorbidity.

Author Contributions: Conceptualization, A.D.-Ś., J.S., E.P.-R. and L.T.; methodology, J.S., E.P.-R., M.K., B.B., S.M., M.J. and L.T.; validation, M.J., S.M., B.B. and L.T.; formal analysis, L.T. and M.K.; investigation, J.B., A.Z., B.B., K.J., N.P., M.K., M.J., A.T. and S.M.; writing—original draft preparation, L.T.; writing—review and editing, B.B., A.D.-Ś., M.J. and S.M.; visualization, M.K.; supervision, A.D.-Ś. and L.T. All authors have read and agreed to the published version of the manuscript.

Funding: This research received no external funding.

Institutional Review Board Statement: The study was conducted in accordance with the Declaration of Helsinki, and approved by Medical University of Gdańsk Ethical Committee (NKBBN/479-759/2022), 18 November 2022.

Informed Consent Statement: Informed consent was obtained from all subjects involved in the study.

Data Availability Statement: The data are available from the corresponding authors upon reasonable request.

Conflicts of Interest: The authors declare no conflicts of interest.

References

1. Lang, T.; Zawada, A.M.; Theis, L.; Braun, J.; Ottilinger, B.; Kopperschmidt, P.; Gagel, A.; Kotanko, P.; Stauss-Grabo, M.; Kennedy, J.P.; et al. Hemodiafiltration: Technical and Medical Insights. *Bioengineering* **2023**, *10*, 145. [CrossRef] [PubMed]
2. Pedreros-Rosales, C.; Jara, A.; Lorca, E.; Mezzano, S.; Pecoits-Filho, R.; Herrera, P. Unveiling the Clinical Benefits of High-Volume Hemodiafiltration: Optimizing the Removal of Medium-Weight Uremic Toxins and Beyond. *Toxins* **2023**, *15*, 531. [CrossRef] [PubMed]
3. Zhang, Z.; Yang, T.; Li, Y.; Li, J.; Yang, Q.; Wang, L.; Jiang, L.; Su, B. Effects of Expanded Hemodialysis with Medium Cut-Off Membranes on Maintenance Hemodialysis Patients: A Review. *Membranes* **2022**, *12*, 253. [CrossRef] [PubMed]
4. Davenport, A.; Peters, S.A.; Bots, M.L.; Canaud, B.; Grooteman, M.P.; Asci, G.; Locatelli, F.; Maduell, F.; Morena, M.; Nubé, M.J.; et al. Higher convection volume exchange with online hemodiafiltration is associated with survival advantage for dialysis patients: The effect of adjustment for body size. *Kidney Int.* **2016**, *89*, 193–199. [CrossRef] [PubMed]
5. Kikuchi, K.; Hamano, T.; Wada, A.; Nakai, S.; Masakane, I. Predilution online hemodiafiltration is associated with improved survival compared with hemodialysis. *Kidney Int.* **2019**, *95*, 929–938. [CrossRef] [PubMed]
6. Blankestijn, P.J.; Vernooij, R.W.M.; Hockham, C.; Strippoli, G.F.M.; Canaud, B.; Hegbrant, J.; Barth, C.; Covic, A.; Cromm, K.; Cucui, A.; et al. Effect of Hemodiafiltration or Hemodialysis on Mortality in Kidney Failure. *N. Engl. J. Med.* **2023**, *389*, 700–709. [CrossRef] [PubMed]
7. Piccoli, G.B.; Nielsen, L.; Gendrot, L.; Fois, A.; Cataldo, E.; Cabiddu, G. Prescribing Hemodialysis or Hemodiafiltration: When One Size Does Not Fit All the Proposal of a Personalized Approach Based on Comorbidity and Nutritional Status. *J. Clin. Med.* **2018**, *7*, 331. [CrossRef]
8. Zawierucha, J.; Małyszko, J.; Dębska-Ślizień, A.; Durlik, M.; Krajewska, M.; Chmiel, G.; Ciechanowski, K.; Klinger, M.; Małyszko, J.; Nowicki, M.; et al. Expert panel position statement on indication for hemodiafiltration (hdf) therapy in end stage renal disease patients. *Nefrol. Dial. Pol.* **2018**, *22*, 9–12.
9. Schiffl, H. Online hemodiafiltration and mortality risk in end-stage renal disease patients: A critical appraisal of current evidence. *Kidney Res. Clin. Pract.* **2019**, *38*, 159–168. [CrossRef]
10. Marcelli, D.; Scholz, C.; Ponce, P.; Sousa, T.; Kopperschmidt, P.; Grassmann, A.; Pinto, B.; Canaud, B. High-Volume Postdilution Hemodiafiltration Is a Feasible Option in Routine Clinical Practice. *Artif. Organs* **2015**, *39*, 142–149. [CrossRef]
11. Smith, J.R.; Zimmer, N.; Bell, E.; Francq, B.G.; McConnachie, A.; Mactier, R. A Randomized, Single-Blind, Crossover Trial of Recovery Time in High-Flux Hemodialysis and Hemodiafiltration. *Am. J. Kidney Dis.* **2017**, *69*, 762–770. [CrossRef] [PubMed]
12. Lindsay, R.M.; Heidenheim, P.A.; Nesrallah, G.; Garg, A.X.; Suri, R.; on behalf of the Daily Hemodialysis Study Group London Health Sciences Centre. Minutes to Recovery after a Hemodialysis Session. *Clin. J. Am. Soc. Nephrol.* **2006**, *1*, 952–959. [CrossRef] [PubMed]
13. Scherhag, A.; Kaden, J.J.; Kentschke, E.; Sueselbeck, T.; Borggrefe, M. Comparison of Impedance Cardiography and Thermodilution-Derived Measurements of Stroke Volume and Cardiac Output at Rest and During Exercise Testing. *Cardiovasc. Drugs Ther.* **2005**, *19*, 141–147. [CrossRef] [PubMed]
14. Moissl, U.M.; Wabel, P.; Chamney, P.W.; Bosaeus, I.; Levin, N.W.; Bosy-Westphal, A.; Korth, O.; Müller, M.J.; Ellegård, L.; Malmros, V.; et al. Body fluid volume determination via body composition spectroscopy in health and disease. *Physiol. Meas.* **2006**, *27*, 921–933. [CrossRef]
15. Shroff, R.; Basile, C.; van der Sande, F.; Mitra, S.; EuDial Working Group of the European Renal Association. Haemodiafiltration for all: Are we convinced? *Nephrol. Dial. Transplant.* **2023**, *38*, 2663–2665. [CrossRef]
16. Merkus, M.P.; Jager, K.J.; Dekker, F.W.; Boeschoten, E.W.; Stevens, P.; Krediet, R.T. Quality of life in patients on chronic dialysis: Self-assessment 3 months after the start of treatment. *Am. J. Kidney Dis.* **1997**, *29*, 584–592. [CrossRef]
17. Bello, A.K.; Okpechi, I.G.; Osman, M.A.; Cho, Y.; Htay, H.; Jha, V.; Wainstein, M.; Johnson, D.W. Epidemiology of haemodialysis outcomes. *Nat. Rev. Nephrol.* **2022**, *18*, 378–395. [CrossRef]
18. Puchalska-Reglińska, E.; Dębska-Ślizień, A.; Biedunkiewicz, B.; Tylicki, P.; Polewska, K.; Jagodziński, P.; Rutkowski, B.; Gellert, R.; Tylicki, L. Extremely high mortality in COVID-19 hemodialyzed patients in before anty-SARS-CoV-2 vaccination era. The first large database from Poland. *Pol. Arch. Intern. Med.* **2021**, *131*, 643–648. [CrossRef]
19. Monardo, P.; Lacquaniti, A.; Campo, S.; Bucca, M.; Casuscelli di Tocco, T.; Rovito, S.; Ragusa, A.; Santoro, A. Updates on hemodialysis techniques with a common denominator: The personalization of the dialytic therapy. *Semin. Dial.* **2021**, *34*, 183–195. [CrossRef]
20. Flythe, J.E.; Dorough, A.; Narendra, J.H.; Forfang, D.; Hartwell, L.; Abdel-Rahman, E. Perspectives on symptom experiences and symptom reporting among individuals on hemodialysis. *Nephrol. Dial. Transplant.* **2018**, *33*, 1842–1852. [CrossRef]
21. Caplin, B.; Alston, H.; Davenport, A. Does Online Haemodiafiltration Reduce Intra-Dialytic Patient Symptoms? *Nephron. Clin. Pract.* **2013**, *124*, 184–190. [CrossRef] [PubMed]
22. Jhamb, M.; Argyropoulos, C.; Steel, J.L.; Plantinga, L.; Wu, A.W.; Fink, N.E.; Powe, N.R.; Meyer, K.B.; Unruh, M.L.; Mark, L.; et al. Correlates and Outcomes of Fatigue among Incident Dialysis Patients. *Clin. J. Am. Soc. Nephrol.* **2009**, *4*, 1779–1786. [CrossRef]
23. Alvarez, L.; Brown, D.; Hu, D.; Chertow, G.M.; Vassalotti, J.A.; Prichard, S. Intradialytic Symptoms and Recovery Time in Patients on Thrice-Weekly In-Center Hemodialysis: A Cross-sectional Online Survey. *Radiology* **2020**, *2*, 125–130. [CrossRef]

24. Rayner, H.C.; Zepel, L.; Fuller, D.S.; Morgenstern, H.; Karaboyas, A.; Culleton, B.F.; Mapes, D.L.; Lopes, A.A.; Gillespie, B.W.; Hasegawa, T.; et al. Recovery Time, Quality of Life, and Mortality in Hemodialysis Patients: The Dialysis Outcomes and Practice Patterns Study (DOPPS). *Am. J. Kidney Dis.* **2014**, *64*, 86–94. [CrossRef] [PubMed]
25. Morena, M.; Jaussent, A.; Chalabi, L.; Leray-Moragues, H.; Chenine, L.; Debure, A.; Thibaudin, D.; Azzouz, L.; Patrier, L.; Maurice, F.; et al. Treatment tolerance and patient-reported outcomes favor online hemodiafiltration compared to high-flux hemodialysis in the elderly. *Kidney Int.* **2017**, *91*, 1495–1509. [CrossRef] [PubMed]
26. Schiffl, H. High-volume online haemodiafiltration treatment and outcome of end-stage renal disease patients: More than one mode. *Int. Urol. Nephrol.* **2020**, *52*, 1501–1506. [CrossRef] [PubMed]
27. Maduell, F.; Moreso, F.; Pons, M.; Ramos, R.; Mora-Macià, J.; Carreras, J.; Soler, J.; Torres, F.; Campistol, J.M.; Martinez-Castelao, A.; et al. High-Efficiency Postdilution Online Hemodiafiltration Reduces All-Cause Mortality in Hemodialysis Patients. *J. Am. Soc. Nephrol.* **2013**, *24*, 487–497. [CrossRef]
28. Ethier, I.; Nevis, I.; Suri, R.S. Quality of Life and Hemodynamic Effects of Switching from Hemodialysis to Hemodiafiltration: A Canadian Controlled Cohort Study. *Can. J. Kidney Health Dis.* **2021**, *8*, 1–9. [CrossRef]
29. Locatelli, F.; Mastrangelo, F.; Redaelli, B.; Ronco, C.; Marcelli, D.; La Greca, G.; Orlandini, G. The Italian Cooperative Dialysis Study Group Effects of different membranes and dialysis technologies on patient treatment tolerance and nutritional parameters. *Kidney Int.* **1996**, *50*, 1293–1302. [CrossRef]
30. Park, H.C.; Lee, Y.K. Who is the winner, pre-, post-, or mixed-dilution hemodiafiltration? *Kidney Res. Clin. Pract.* **2021**, *40*, 332–334. [CrossRef]
31. Donauer, J.; Schweiger, C.; Rumberger, B.; Krumme, B.; Böhler, J. Reduction of hypotensive side effects during online-haemodiafiltration and low temperature haemodialysis. *Nephrol. Dial. Transplant.* **2003**, *18*, 1616–1622. [CrossRef] [PubMed]
32. Locatelli, F.; Altieri, P.; Andrulli, S.; Bolasco, P.; Sau, G.; Pedrini, L.A.; Basile, C.; David, S.; Feriani, M.; Montagna, G.; et al. Hemofiltration and Hemodiafiltration Reduce Intradialytic Hypotension in ESRD. *J. Am. Soc. Nephrol.* **2010**, *21*, 1798–1807. [CrossRef] [PubMed]
33. Park, K.S.; Kang, E.W.; Chang, T.I.; Jo, W.; Park, J.T.; Yoo, T.-H.; Kang, S.-W.; Han, S.H. Mixed- versus predilution hemodiafiltration effects on convection volume and small and middle molecule clearance in hemodialysis patients: A prospective randomized controlled trial. *Kidney Res. Clin. Pract.* **2021**, *40*, 445–456. [CrossRef] [PubMed]
34. Bolton, S.; Gair, R.; Nilsson, L.-G.; Matthews, M.; Stewart, L.; McCullagh, N. Clinical Assessment of Dialysis Recovery Time and Symptom Burden: Impact of Switching Hemodialysis Therapy Mode. *Patient Relat. Outcome Meas.* **2021**, *12*, 315–321. [CrossRef] [PubMed]
35. Pongsittisak, W.; Satpanich, P.; Jaturapisanukul, S.; Keawvichit, R.; Prommool, S.; Trakranvanich, T.; Ngamvichukorn, T.; Kurathong, S. Medium Cut-Off versus Low-Flux Dialyzers in Hemodialysis Patients with COVID-19: Clinical Outcomes and Reduction in Interleukin-6. *Blood Purif.* **2023**, *52*, 591–599. [CrossRef] [PubMed]
36. Alarcon, J.C.; Bunch, A.; Ardila, F.; Zuñiga, E.; Vesga, J.I.; Rivera, A.; Sánchez, R.; Sanabria, R.M.; on behalf of the Colombian Registry of Expanded Hemodialysis Investigators. Impact of Medium Cut-Off Dialyzers on Patient-Reported Outcomes: Corexh Registry. *Blood Purif.* **2021**, *50*, 110–118. [CrossRef] [PubMed]
37. Penny, J.D.; Salerno, F.R.; Akbari, A.; McIntyre, C.W. Pruritus: Is there a grain of salty truth? *Hemodial. Int.* **2021**, *25*, E10–E14. [CrossRef]
38. Jankowska, M.; Cobo, G.; Lindholm, B.; Stenvinkel, P. Inflammation and protein-energy wasting in the uremic milieu. *Contrib. Nephrol.* **2017**, *191*, 58–71. [CrossRef]
39. Hadad-Arrascue, F.; Nilsson, L.G.; Rivera, A.S.; Bernardo, A.A.; Cabezuelo Romero, J.B. Expanded hemodialysis as effective alternative to on-line hemodiafiltration: A randomized mid-term clinical trial. *Ther. Apher. Dial.* **2022**, *26*, 37–44. [CrossRef]
40. Kawai, Y.; Maeda, K.; Moriishi, M.; Kawanishi, H.; Masaki, T. Comparison of the pre-dilution and post-dilution methods for online hemodiafiltration. *J. Artif. Organs* **2023**, *Online ahead of print*. [CrossRef]
41. Lee, Y.; Jang, M.-J.; Jeon, J.; Lee, J.E.; Huh, W.; Choi, B.S.; Park, C.W.; Chin, H.J.; Kang, C.L.; Kim, D.K.; et al. Cardiovascular Risk Comparison between Expanded Hemodialysis Using Theranova and Online Hemodiafiltration (CARTOON): A Multicenter Randomized Controlled Trial. *Sci. Rep.* **2021**, *11*, 10807. [CrossRef] [PubMed]
42. Doenyas-Barak, K.; de Abreu, M.H.F.G.; Borges, L.E.; Filho, H.A.T.; Yunlin, F.; Yurong, Z.; Levin, N.W.; Kaufman, A.M.; Efrati, S.; Pereg, D.; et al. Non-invasive hemodynamic profiling of patients undergoing hemodialysis—A multicenter observational cohort study. *BMC Nephrol.* **2019**, *20*, 347. [CrossRef] [PubMed]
43. Elsayed, M.M.; Zeid, M.M.; Hamza, O.M.R.; Elkholy, N.M. Dialysis recovery time: Associated factors and its association with quality of life of hemodialysis patients. *BMC Nephrol.* **2022**, *23*, 298. [CrossRef] [PubMed]
44. Davenport, A.; Guirguis, A.; Almond, M.; Day, C.; Chilcot, J.; Gane, M.D.S.; Fineberg, N.; Friedl, K.; Spencer, B.; Wellsted, D.; et al. Postdialysis recovery time is extended in patients with greater self-reported depression screening questionnaire scores. *Hemodial. Int.* **2018**, *22*, 369–376. [CrossRef] [PubMed]
45. Bossola, M.; Di Stasio, E.S.; Giungi, S.; Rosa, F.; Tazza, L. Fatigue Is Associated with Serum Interleukin-6 Levels and Symptoms of Depression in Patients on Chronic Hemodialysis. *J. Pain Symptom Manag.* **2015**, *49*, 578–585. [CrossRef]

46. Yoowannakul, S.; Vongsanim, S.; Tangvoraphonkchai, K.; Davenport, A. Do patients dialysing with higher ultrafiltration rates report more intradialytic symptoms and longer postdialysis recovery times? *Artif. Organs* **2023**. *Online ahead of print.* [CrossRef]

47. Vinson, A.J.; Collister, D.; Ahmed, S.; Tennankore, K. Underrepresentation of Women in Recent Landmark Kidney Trials: The Gender Gap Prevails. *Kidney Int. Rep.* **2022**, *7*, 2526–2529. [CrossRef]

Disclaimer/Publisher's Note: The statements, opinions and data contained in all publications are solely those of the individual author(s) and contributor(s) and not of MDPI and/or the editor(s). MDPI and/or the editor(s) disclaim responsibility for any injury to people or property resulting from any ideas, methods, instructions or products referred to in the content.

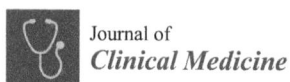

Article

Predictors for Unsuccessful Reductions in Hemodialysis Frequency during the Pandemic

Suthiya Anumas [1], Sithichai Kunawathanakul [2], Pichaya Tantiyavarong [2,3], Pajaree Krisanapan [2] and Pattharawin Pattharanitima [2,*]

1. Chulabhorn International College of Medicine, Thammasat University, Pathum Thani 12120, Thailand
2. Division of Nephrology, Department of Medicine, Faculty of Medicine, Thammasat University, Pathum Thani 12120, Thailand
3. Department of Clinical Epidemiology, Faculty of Medicine, Thammasat University, Pathum Thani 12120, Thailand
* Correspondence: pattharawin@hotmail.com

Abstract: Background and Objectives: Patients receiving in-center hemodialysis are at a high risk of coronavirus disease 2019 (COVID-19) infection. A reduction in hemodialysis frequency is one of the proposed measures for preventing COVID-19 infection. However, the predictors for determining an unsuccessful reduction in hemodialysis frequency are still lacking. Materials and Methods: This retrospective observational study enrolled patients who were receiving long-term thrice-weekly hemodialysis at the Thammasat University Hospital in 2021 and who decreased their dialysis frequency to twice weekly during the COVID-19 outbreak. The outcomes were to determine the predictors and a prediction model of unsuccessful reduction in dialysis frequency at 4 weeks. Bootstrapping was performed for the purposes of internal validation. Results: Of the 161 patients, 83 patients achieved a dialysis frequency reduction. Further, 33% and 82% of the patients failed to reduce their dialysis frequency at 4 and 8 weeks, respectively. The predictors for unsuccessful reduction were diabetes, congestive heart failure (CHF), pre-dialysis overhydration, set dry weight (DW), DW from bioelectrical impedance analysis, and the mean pre- and post-dialysis body weight. The final model including these predictors demonstrated an AUROC of 0.763 (95% CI 0.654–0.866) for the prediction of an unsuccessful reduction. Conclusions: The prediction score involving diabetes, CHF, pre-dialysis overhydration, DW difference, and net ultrafiltration demonstrated a good performance in predicting an unsuccessful reduction in hemodialysis frequency at 4 weeks.

Keywords: COVID-19; hemodialysis; reduction dialysis frequency; prediction

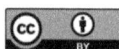

1. Introduction

Coronavirus disease 2019 (COVID-19) was declared a pandemic on 11 March 2020 [1] by the World Health Organization (WHO), and it has affected millions worldwide. The mortality-related risk factors of COVID-19 are chronic comorbidities, including diabetes, hypertension, chronic obstructive pulmonary disease (COPD), cardiovascular disease, obesity, cancer, and chronic kidney disease, especially in those who were suffering from end-stage kidney disease (ESKD) and receiving dialysis treatment [2–4].

COVID-19 spreads via droplet transmission from coughing, sneezing, speaking, and breathing [5]. It also spreads via direct contact with the eyes, nose, and mouth, or through the air over a short range (short-range airborne transmission). However, in a crowded indoor setting where people spend time for extended periods and/or in a poorly ventilated environment, infectious particles remain in the air for a longer duration of time and travel farther than usual, thus resulting in long-range airborne transmission [5]. A dialysis unit is compatible with the aforementioned setting, which thus results in a higher risk of COVID-19 infection in hemodialysis patients.

Reducing hemodialysis frequency might diminish COVID-19 exposure in either patients or dialysis staff, reduce dialysis staff work, increase the space between patients, reduce the amount of public transportation used, and conserve personal protective equipment (PPE) [6]. Although a reduced long-term hemodialysis frequency may result in an inadequate dialysis, especially in patients with a residual renal urea clearance of less than 2 mL/min/1.73 m^2 [7], a reduced short-term hemodialysis frequency during a pandemic might be beneficial. Some guidance has suggested consideration of a reduction in hemodialysis frequency from thrice to twice weekly in patients who are able to tolerate this reduction as one of measures for managing hemodialysis patients during the COVID-19 pandemic [8]. However, there has been limited evidence by which to determine the effect of reducing short-term dialysis frequency and the predictors for an unsuccessful reduction in dialysis frequency during the pandemic. Thus, we conducted this study to determine the predictors of unsuccessful reduction and to develop a clinical prediction score in order to determine the risk of unsuccessfully reducing dialysis frequency in a pandemic setting.

2. Materials and Methods

This retrospective observational study utilized data from the dialysis unit at the Thammasat University Hospital, Thailand. Ethical approval was granted by The Human Research Ethics Committee of Thammasat University: Medicine (111/2565). All adult ESKD patients who were receiving thrice-weekly hemodialysis in 2021 for at least one week before a decrease in dialysis frequency to twice-weekly hemodialysis were included in the study. The exclusion criteria were patients who (1) received the first hemodialysis session after 5 July 2021, which was the date of starting a reduction in dialysis frequency; (2) received their last hemodialysis session before 5 July 2021; and (3) had no dialysis data within one week prior to decreasing their dialysis frequency.

The primary outcome was determining the predictors of an unsuccessful reduction in hemodialysis frequency at 4 weeks, which was defined as a failure to maintain twice-weekly hemodialysis sessions for 4 weeks and the need to transfer back to thrice-weekly hemodialysis for any reason. The secondary outcome was to determine a prevalence of unsuccessfully reducing dialysis frequency at 4 and 8 weeks as well as to create a clinical prediction model score for the unsuccessful reductions in dialysis frequency.

All hemodialysis patients who met the eligibility criteria were identified from an electronic hemodialysis database. We retrieved demographics, laboratory data, and dialysis parameter records. The baseline demographic variables, including age, sex, vascular access, and comorbidities, were retrieved. The latest laboratory data within 90 days prior to dialysis frequency reduction, including hemoglobin, electrolytes, calcium, phosphate, parathyroid hormones, albumin, dialysis adequacy parameters, and last dry weight (as measured by bioelectrical impedance (BIA) within 90 days before decreasing frequency), were included. Pre-dialysis overhydration was defined as the mean of pre-dialysis body weight minus the dry weight from BIA. Post-dialysis overhydration was defined as the mean of post-dialysis body weight minus the dry weight from BIA. The mean value of dialysis parameters—including net ultrafiltration, pre- and post-dialysis body weight, blood pressure, and heart rate within one week prior to decreasing dialysis frequency—were included. All patients were provided with education for fluid and protein-restricted diets; additionally, diuretics were given to those patients who had residual urine outputs. All patients were prescribed 4-h dialysis treatment times, with a dialysis prescription at the discretion of the attending nephrologists. The causes of unsuccessful reductions in dialysis frequency were reported.

2.1. Statistical Analysis

The categorical data were presented in frequency and percentage. The numerical data were presented in the median and interquartile range (IQR). The medians were compared using a Wilcoxon rank-sum test, whereas the proportions were compared using Fisher's exact test. The logistic regression analysis was performed to determine the predictors for an unsuccessful reduction in dialysis frequency. Non-missing variables with a p-value of

≤0.1 from a univariate logistic regression analysis were included in a multivariate logistic regression analysis. The strength of association between the predictors and outcome was reported as an odds ratio (OR) and a 95% confidence interval (95% CI). A two-sided p-value of <0.05 was considered statistically significant. All statistical analyses were performed using the STATA version 17.0/BE.

2.2. Model Development

The predictors from the multivariate logistic regression analysis were included in a developed model. The internal validation was assessed by a bootstrapping procedure [9], with a 500-bootstrap sample in order to quantify the optimism of the developed model. The model was then adjusted by a shrinkage factor to create a final model. The log odds from the final model were used to create a prediction score. The area under the receiver operating characteristics curve (AUROC) was calculated to determine the performance of the developed model, final model, and the prediction scores.

3. Results

3.1. Baseline Characteristics

Of the 161 hemodialysis patients in the dialysis unit at Thammasat University Hospital in 2021, 78 patients were excluded: 19 patients received their first hemodialysis session after 5 July 2021, 6 patients received their last hemodialysis session before 5 July 2021, 4 patients had no data within one week prior to their decreasing frequency, 18 patients received hemodialysis twice a week, and 31 patients continued hemodialysis thrice a week due to the treating physician's decision. Of the 83 included patients, 56 patients successfully reduced their hemodialysis frequency (67%) for 4 weeks.

The median (IQR) age of the included patients was 69.6 (63.1–80.4) years. Further, 53% of the patients were female. The most common vascular access was via the arteriovenous fistula (65.1%). Hypertension, dyslipidemia, and diabetes mellitus (DM) were found in 96.4, 66.3, and 57.8% of patients, respectively. There was significantly higher proportion of DM patients in the unsuccessful group (77.8%) than in the successful group (48.2%). In addition, a numerically higher proportion of patients with congestive heart failure (CHF) was observed in the unsuccessful group (14.8%) than in the successful group (3.6%). The median bicarbonate and intact parathyroid hormone (iPTH) level was found to be lesser in the unsuccessful group; however, the data were not available for some patients. The dialysis adequacy was not significantly different in both groups. However, pre-dialysis overhydration was significantly greater in the unsuccessful group. The dry weight from BIA, actual set dry weight, and the pre- and post-dialysis body weight were numerically higher in the unsuccessful group (Table 1).

Table 1. Baseline characteristics of the hemodialysis patients.

Characteristics	Successful (n = 56)	Non-Successful (n = 27)	Total (n = 83)	p-Value
Age, year, median (IQR)	70.65 (64.0–81.2)	68.3 (60.3–78.6)	69.6 (63.1–80.4)	0.24
Female, n (%)	30 (53.6)	14 (51.2)	44 (53.0)	1.00
Vascular access, n (%)				0.86
Fistula	36 (64.3)	18 (66.7)	54 (65.1)	
Graft	5 (8.9)	1 (3.7)	6 (7.2)	
Permanent catheter	15 (26.8)	8 (29.6)	23 (27.7)	
comorbidity, n (%)				
Diabetes mellitus	27 (48.2)	21 (77.8)	48 (57.8)	0.02
Hypertension	55 (98.2)	25 (92.6)	80 (96.4)	0.25
Dyslipidemia	35 (62.5)	20 (74.1)	55 (66.3)	0.33
Congestive heart failure	2 (3.6)	4 (14.8)	6 (7.2)	0.08
Ischemic heart disease	14 (25.0)	10 (37.0)	24 (28.9)	0.31
Cerebrovascular disease	10 (17.9)	6 (22.2)	16 (19.3)	0.77

Table 1. Cont.

Characteristics	Successful (n = 56)	Non-Successful (n = 27)	Total (n = 83)	p-Value
Dialysis vintage, year, median (IQR)	4.7 (2.5–7.4)	4.5 (3.0–7.9)	4.5 (2.8–7.5)	0.83
Laboratory, median (IQR)				
Hemoglobin, g/dL	10.9 (10.1–11.6)	10.4 (9.8–11.1)	10.8 (10–11.6)	0.22
White blood cell [a], $10^3/\mu L$	5.7 (5.0–6.9)	5.8 (5.1–7.3)	5.7 (5.0–6.9)	0.70
Platelet, $10^3/\mu L$	193 (158–227)	197 (131–236)	193 (147–232)	0.83
Sodium [b], mmol/L	137 (135–139)	136 (134–139)	137 (134–139)	0.69
Potassium [b], mmol/L	4.1 (3.7–4.7)	4.1 (3.8–4.5)	4.1 (3.7–4.5)	0.85
Chloride [b], mmol/L	98 (97–100)	98 (96–100)	98 (97–100)	0.89
Bicarbonate [b], mmol/L	25 (24–27)	24 (23–25)	25 (23–26)	0.049
Calcium [c], mg/dL	9.1 (8.3–9.7)	8.8 (8.1–9.2)	8.9 (8.3–9.5)	0.14
Phosphate [c], mg/dL	3.8 (3.2–4.9)	4.3 (3.5–6.1)	3.9 (3.3–5.1)	0.13
iPTH [d], pg/mL	582 (385–805)	442 (322–537)	536 (348–735)	0.04
Albumin [e], g/dL	3.7 (3.4–3.9)	3.6 (3.45–3.8)	3.6 (3.4–3.9)	0.63
Dialysis adequacy, median (IQR)				
spKt/V	1.91 (1.66–2.09)	1.85 (1.67–2.04)	1.88 (1.67–2.07)	0.52
URR (%)	80.5 (75.7–83.1)	77.8 (75.4–83.3)	80.0 (75.4–83.3)	0.32
nPCR (g/kg/d)	0.99 (0.87–1.26)	1.08 (0.98–1.17)	1.02 (0.88–1.21)	0.32
eqKt/V	1.67 (1.45–1.82)	1.61 (1.46–1.76)	1.65 (1.45–1.81)	0.55
stdKt/V	2.83 (2.42–3.27)	2.9 (2.47–3.13)	2.84 (2.42–3.17)	0.88
Dry weight, kg, median (IQR)				
Dry weight from BIA	56.2 (49.0–65.1)	60.7 (52.7–73.8)	58.2 (50.3–68.7)	0.06
Set dry weight	57.3 (48.5–65.3)	61.5 (52.5–73.5)	58.5 (50.0–69.0)	0.06
Pre-dialysis parameter, median (IQR)				
Pre-dialysis body weight, kg	58.8 (50.5–67.1)	63.5 (54.5–75.3)	60.0 (51.2–71.3)	0.054
Pre-dialysis overhydration, L	1.9 (1.0–2.5)	2.3 (1.6–3.1)	2 (1.3–2.6)	0.01
Interdialytic weight gain, %	3.4 (2.5–4.0)	3.1 (2.6–3.9)	3.3 (2.5–4.0)	0.92
SBP, mmHg	138.2 (126.8–152.9)	146.7 (127.7–158.0)	140 (127.3–155.3)	0.28
DBP, mmHg	61.3 (54.7–68.0)	61.3 (49.3–74.7)	61.3 (53.7–69.0)	0.98
Heart rate, bpm	69.0 (64.2–76.8)	74.0 (65.3–79.3)	71.3 (64.7–78.3)	0.24
Post-dialysis parameter, median (IQR)				
Post-dialysis body weight, kg	57.2 (49.0–65.2)	61.4 (53.1–74.1)	58.4 (49.9–69.0)	0.06
Post-dialysis overhydration, L	0.2 ((−0.6)–0.8)	−0.2 ((−0.6)–0.4)	0 ((−0.6)–0.6)	0.27
SBP, mmHg	151.9 (139.9–162.7)	154.7 (145.7–163.0)	153.3 (140.7–162.7)	0.70
DBP, mmHg	67.0 (60.7–73.7)	68.0 (59.7–73.7)	67.0 (60.7–73.7)	0.76
Heart rate, bpm	67.9 (60.7–74.0)	69.3 (59.7–76.0)	68.0 (60.7–74.3)	0.99
Ultrafiltration, L	1.8 (1.4–2.2)	2.0 (1.5–2.4)	1.9 (1.5–2.2)	0.15
Ultrafiltration rate, mL/kg/h	8.1 (6.0–9.8)	7.5 (6.7–9.1)	8.0 (6.4–9.8)	0.85

Abbreviations: BIA, bioelectrical impedance analysis; iPTH, intact parathyroid hormone; spKt/V, single pool Kt/V; URR, urea reduction ratio; nPCR, normalized protein catabolic rate; eqKt/V, equilibrated Kt/V; stdKt/V, standard Kt/V; SBP, systolic blood pressure; DBP, diastolic blood pressure. [a] The missing 5 patients in the success group and 5 patients in the unsuccessful group. [b] The missing 4 patients in the success group. [c] The missing 6 patients in the successful group. [d] The missing 25 patients in the success group and 12 patients in the failure group. [e] The missing 15 patients in the successful group and 3 patients in the unsuccessful group. Pre-dialysis overhydration = pre-dialysis body weight—DW from the BIA; post-dialysis overhydration = post-dialysis body weight—DW from the BIA.

Of the hemodialysis patients, the rates of unsuccessfully reducing the dialysis frequency at 4 and 8 weeks were 33% and 88%, respectively. In the successful group at 4 weeks, 41 (73%) patients failed to maintain a reduction in hemodialysis frequency throughout 8 weeks, and most of them failed at the fifth week. There were some differences observed among the baseline characteristics of patients who were unsuccessful in reducing their hemodialysis frequency over 4 weeks and over 8 weeks, and who were successful in reducing hemodialysis frequency over 8 weeks. However, the results of the Bonferroni multiple-comparison test were not significantly different (Table S1).

The most common cause for an unsuccessful reduction in dialysis frequency at 4 weeks was in volume overload (48.15%) (Figure 1).

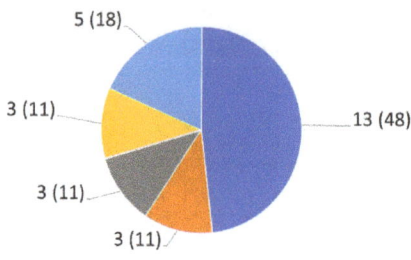

Figure 1. The causes of unsuccessful reductions in hemodialysis frequency. Other causes included uremic symptoms (two patients), alterations of consciousness during dialysis (two patients), and an uncomfortable feeling after the dialysis session (one patient).

3.2. Predictors of Unsuccessful Reductions in Hemodialysis Frequency

The univariate logistic regression analysis showed that the predictors of an unsuccessful reduction in dialysis frequency were diabetes mellitus, iPTH level, and pre-dialysis overhydration (i.e., the pre-dialysis body weight minus the dry weight from the BIA) (Table 2).

Table 2. The univariate analyses for unsuccessful reductions in hemodialysis frequency.

	Univariate OR (95% C.I.)	p-Value
Age (year)	0.98 (0.94–1.02)	0.32
Female	0.93 (0.37–2.34)	0.88
Comorbidity		
Diabetes mellitus	3.76 (1.32–10.72)	0.01
Hypertension	0.23 (0.02–2.62)	0.24
Dyslipidemia	1.71 (0.63–4.74)	0.30
Congestive heart failure	4.70 (0.80–27.46)	0.09
Ischemic heart disease	1.76 (0.66–4.74)	0.26
Cerebrovascular disease	1.31 (0.42–4.09)	0.64
Laboratory data		
Hemoglobin (g/dL)	0.88 (0.63–1.24)	0.47
Sodium [a], mmol/L	0.98 (0.85–1.14)	0.84
Potassium [a], mmol/L	0.83 (0.41–1.68)	0.61
Bicarbonate [a], mmol/L	0.84 (0.69–1.03)	0.09
Calcium [b], mg/dL	0.86 (0.53–1.40)	0.55
Phosphate [b], mg/dL	1.25 (0.94–1.68)	0.13
iPTH [c], pg/mL	1.00 (0.99–1.00)	0.048
Albumin [d], g/dL	0.69 (0.12–3.99)	0.68
Dialysis adequacy		
spKt/V	0.54 (0.10–2.81)	0.46
URR, %	0.94 (0.85–1.04)	0.23
nPCR, g/kg/d	1.50 (0.24–9.39)	0.66
stdKt/V	1.25 (0.64–2.47)	0.51
Dialysis vintage, year	0.98 (0.87–1.09)	0.69
Pre-dialysis overhydration, L	1.82 (1.12–2.96)	0.02
Post-dialysis overhydration, L	0.86 (0.52–1.42)	0.55
Dry weight BIA, kg	1.03 (1.00–1.07)	0.07
Set dry weight, kg	1.03 (1.00–1.07)	0.06

Table 2. Cont.

	Univariate OR (95% C.I.)	p-Value
Ultrafiltration, L	1.00 (1.00–1.00)	
Ultrafiltration rate, mL/kg/hour	1.00 (0.83–1.20)	
Pre-dialysis parameter		
Body weight, kg	1.03 (1.00–1.07)	0.06
Interdialytic weight gain, %	1.02 (0.68–1.53)	0.94
SBP, mmHg	1.01 (0.99–1.04)	0.37
DBP, mmHg	1.00 (0.96–1.04)	0.92
Heart rate, bpm	1.03 (0.99–1.08)	0.15
Post-dialysis parameter		
Body weight, kg	1.03 (1.00–1.07)	0.06
SBP, mmHg	1.00 (0.97–1.03)	0.89
DBP, mmHg	0.99 (0.96–1.03)	0.76

Abbreviations: BIA, bioelectrical impedance analysis; iPTH, intact parathyroid hormone; spKt/V, single pool Kt/V; URR, urea reduction ratio; nPCR, normalized protein catabolic rate; eqKt/V, equilibrated Kt/V; stdKt/V, standard Kt/V; SBP, systolic blood pressure; DBP, diastolic blood pressure. [a] The missing 4 patients in the successful group. [b] The missing 6 patients in the successful group. [c] The missing 25 patients in the successful group and 12 patients in the unsuccessful group. [d] The missing 15 patients in the successful group and 3 patients in the unsuccessful group.

The multivariate logistic regression analysis demonstrated that the DM (OR 4.37; 95% CI 1.13–16.83; p-value = 0.032), CHF (OR 9.71; 95% CI 1.16–81.43; p-value = 0.036), pre-dialysis overhydration (OR 2.97; 95% CI 1.23–7.19; p-value = 0.016), and dry weight from the BIA (OR 3.41; 95% CI 1.01–11.49; p-value = 0.047) were predictors of an unsuccessful reduction in hemodialysis frequency (Table 3).

Table 3. The multivariate analyses of the risk factors of unsuccessful reduction in hemodialysis frequency.

Predictors	Univariate OR (95% C.I.)	p-Value	Multivariate OR (95% C.I.)	p-Value
Diabetes mellitus	3.76 (1.32–10.72)	0.01	4.37 (1.13–16.83)	0.03
Congestive heart failure	4.70 (0.80–27.46)	0.09	9.71 (1.16–81.43)	0.04
Pre-dialysis overhydration (L)	1.82 (1.12–2.96)	0.02	2.97 (1.23–7.19)	0.02
Dry weight BIA (kg)	1.03 (1.00–1.07)	0.07	3.41 (1.01–11.49)	0.047
Dry weight (kg)	1.03 (1.00–1.07)	0.06	0.32 (0.06–1.74)	0.19
Pre-dialysis body weight (kg)	1.03 (1.00–1.07)	0.06	0.50 (0.14–1.72)	0.27
Post-dialysis body weight (kg)	1.03 (1.00–1.07)	0.06	1.88 (0.38–9.25)	0.44

Abbreviations: BIA, bioelectrical impedance analysis.

3.3. Clinical Prediction Score

The linear equation was log odds (failure reducing hemodialysis frequency) = −3.24 + 1.47 (DM) + 2.27 (CHF) + 1.09 (pre-dialysis overhydration) + 1.23 (dry weight from BIA) − 1.15 (set dry weight) − 0.70 (pre-dialysis body weight) + 0.63 (post-dialysis body weight). The Hosmer–Lemeshow test was performed to test the goodness of fit, which demonstrated a p-value of 0.54. The E:O ratio and the AUROC of the developed model were 1.000 and 0.798 (95% CI 0.704–0.893), respectively (Table 4).

For the purposes of internal validation, bootstrapping was performed with a 500-bootstrap sample. The coefficients from the developed model were multiplied by the shrinkage factors of 0.65 (optimism adjusted) (Table 4). The optimism-adjusted linear equation was log odds (failure reducing hemodialysis frequency) = −2.3 + 0.95 (DM) + 1.47 (CHF) + 0.71 (pre-dialysis overhydration) + 0.80 (dry weight from BIA) − 0.75 (set dry weight) − 0.46 (pre-dialysis body weight) + 0.41 (post-dialysis body weight). For the calibration, the E:O ratio and the AUROC of the optimism-adjusted model were 0.997 and 0.728 (95% CI 0.637–0.828), respectively (Table 4).

Table 4. The multiple correlation coefficient of the risk factors for unsuccessful reductions in hemodialysis frequency.

	Multivariate Coeff. (95% CI) [a]	*p*-Value	Multivariate Coeff. (95% CI) [b]	*p*-Value
Diabetes mellitus	1.47 (0.13 to 2.82)	0.03	0.95 (0.08 to 1.83)	0.03
Congestive heart failure	2.27 (0.15 to 4.40)	0.04	1.47 (0.09 to 2.86)	0.03
Pre-dialysis overhydration (L)	1.09 (0.21 to 1.97)	0.02	0.70 (0.13 to 1.28)	0.02
Dry weight BIA (kg)	1.23 (0.01 to 2.44)	0.047	0.80 (0.01 to 1.58)	0.047
Dry weight (kg)	−1.15 (−2.85 to −0.55)	0.19	−0.75 (−1.85 to 0.36)	0.18
Pre-dialysis body weight (kg)	−0.70 (−0.96 to 2.22)	0.27	−0.46 (−1.26 to 0.35)	0.27
Post-dialysis body weight (kg)	0.63 (−0.96 to −2.22)	0.44	0.41 (−0.62 to 1.44)	0.44

[a] Developed model; [b] optimism-adjusted model. Abbreviations: BIA, bioelectrical impedance analysis.

The lowest coefficient of 0.45 was used as a denominator for the other predictors' coefficients. The results were rounded to integers and used for predicting the score. The weighting scores were assigned as 2 points for a patient with DM, 3 points for a patient with CHF, 2 points per pre-dialysis overhydration in a liter, 2 points per dry weight difference (dry weight from BIA − dry weight in actual dialysis setting) in kilograms, and −1 point for a net ultrafiltration in a liter (post-dialysis body weight − pre-dialysis body weight). The AUROC of the prediction score was 0.760 (95% CI 0.654–0.866) (Table 5, Figure 2).

Table 5. The final model of the prediction score for unsuccessful reductions in hemodialysis frequency.

Prediction Factors	Point
Diabetes mellitus	2
Congestive heart failure	3
Pre-dialysis overhydration (per L)	2
Dry weight difference (per kg)	2
Net ultrafiltration (per kg)	−1

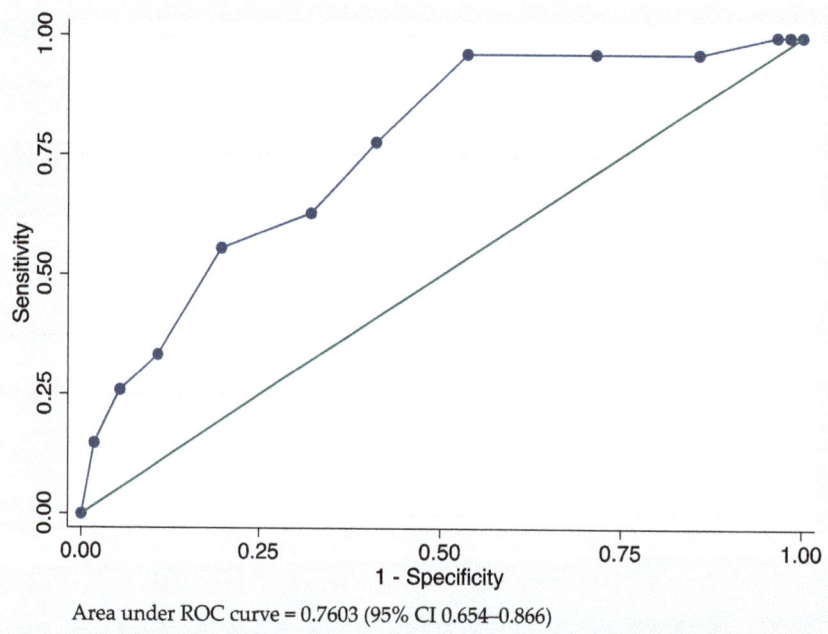

Area under ROC curve = 0.7603 (95% CI 0.654–0.866)

Figure 2. The receiver operating characteristic (ROC) curves and the area under the ROC (AUROC) of the final prediction model for unsuccessful reductions in hemodialysis frequency.

The score from the final model of 5 or less, 6–8, and 9 or more demonstrated an unsuccessful rate of 3.7%, 36.7%, and 57.7%, respectively (Figure 3).

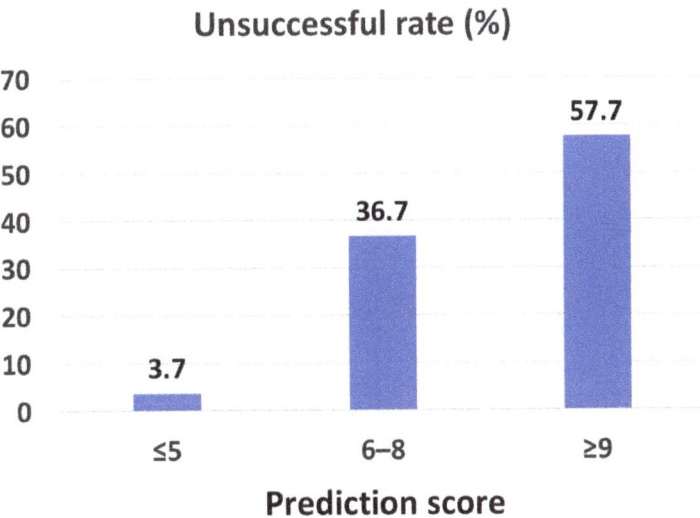

Figure 3. The rate of unsuccessful reductions in hemodialysis frequency at 4 weeks according to the score from the final prediction model.

4. Discussion

This study showed the predictors of unsuccessful reductions in hemodialysis frequency from thrice to twice weekly at 4 weeks during the COVID-19 pandemic, which included DM, CHF, pre-dialysis overhydration, and dry weights that were calculated by BIA. The developed, validated, and final model using these predictors showed a good performance for predicting non-success in terms of reducing hemodialysis frequency.

This study showed that the prevalence of success in reducing dialysis frequency at 4 weeks was about two-thirds. However, only 18% of these patients could achieve this over 8 weeks. Therefore, reducing hemodialysis frequency could theoretically reduce COVID-19 infection transmission for both patients and dialysis staff [6]; however, a reduction in hemodialysis frequency of more than 4 weeks is usually unfeasible.

In one study, Lodge MDS [10] demonstrated that safe detection could be achieved by temporarily reducing hemodialysis frequency in a pandemic setting. Thrice-weekly hemodialysis patients converted to twice weekly for 4 weeks with no definitive inclusion criteria; suitability was determined by the attending nephrologists. They showed that 68% of patients were able to continue twice-weekly dialysis for a 4-week period. This percentage of successfully reducing hemodialysis frequency was comparable to our study. A retrospective survey of the clinicians suggests that temporarily reducing hemodialysis was preferred for patients with a greater age, lower ultrafiltration requirement, higher residual renal function, pre-dialysis potassium and/or phosphate levels within the normal range, and in patients who were willing to decrease the dialysis frequency. However, the potassium and phosphate levels in our study were not significantly different between the two groups.

The predictors of unsuccessful reductions in hemodialysis frequency in this study can be categorized into non-modifiable factors—which include diabetes mellitus and congestive heart failure—and modifiable factors, which are mostly associated with patients' hydration status. Therefore, we would suggest that reducing hemodialysis frequency should be cautiously performed in patients who have any of these two comorbidities, especially congestive heart failure and/or previous requirement of high ultrafiltration volume. Moreover, this study also showed that hypervolemic-associated conditions, e.g., volume overload and uncontrolled hypertension, were major causes (81.5%) of failure in reducing dialysis frequency. Thus, a strict control of sodium and water intake should be advised for patients who are in a period of reducing dialysis sessions.

This is the first study to use predictor factors to develop a prediction model of unsuccessful reduction of hemodialysis frequency in a pandemic. The presented model demonstrated good discrimination. Although the COVID-19 infection rate has gradually subsided, this model is still beneficial in other situations where dialysis availability is limited, for example, during a natural disaster, war, or another pandemic. In the aforementioned circumstances, this model can guide clinicians in selecting hemodialysis patients who may encounter fewer complications from hemodialysis frequency reduction.

There were some limitations in this study. First, this study was a single-center study; therefore, the results might not be representative for other populations, and the predicting risk score might have a limit in terms of its generalizability. Second, the residual urine output, which is an essential factor for volume control, is not available, and this factor might affect the predictability of the model. However, the median dialysis vintage was quite long (4.5 years), and the residual urine output in these patients would likely be small, having a minor effect on the model. Finally, the dry weight being measured by BIA might not be widely available in every dialysis unit. Using other methods to determine the dry weight may not be applicable with respect to this predictive score.

5. Conclusions

The prediction score using diabetes mellitus, congestive heart failure, pre-dialysis overhydration, dry weight difference, and net ultrafiltration demonstrated a good performance in predicting unsuccessful hemodialysis frequency reduction at 4 weeks. Our risk prediction score may support physicians' decisions in choosing a patient who is eligible for hemodialysis frequency reduction.

Supplementary Materials: The following supporting information can be downloaded at: https://www.mdpi.com/article/10.3390/jcm12072550/s1, Table S1: Baseline characteristics of the hemodialysis patients compared between patients who were unsuccessful in reducing hemodialysis frequency over 4 weeks, over 8 weeks and who were successful in reducing hemodialysis frequency over 8 weeks.

Author Contributions: Conceptualization, S.A., P.K., S.K. and P.P.; methodology, S.A. and P.P.; software, S.A., P.T. and P.P.; validation, P.K., P.P. and S.A.; formal analysis, S.A., P.T. and P.P.; investigation, P.K., S.K., S.A. and P.P.; resources, S.A., P.K., S.K. and P.P.; data curation, S.A. and P.P.; writing—original draft preparation, S.A., S.K. and P.P.; writing—review and editing, S.A. and P.P.; visualization, S.A. and P.P.; supervision, S.A. and P.P.; project administration, S.A. and P.P. All authors have read and agreed to the published version of the manuscript.

Funding: This research received no external funding.

Institutional Review Board Statement: This study was granted permission from the Human Research Ethics Committee of Thammasat University Hospital, Thailand (COA number 111/2565).

Informed Consent Statement: Patient consent was waived because (1) the research protocol being less than the minimal risk; (2) the research could not be carried out practically without the waiver or alteration; and (3) the waiver or alteration had no impact on the rights and wellbeing of the research participants.

Data Availability Statement: Data are available from the corresponding author (PP) upon reasonable request.

Acknowledgments: This study was supported by the Research Group in Nephrology and Renal Replacement Therapy from the Faculty of Medicine, Thammasat University.

Conflicts of Interest: The authors declare no conflict of interest.

References

1. World Health Organization (WHO). Coronavirus Disease 2019 (COVID-19) Situation Report—52. 2020. Available online: https://www.who.int/docs/default-source/coronaviruse/situation-reports/20200312-sitrep-52-covid-19.pdf (accessed on 28 February 2023).
2. Dessie, Z.G.; Zewotir, T. Mortality-Related Risk Factors of COVID-19: A Systematic Review and Meta-Analysis of 42 Studies and 423,117 Patients. *BMC Infect. Dis.* **2021**, *21*, 855. [CrossRef] [PubMed]
3. Ghonimi, T.A.L.; Alkad, M.M.; Abuhelaiqa, E.A.; Othman, M.M.; Elgaali, M.A.; Ibrahim, R.A.M.; Joseph, S.M.; Al-Malki, H.A.; Hamad, A.I. Mortality and Associated Risk Factors of COVID-19 Infection in Dialysis Patients in Qatar: A Nationwide Cohort Study. *PLoS ONE* **2021**, *16*, e0254246. [CrossRef] [PubMed]
4. Jdiaa, S.S.; Mansour, R.; El Alayli, A.; Gautam, A.; Thomas, P.; Mustafa, R.A. COVID-19 and Chronic Kidney Disease: An Updated Overview of Reviews. *J. Nephrol.* **2022**, *35*, 69–85. [CrossRef] [PubMed]
5. Coronavirus Disease (COVID-19): How Is It Transmitted? Available online: https://www.who.int/news-room/questions-and-answers/item/coronavirus-disease-covid-19-how-is-it-transmitted (accessed on 26 February 2023).
6. Meyer, T.W.; Hostetter, T.H.; Watnick, S. Twice-Weekly Hemodialysis Is an Option for Many Patients in Times of Dialysis Unit Stress. *J. Am. Soc. Nephrol.* **2020**, *31*, 1141–1142. [CrossRef] [PubMed]
7. Daugirdas, J.T.; Depner, T.A.; Inrig, J.; Mehrotra, R.; Rocco, M.V.; Suri, R.S.; Weiner, D.E.; Greer, N.; Ishani, A.; MacDonald, R.; et al. KDOQI Clinical Practice Guideline for Hemodialysis Adequacy: 2015 Update. *Am. J. Kidney Dis.* **2015**, *66*, 884–930. [CrossRef]
8. Kliger, A.S.; Cozzolino, M.; Jha, V.; Harbert, G.; Ikizler, T.A. Managing the COVID-19 Pandemic: International Comparisons in Dialysis Patients. *Kidney Int.* **2020**, *98*, 12–16. [CrossRef] [PubMed]
9. Fernandez-Felix, B.M.; García-Esquinas, E.; Muriel, A.; Royuela, A.; Zamora, J. Bootstrap Internal Validation Command for Predictive Logistic Regression Models. *Stata J.* **2021**, *21*, 498–509. [CrossRef]
10. Lodge, M.D.S.; Abeygunaratne, T.; Alderson, H.; Ali, I.; Brown, N.; Chrysochou, C.; Donne, R.; Erekosima, I.; Evans, P.; Flanagan, E.; et al. Safely Reducing Haemodialysis Frequency during the COVID-19 Pandemic. *BMC Nephrol.* **2020**, *21*, 532. [CrossRef] [PubMed]

Disclaimer/Publisher's Note: The statements, opinions and data contained in all publications are solely those of the individual author(s) and contributor(s) and not of MDPI and/or the editor(s). MDPI and/or the editor(s) disclaim responsibility for any injury to people or property resulting from any ideas, methods, instructions or products referred to in the content.

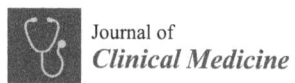

Article

Prevalence of Impaired Physical Mobility in Dialysis Patients: A Single-Centre Cross-Sectional Study

Špela Bogataj [1], Jernej Pajek [1,2], Blaž Slonjšak [1] and Vanja Peršič [1,2,*]

[1] Department of Nephrology, University Medical Centre Ljubljana, 1000 Ljubljana, Slovenia; spela.bogataj@kclj.si (Š.B.); jernej.pajek@mf.uni-lj.si (J.P.); blaz.slonjsak@kclj.si (B.S.)
[2] Faculty of Medicine, University of Ljubljana, 1000 Ljubljana, Slovenia
* Correspondence: vanja.persic@kclj.si

Abstract: Impaired physical mobility in hemodialysis (HD) patients is considered an important modifiable risk factor of increased all-cause morbidity and mortality. To our knowledge, no study to date has determined the overall burden of limited physical mobility in prevalent HD patients. The aim of this research is to investigate impaired physical mobility and its clinical correlates. We conducted a cross-sectional observational study in all patients of the Centre for Acute and Complicated Dialysis at the University Medical Centre of Ljubljana, where the most complex patients receive HD on average three times per week. The data were collected through interviews based on a prepared questionnaire and medical history review. A total of 205 patients were included in this study (63.9 ± 15.4 years). Sixty percent (122/205) of the patients had little or no physical mobility impairment, and others were categorized with a minor or severe mobility limitation. A minor mobility impairment was found in 21% (43/205) of patients: 10 patients (5%) used a mobility aid in the form of a crutch, 9 patients (4%) were dependent on two crutches or a walker, and 24 patients (12%) were temporarily dependent on the assistance of a third person. Severe mobility limitations were observed in 22% (40/205) of patients, ranging from being confined to bed (19/205, 9%), confined to bed but able to perform some movements (19/205, 9%), and ambulatory but dependent on the assistance of a third person for locomotion (2/205, 1%). The most common causes of the limitation of mobility were neurological (19/40, 47.5%), cardiovascular (9/40, 22.5%), musculoskeletal (8/40, 20%), and other causes (4/40, 10%). A significant, moderate positive correlation was observed between mobility problems and the age of the participants (r = 0.36, $p < 0.001$), while a significant, small positive correlation was obtained between the mobility problems and C-reactive protein (r = 0.15, $p = 0.044$). Moreover, mobility problems had a small but significant negative correlation with albumin levels (r = −0.15, $p = 0.042$). When controlling for age, results yield no significant correlations, and, in regression analysis, only the age ($p < 0.001$) and male gender ($p = 0.007$) of the participants were independent predictors of mobility impairment. We conclude that impaired mobility has a high overall prevalence among chronic HD patients. Strategies to prevent and improve mobility limitations are strongly needed.

Keywords: physical mobility; impairment; chronic kidney disease; hemodialysis; morbidity

Citation: Bogataj, Š.; Pajek, J.; Slonjšak, B.; Peršič, V. Prevalence of Impaired Physical Mobility in Dialysis Patients: A Single-Centre Cross-Sectional Study. J. Clin. Med. 2023, 12, 6634. https://doi.org/10.3390/jcm12206634

Academic Editors: Shuzo Kobayashi and Takayasu Ohtake

Received: 4 September 2023
Revised: 16 October 2023
Accepted: 18 October 2023
Published: 20 October 2023

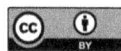

Copyright: © 2023 by the authors. Licensee MDPI, Basel, Switzerland. This article is an open access article distributed under the terms and conditions of the Creative Commons Attribution (CC BY) license (https://creativecommons.org/licenses/by/4.0/).

1. Introduction

Chronic kidney disease (CKD) is a condition characterized by the gradual loss of kidney function over time, leading to a decrease in the organ's ability to filter waste products from the blood and regulate essential bodily functions [1]. Patients with CKD are often less physically active and less physically capable compared to their healthy counterparts [2]. Physical inactivity is thought to be a contributing factor to the increased mortality seen in this population [3]. It can lead to a worsening of other comorbidities such as diabetes, hypertension, and cardiovascular disease [4], and it can have a number of negative consequences for patients with CKD, including muscle wasting, decreased cardiovascular fitness, and impaired mobility [5]. Additionally, a substantial and continuous decline in physical function is noticed at the initiation of dialysis. This decline is a progressive process with further worsening of physical function during hospitalizations and acute illnesses [6]. The final result of the aforementioned deterioration often leads to irreversibly impaired physical mobility with dependence on the caregivers. Recent research [7] has highlighted the importance of understanding the factors influencing mobility decline during the induction phase of dialysis. This phase, which often involves emergency dialysis start, has been associated with a significant decline in walking independence among CKD patients. Therefore, a comprehensive examination of physical mobility in CKD patients is essential for improving their overall quality of life and informing early rehabilitation strategies.

Impaired mobility can be a temporary or permanent condition (it can have both physical and psychological consequences), and it can be caused by a variety of modifiable and non-modifiable risk factors [8]. Besides physical inactivity and the initiation of renal replacement therapy, reduced mobility can have a range of other causes in CKD patients. Musculoskeletal disorders, cardiovascular diseases, neurological disorders, cognitive disorders, and acute illnesses are all common modifiable risk factors that can contribute to impaired mobility [9,10]. Terminal musculoskeletal, cardiovascular, and neurological diseases are common non-modifiable risk factors that can lead to permanent impairment [10,11]. Limited mobility can also have negative physical consequences, such as osteoporosis, hypercalcemia, obesity, pain, and decubitus ulcers, as well as psychological consequences such as sleep disturbances and depression [12–14].

It is also important to consider the potential impact of blood parameters on physical mobility in HD patients. For example, high levels of inflammation, such as C-reactive protein (CRP), have been linked to decreased physical function in HD patients [15]. Similarly, low levels of hemoglobin and erythrocyte mass can also contribute to impaired physical mobility due to anemia [16].

Since only in-center HD is currently available in Slovenia, patients have to commute to dialysis facilities usually three times a week; therefore, this complex situation causes a considerable burden on the patients, patient's relatives, and healthcare providers, especially in patients with impaired mobility. To the best of our knowledge, no study had comprehensively investigated the overall burden of limited physical mobility in prevalent HD patients. Therefore, our research aimed to fill this gap by assessing the prevalence, causes, and clinical correlations of impaired physical mobility in HD patients in Slovenia.

2. Materials and Methods

2.1. Patients and Study Design

We conducted a cross-sectional observational study of all patients from the Centre for Acute and Complicated Dialysis at the University Medical Centre of Ljubljana. We employed a consecutive enrollment approach, where all patients receiving hemodialysis at the center were enrolled. The sample size of 205 patients was deemed sufficient for our study objectives, as it allowed us to comprehensively investigate the prevalence, causes, and clinical correlates of impaired physical mobility in our specific population of hemodialysis patients in Slovenia. Data were collected through interviews based on a pre-prepared questionnaire (Appendix A), based on files filled by nephrologists and dialysis nurses, and a review of the medical history.

Included patients received hemodialysis for 4–5 h, three times per week. Dialysis procedures were performed with a standard bicarbonate-based dialysate and using a high-flux HD membrane: polyamide high-flux hemodialyzer (Polyflux 140 H, 170 H, 210 H; Gambro Dialysatoren GmbH, Hechingen, Germany) or polysulfone high-flux hemodialyzer (Fx 60, Fx 80, Fx 100; Fresenius, Bad Homburg, Germany).

Patients were classified into three mobility problem groups: (1) no or inconsiderable impairment of physical mobility, (2) minor mobility impairment, and (3) severe mobility impairment. We defined minor mobility impairment as a need for mobility aid in the form of one or two crutches or a walking frame. Severe mobility impairment was defined in three levels: being confined to bed, confined to bed but able to perform some movements, and ambulatory but dependent on the assistance of a third person for locomotion. The causes of impaired mobility were classified as neurological (ischemic brain injury, intracerebral hemorrhage, traumatic brain injury, dementia, parkinsonism...), cardiovascular (ischemic heart disease, heart failure, peripheral arterial disease...), musculoskeletal (age-related losses of muscle mass, amputation, osteoporosis with fractures, spine injury...), and others.

Data collection included demographics, dialysis vintage, leucocyte count, hemoglobin levels, thrombocyte count, serum calcium, phosphate, intact parathormone (iPTH), albumin concentrations, and CRP levels.

This study was performed in compliance with the Declaration of Helsinki (as revised in Fortaleza 2013) and was approved by the National Medical Ethics Committee (0120-280/2018); patient consent was waived due to the observational nature of this study.

2.2. Statistical Analysis

Statistical analysis was performed using IBM SPSS statistics program (version 28.0; Chicago, IL, USA). The normality of the data was assessed with the Kolmogorov–Smirnov test. Data are reported as a mean ± standard deviation (SD), absolute frequency, or percentage. Spearman's correlations were used to calculate relationships between mobility problems, dialysis vintage, and blood parameters (hemoglobin, calcium, phosphate, iPTH, albumin, CRP). Additionally, correlation analysis was conducted while controlling for age. Correlation strength was interpreted as r = 0 to 0.3, or 0 to −0.3, small; 0.31 to 0.49, or −0.31 to −0.49, moderate; 0.5 to 0.69, or −0.5 to −0.69, large; 0.7 to 0.89, or −0.7 to −0.89, very large; and 0.9 to 1, or −0.9 to −1, perfect correlation [17]. Furthermore, a multivariate linear regression analysis was performed to assess the combined influence of all independent variables on the extent of mobility impairment. A p-value of <0.05 was considered statistically significant.

3. Results

3.1. Patients' Characteristics

The demographic and clinical characteristics of the patients are described in Table 1.

Table 1. Demographic and clinical characteristics of patients. Data are presented as mean ± standard deviation (range) or percentage.

Parameter	Value
N	205
Age [years], range	63.9 ± 15.4 (24–92)
Male gender	119 (58%)
Dialysis vintage [years], range	7.3 ± 9.0 (1–44)
Comorbidities	
Diabetes mellitus	77 (38%)
Arterial hypertension	193 (95%)
Peripheral vascular disease	55 (27%)
Laboratory values	
Leucocytes (10 * 9/L)	6.4 ± 2.3
Hemoglobin (g/L)	117 ± 13
Thrombocytes (10 * 9/L)	185.4 ± 60.5
Calcium (mmol/L)	2.2 ± 0.3
Phosphate (mmol/L)	1.4 ± 0.4
iPTH (ng/L)	430.4 ± 488.1
Albumin (g/L)	37 ± 4
CRP (mg/L)	12 ± 18

Abbreviations: N, number of subjects; CRP, C-reactive protein; iPTH, intact parathormone.

3.2. Impaired Physical Mobility

Most patients showed no or inconsiderable impairment of physical mobility (122/205, 60%); details are reported in Table 2. The common causes of mobility impairment were as follows: neurological (19/40, 47.5%), cardiovascular (9/40, 22.5%), musculoskeletal (8/40, 20%), and others (4/40, 10%).

Table 2. Prevalence of different stages of immobility (N = 205).

Physical Mobility	Value (n (%))
No or inconsiderable impairment (%)	122 (60)
Minor mobility impairment (%)	43 (21)
A crutch	10 (5)
Two crutches or a walking frame	9 (4)
Intermittent help of a third person	24 (12)
Severe mobility impairment (%)	40 (19)
Confined to bed	19 (9)
Confined to bed but able to perform some movements	19 (9)
Dependent on assistance of a third person	2 (1)

The results of Spearman's correlations for the selected variables are presented in Table 3.

Table 3. Correlation coefficients between clinical and demographic parameters variables and mobility impairment.

Variable	Mobility Impairment	
	r	p
Age	0.36 **	<0.001
Dialysis vintage	0.01	0.922
Hemoglobin	−0.04	0.569
Calcium	0.02	0.836
Phosphate	−0.03	0.671
iPTH	−0.05	0.490
Albumin	−0.15 *	0.042
C-reactive protein	0.15 *	0.044

Note: **, significance at $p < 0.001$ level; *, significance at $p < 0.05$ level. Abbreviations: iPTH, intact parathormone.

A significant, moderate positive correlation was observed between mobility problems and the age of the participants (r = 0.36, $p < 0.001$), while a significant, small positive correlation was obtained between the mobility problems and CRP (r = 0.15, $p = 0.044$). Moreover, mobility problems had a small but significant negative correlation with albumin levels (r = −0.15, $p = 0.042$). Twenty-seven percent of patients had an albumin level of 35 g/L or lower. Finally, no statistically significant correlations were found between other selected variables (dialysis vintage, hemoglobin, calcium, phosphate, and iPTH) and mobility impairments.

Furthermore, we examined the correlation between clinical parameters and mobility impairment while controlling for the age of participants (Table 4).

Table 4. Correlation coefficients between clinical parameters variables and mobility impairment controlled for age.

Variable	Mobility Impairment	
	r	p
Dialysis vintage	0.065	0.375
Hemoglobin	0.093	0.207
Calcium	0.000	0.995
Phosphate	−0.039	0.593
iPTH	0.003	0.965
Albumin	−0.103	0.161
C-reactive protein	0.022	0.767

Abbreviations: iPTH, intact parathormone.

After controlling for the age, the analysis did not reveal any statistically significant correlations between these clinical parameters (dialysis vintage, hemoglobin, calcium, phosphate, iPTH, albumin, and CRP) and mobility impairment in the studied population.

Additionally, Table 5 presents the results of the regression analysis, highlighting the predictors of mobility impairment and their corresponding coefficients, standardized coefficients, t-values, and significance levels.

Table 5. Regression analysis results for mobility impairment predictors.

Independent Variable	Regression Coefficient	Standardized Regression Coefficient Beta	t	p	95% CI	Coefficient of Determination R^2	F	p
Age	0.013	0.316	4.077	<0.001	0.007–0.019			
Gender	0.238	0.193	2.601	0.010	0.057–0.418			
Dialysis vintage	0.007	0.099	1.338	0.183	−0.003–0.017			
Hemoglobin	0.003	0.075	1.017	0.311	−0.003–0.009			
Calcium	0.091	0.032	0.416	0.678	−0.340–0.522	0.137	3.018	0.002
Phosphate	0.000	0.000	0.005	0.996	−0.176–0.177			
iPTH	-1.423×10^{-5}	−0.010	−0.136	0.892	0.000–0.000			
Albumin	−0.024	−0.147	−1.688	0.093	−0.051–0.004			
C-reactive protein	−0.002	−0.047	−0.557	0.579	−0.007–0.004			

Abbreviations: iPTH, intact parathormone; CI, confidence interval.

The model explains a moderate portion (13.7%) of the variance in mobility problems when controlling for multiple independent variables. The adjusted R-squared coefficient indicates that about 9.2% of this variance is explained when accounting for the number of predictors in the model. The regression model is statistically significant, as indicated by the low p-value (0.002). This suggests that at least one of the predictor variables significantly contributes to explaining the variance in mobility problems. Age has a significant positive effect on mobility problems, with a standardized coefficient (Beta) of 0.316. This indicates that as a patient's age increases, mobility problems tend to increase as well. Gender also has a significant positive effect, with a Beta of 0.193. This suggests that being male is associated with higher levels of mobility problems. None of the other variables show significant effects on mobility problems as their p-values are greater than the significance level of 0.05.

4. Discussion

It is well established that impaired physical mobility is a common problem among hemodialysis (HD) patients [18], and it is associated with increased morbidity and mortality [19,20]. To our knowledge, this is the first study of the prevalence and causes of impaired physical mobility in HD patients. In our cross-sectional observational study, 60% of all patients had no or little physical impairment; however, a significant proportion (40%) showed at least some degree of mobility impairment. Nineteen percent expressed a severe mobility limitation, similar to those reported by Van Loon [21] and Shimoda [22]. Patients with severe mobility impairment are unable to live on their own since they are dependent on a third person for the majority of time. Slightly higher mobility impairment was observed in a study from 2008 [23], where 57% of older adults receiving HD had some limitations in mobility. Furthermore, we observed a significant positive correlation between CRP levels and the age of patients in relation to mobility problems, along with a negative correlation between mobility problems and albumin levels. Our findings align with a related study conducted by Hirano et al. [7], which focused on the induction phase of dialysis. They observed a decline in walking independence during this phase, with age, high Charlson comorbidity index, CRP, and emergency dialysis start to be significant predictors of decreased walking independence. While our study provides valuable insights into the prevalence and causes of impaired mobility in HD patients in Slovenia, the study by Hirano et al. emphasizes the significance of addressing mobility decline during the dialysis induction phase. Combining our findings highlights the global nature of the issue and underscores the need for comprehensive strategies to prevent and manage impaired mobility in CKD patients undergoing dialysis.

In general, high prevalence of impaired mobility in dialysis patients can be at least partially explained by illnesses with a high impact on reduced mobility: cardiovascular diseases [24,25], neurological complications [24,26], and musculoskeletal disorders [18]. In line with these findings, the most common causes of mobility impairment in our cohort were neurological (47.5%), cardiovascular (22.5%), and musculoskeletal disorders (20%). Besides chronic illnesses, impaired mobility can be a consequence of age-related losses of muscle mass or acute events [27]. As expected, the age of HD patients had a significant positive correlation, and it was as an independent predictor for mobility impairment. In our cohort, patients were relatively young (mean age 63.9 ± 15.4 years) compared to the European population, and since the median age of patients starting renal replacement therapy in Europe in 2019 was 67.9 years [28], we could expect even more patients with reduced mobility in the near future with an additional high burden on medical staff.

We performed correlation analyses between mobility impairment and some laboratory data that were likely to have an impact on mobility. We measured CRP levels, since elevated CRP is associated with poorer physical function in the elderly with various comorbidities [29]. A significant, but small positive correlation was obtained between mobility impairment and CRP levels in our patients. We also confirmed a small but significant negative correlation between mobility impairment and albumin levels. In dialysis patients, the causes of hypoalbuminemia are multifactorial—a result of imbalance between albumin loss into dialysate, catabolism, and albumin synthesis [30]. Serum albumin concentration in our cohort was 37 ± 4 g/L; however, a total of 27% of patients had serum albumin levels below 35 g/L. When controlled for the age, those two parameters were not significantly correlated. Nevertheless, other studies showed that a low level of serum albumin was an independent predictor of adverse outcomes, such as mobility impairment [31] and even mortality [32]; therefore, improving the nutritional status and albumin levels is of special importance in chronic hemodialysis patients.

Deranged calcium–phosphate metabolism is a very common finding in patients with end-stage renal disease. It has been associated with disorders of bone turnover as well as with vascular and soft tissue calcification [33]. Renal osteodystrophy may occur alongside bone pain or fractures, leading to impaired physical mobility, and vice versa, and immobility can lead to osteoporosis and hypercalcemia [34]. Vascular calcifications lead to arterial stiffening, damaged microcirculatory beds, and an increase in cardiac afterload, and contributes to the development of left ventricular hypertrophy, cardiac dysfunction, and, consequently, impaired physical mobility [35]. We found no association with parameters of

CKD-mineral bone disease. That finding could be partially explained by the fact that, in our patients, calcium concentration in iPTH levels were very tightly controlled.

We expected to find an association between lower hemoglobin levels and impaired physical mobility, since common symptoms of anemia are fatigue, dyspnea, and decreased physical function. According to our results, we found no such correlation. One of the possible explanations for this unpredicted finding could be that the majority (83%) of our patients had hemoglobin levels above 100 g/L, which are associated with few specific clinical symptoms. Similarly, there was no correlation between dialysis vintage and impaired mobility, even though dialysis vintage is an independent predictor of osteoporosis [36] and is associated with somatic symptoms (e.g., fatigue) [37]. Gender also played a significant role, with male patients showing a higher degree of mobility impairment compared to their female counterparts.

Our study has several strengths: (1) Comprehensive data collection—this study collected data through interviews, medical history reviews, and questionnaire-based assessments, providing a comprehensive understanding of the patients' mobility status and associated factors. (2) Representative sample—this study included all patients from the Centre for Acute and Complicated Dialysis at the University Medical Centre of Ljubljana, which enhances the representativeness of the findings and allows for generalization to a similar population. (3) Clear classification of mobility impairment—this study classified patients into three mobility impairment groups based on specific criteria, providing clear categories to analyze and compare the levels of impairment.

This study has five main limitations: (1) Cross-sectional design—as a cross-sectional study, the findings only provide a snapshot of the patients' mobility and associated factors at a specific point in time. Longitudinal studies would be required to establish causal relationships and observe changes over time. (2) Limited generalizability—this study was conducted at a single medical center in Ljubljana, Slovenia, which may limit the generalizability of the findings to other populations or settings. Further research involving diverse populations would help validate the results. (3) Self-reporting bias—data collection relied on interviews and medical history reviews, which could be subject to recall bias or misreporting by patients or healthcare professionals. Objective measures or additional assessment tools could strengthen the validity of the findings. (4) Limited scope of variables—this study focused on a specific set of variables, such as demographics, dialysis vintage, blood parameters, and causes of impaired mobility. Other potential contributing factors, such psychosocial factors, were not considered, limiting the comprehensive understanding of mobility impairment in hemodialysis patients. (5) Another significant limitation of our study is the absence of a control group for comparison, particularly in terms of assessing the mobility and physical disability of HD patients versus those in the early stages of CKD. Including such a control group would have allowed for a more comprehensive evaluation of the impact of HD on physical mobility and a better understanding of how mobility changes across different stages of CKD. Future research endeavors should consider incorporating control groups to address this aspect and provide a more holistic perspective on the mobility challenges faced by CKD patients.

From our data, it is clear that the prevalence of mobility impairment is large and therefore it is important to assess and address this as a part of high-quality holistic dialysis care. The possible underlying causes of impaired mobility (neurological, cardiovascular, and musculoskeletal disorders) may be amenable to preventive interventions [38]. In addition, exercise interventions with a physical therapist or other healthcare provider should be incorporated to improve muscle strength and function—with intradialytic exercise being the first obvious opportunity, which may significantly improve physical performance (e.g., intra-dialysis exercise [39]). It is also important to address any psychological and cognitive consequences of hemodialysis treatment and intervene to limit these influences [40].

5. Conclusions

In conclusion, our study highlights the high prevalence of impaired mobility among chronic hemodialysis patients. Neurological, cardiovascular, and musculoskeletal diseases were identified as the most common causes of mobility limitations in this population. Only the age and male gender of the participants were found to be independent predictors of impaired mobility. Further investigations are warranted to identify additional risk factors and develop effective strategies to mitigate the burden of immobility on patients, their families, and healthcare providers. By addressing these factors, we can potentially enhance the quality of life and clinical outcomes in HD patients.

Author Contributions: Conceptualization, J.P. and V.P.; methodology, Š.B.; investigation, B.S.; writing—original draft preparation, Š.B. and V.P.; writing—review and editing, J.P. and B.S. All authors have read and agreed to the published version of the manuscript.

Funding: This study was funded by Slovenian Research and Innovation Agency (Grant number: Z3-3212, Grant recipient: Špela Bogataj).

Institutional Review Board Statement: The study was conducted according to the guidelines of the Declaration of Helsinki, and was approved by the National Medical Ethics Committee (0120-280/2018).

Informed Consent Statement: Informed consent was waived due to the observational nature of this study.

Data Availability Statement: The datasets generated and/or analyzed during this study are available from the corresponding author upon reasonable request.

Conflicts of Interest: The authors declare no conflict of interest.

Appendix A

Questionnaire for hemodialysis patients regarding physical mobility

Name and surname:
Date of birth:
Phone number:
Name of dialysis center:

Patient is currently living:
(a) at home – by himself/herself
(b) at home – with other family members
(c) in a retirement home
(d) other:

Hemodialysis schedule: in the morning   in the afternoon
(a) Monday, Wednesday, Friday
(b) Tuesday, Thursday, Saturday

Cause of kidney failure:

Date of first hemodialysis procedure:

Current mobility capacity:
(a) no impairment (e.g. walks by himself/herself, needs no assistance)
(b) minor impairment – please specify:
   one crutch
   two crutches
   walker
   occasional assistance of third person
(c) severe impairment – please specify:
   completely dependent upon third person assistance
   confined to bed – capable of miniscule movements
   confined to bed – unable to perform miniscule movements

Previous partial or complete limb amputation: yes no (if you answered yes please mark accordingly)

References

1. Levey, A.S.; Becker, C.; Inker, L.A. Glomerular Filtration Rate and Albuminuria for Detection and Staging of Acute and Chronic Kidney Disease in Adults: A Systematic Review. *JAMA* **2015**, *313*, 837–846. [CrossRef]
2. Bučar Pajek, M.; Pajek, J. Characterization of Deficits across the Spectrum of Motor Abilities in Dialysis Patients and the Impact of Sarcopenic Overweight and Obesity. *Clin. Nutr.* **2018**, *37*, 870–877. [CrossRef]
3. Stack, A.G.; Molony, D.A.; Rives, T.; Tyson, J.; Murthy, B.V.R. Association of Physical Activity with Mortality in the US Dialysis Population. *Am. J. Kidney Dis.* **2005**, *45*, 690–701. [CrossRef]
4. Gaetano, A. Relationship between Physical Inactivity and Effects on Individual Health Status. *J. Phys. Educ. Sport* **2016**, *16*, 1069–1074. [CrossRef]
5. Painter, P.; Marcus, R.L. Assessing Physical Function and Physical Activity in Patients with CKD. *Clin. J. Am. Soc. Nephrol.* **2013**, *8*, 861–872. [CrossRef]
6. Anding, K.; Bär, T.; Trojniak-Hennig, J.; Kuchinke, S.; Krause, R.; Rost, J.M.; Halle, M. A Structured Exercise Programme during Haemodialysis for Patients with Chronic Kidney Disease: Clinical Benefit and Long-Term Adherence. *BMJ Open* **2015**, *5*, e008709. [CrossRef]
7. Hirano, Y.; Fujikura, T.; Kono, K.; Ohashi, N.; Yamaguchi, T.; Hanajima, W.; Yasuda, H.; Yamauchi, K. Decline in Walking Independence and Related Factors in Hospitalization for Dialysis Initiation: A Retrospective Cohort Study. *J. Clin. Med.* **2022**, *11*, 6589. [CrossRef]
8. Zelle, D.M.; Klaassen, G.; van Adrichem, E.; Bakker, S.J.L.; Corpeleijn, E.; Navis, G. Physical Inactivity: A Risk Factor and Target for Intervention in Renal Care. *Nat. Rev. Nephrol.* **2017**, *13*, 152–168. [CrossRef]
9. Ahmad, E.; Sargeant, J.A.; Yates, T.; Webb, D.R.; Davies, M.J.; Ahmad, E.; Sargeant, J.A.; Yates, T.; Webb, D.R.; Davies, M.J. Type 2 Diabetes and Impaired Physical Function: A Growing Problem. *Diabetology* **2022**, *3*, 30–45. [CrossRef]
10. Robinson, S.M.; Jameson, K.A.; Syddall, H.E.; Dennison, E.M.; Cooper, C.; Aihie Sayer, A. Clustering of Lifestyle Risk Factors and Poor Physical Function in Older Adults: The Hertfordshire Cohort Study. *J. Am. Geriatr. Soc.* **2013**, *61*, 1684–1691. [CrossRef]
11. Minetto, M.A.; Giannini, A.; McConnell, R.; Busso, C.; Torre, G.; Massazza, G. Common Musculoskeletal Disorders in the Elderly: The Star Triad. *J. Clin. Med.* **2020**, *9*, 1216. [CrossRef] [PubMed]
12. Penedo, F.; Dahn, J. Exercise and Well-Being: A Review of Mental and Physical Health Benefits Associated with Physical Activity. *Behav. Med.* **2005**, *18*, 189–193. [CrossRef] [PubMed]
13. Asp, M.; Simonsson, B.; Larm, P.; Molarius, A. Physical Mobility, Physical Activity, and Obesity among Elderly: Findings from a Large Population-Based Swedish Survey. *Public Health* **2017**, *147*, 84–91. [CrossRef]
14. Katzman, W.B.; Vittinghoff, E.; Kado, D.M. Age-Related Hyperkyphosis, Independent of Spinal Osteoporosis, Is Associated with Impaired Mobility in Older Community-Dwelling Women. *Osteoporos. Int.* **2011**, *22*, 85–90. [CrossRef] [PubMed]
15. Pajek, M.; Jerman, A.; Osredkar, J.; Ponikvar, J.B.; Pajek, J. Association of Uremic Toxins and Inflammatory Markers with Physical Performance in Dialysis Patients. *Toxins* **2018**, *10*, 403. [CrossRef]
16. Braumann, K.M.; Nonnast-Daniel, B.; Boning, D.; Bocker, A.; Frei, U. Improved Physical Performance after Treatment of Renal Anemia with Recombinant Human Erythropoietin. *Nephron* **1991**, *58*, 129–134. [CrossRef]
17. Hopkins, W. How to Interpret Changes in an Athletic Performance Test. *Sportscience* **2004**, *8*, 1–7.
18. Moorthi, R.N.; Fadel, W.F.; Cranor, A.; Hindi, J.; Avin, K.G.; Lane, K.A.; Thadhani, R.I.; Moe, S.M. Mobility Impairment in Patients New to Dialysis. *Am. J. Nephrol.* **2020**, *51*, 705–714. [CrossRef]
19. Garcia-Canton, C.; Rodenas, A.; Lopez-Aperador, C.; Rivero, Y.; Anton, G.; Monzon, T.; Diaz, N.; Vega, N.; Loro, J.F.; Santana, A.; et al. Frailty in Hemodialysis and Prediction of Poor Short-Term Outcome: Mortality, Hospitalization and Visits to Hospital Emergency Services. *Ren. Fail.* **2019**, *41*, 567–575. [CrossRef]
20. Kutner, N.G.; Zhang, R.; Huang, Y.; Painter, P. Gait Speed and Mortality, Hospitalization, and Functional Status Change among Hemodialysis Patients: A US Renal Data System Special Study. *Am. J. Kidney Dis.* **2015**, *66*, 297–304. [CrossRef]
21. Van Loon, I.N.; Goto, N.A.; Boereboom, F.T.J.; Bots, M.L.; Hoogeveen, E.K.; Gamadia, L.; Van Bommel, E.F.H.; Van De Ven, P.J.G.; Douma, C.E.; Vincent, H.H.; et al. Geriatric Assessment and the Relation with Mortality and Hospitalizations in Older Patients Starting Dialysis. *Nephron* **2019**, *143*, 108–119. [CrossRef] [PubMed]
22. Shimoda, T.; Matsuzawa, R.; Yoneki, K.; Harada, M.; Watanabe, T.; Yoshida, A.; Takeuchi, Y.; Matsunaga, A. Combined Contribution of Reduced Functional Mobility, Muscle Weakness, and Low Serum Albumin in Prediction of All-Cause Mortality in Hemodialysis Patients: A Retrospective Cohort Study. *J. Ren. Nutr.* **2018**, *28*, 302–308. [CrossRef] [PubMed]
23. Cook, W.L.; Jassal, S.V. Functional Dependencies among the Elderly on Hemodialysis. *Kidney Int.* **2008**, *73*, 1289–1295. [CrossRef] [PubMed]
24. Bianchi, L.; Volpato, S. Muscle Dysfunction in Type 2 Diabetes: A Major Threat to Patient's Mobility and Independence. *Acta Diabetol.* **2016**, *53*, 879–889. [CrossRef] [PubMed]
25. Hajjar, I.; Quach, L.; Yang, F.; Chaves, P.H.M.; Newman, A.B.; Mukamal, K.; Longstreth, W.; Inzitari, M.; Lipsitz, L.A. Hypertension, White Matter Hyperintensities and Concurrent Impairments in Mobility, Cognition and Mood: The Cardiovascular Health Study. *Circulation* **2011**, *123*, 858. [CrossRef]
26. Arnold, R.; Issar, T.; Krishnan, A.V.; Pussell, B.A. Neurological Complications in Chronic Kidney Disease. *JRSM Cardiovasc. Dis.* **2016**, *5*, 204800401667768. [CrossRef]

27. Brinkley, T.E.; Leng, X.; Miller, M.E.; Kitzman, D.W.; Pahor, M.; Berry, M.J.; Marsh, A.P.; Kritchevsky, S.B.; Nicklas, B.J. Chronic Inflammation Is Associated with Low Physical Function in Older Adults across Multiple Comorbidities. *J. Gerontol. A Biol. Sci. Med. Sci.* **2009**, *64A*, 455. [CrossRef]
28. Boenink, R.; Astley, M.E.; Huijben, J.A.; Stel, V.S.; Kerschbaum, J.; Ots-Rosenberg, M.; Åsberg, A.A.; Lopot, F.; Golan, E.; Castro De La Nuez, P.; et al. The ERA Registry Annual Report 2019: Summary and Age Comparisons. *Clin. Kidney J.* **2021**, *15*, 452–472. [CrossRef]
29. Beavers, D.P.; Kritchevsky, S.B.; Gill, T.M.; Ambrosius, W.T.; Anton, S.D.; Fielding, R.A.; King, A.C.; Rejeski, W.J.; Lovato, L.; McDermott, M.M.; et al. Elevated IL-6 and CRP Levels Are Associated with Incident Self-Reported Major Mobility Disability: A Pooled Analysis of Older Adults with Slow Gait Speed. *J. Gerontol. A Biol. Sci. Med. Sci.* **2021**, *76*, 2293–2299. [CrossRef]
30. Kalantar-Zadeh, K.; Ficociello, L.H.; Bazzanella, J.; Mullon, C.; Anger, M.S. Slipping Through the Pores: Hypoalbuminemia and Albumin Loss during Hemodialysis. *Int. J. Nephrol. Renov. Dis.* **2021**, *14*, 11–21. [CrossRef]
31. Li, X.; Cao, X.; Ying, Z.; Zhang, J.; Sun, X.; Hoogendijk, E.O.; Liu, Z. Associations of Serum Albumin With Disability in Activities of Daily Living, Mobility and Objective Physical Functioning Regardless of Vitamin D: Cross-Sectional Findings from the Chinese Longitudinal Healthy Longevity Survey. *Front. Nutr.* **2022**, *9*, 809499. [CrossRef] [PubMed]
32. Akirov, A.; Masri-Iraqi, H.; Atamna, A.; Shimon, I. Low Albumin Levels Are Associated with Mortality Risk in Hospitalized Patients. *Am. J. Med.* **2017**, *130*, 1465.e11–1465.e19. [CrossRef] [PubMed]
33. Eddington, H.; Heaf, J.G. Clinical Management of Disturbances of Calcium and Phosphate Metabolism in Dialysis Patients. *NDT Plus* **2009**, *2*, 267–272. [CrossRef]
34. Shah, A.; Aeddula, N.R. Renal Osteodystrophy. *StatPearls* **2022**, *45*, 180–186. [CrossRef]
35. Nitta, K.; Ogawa, T. Vascular Calcification in End-Stage Renal Disease Patients. *Contrib. Nephrol.* **2015**, *185*, 156–167. [CrossRef]
36. Carbonara, C.E.M.; Reis, L.M.D.; Quadros, K.R.d.S.; Roza, N.A.V.; Sano, R.; Carvalho, A.B.; Jorgetti, V.; Oliveira, R.B.d. Renal Osteodystrophy and Clinical Outcomes: Data from the Brazilian Registry of Bone Biopsies—REBRABO. *Braz. J. Nephrol.* **2020**, *42*, 138–146. [CrossRef]
37. Cheng, H.T.; Ho, M.C.; Hung, K.Y. Affective and Cognitive Rather than Somatic Symptoms of Depression Predict 3-Year Mortality in Patients on Chronic Hemodialysis. *Sci. Rep.* **2018**, *8*, 5868. [CrossRef]
38. Bogataj, Š.; Pajek, M.; Pajek, J.; Buturović Ponikvar, J.; Paravlic, A. Exercise-Based Interventions in Hemodialysis Patients: A Systematic Review with a Meta-Analysis of Randomized Controlled Trials. *J. Clin. Med.* **2020**, *9*, 43. [CrossRef]
39. Bogataj, Š.; Pajek, J.; Buturović Ponikvar, J.; Pajek, M. Functional Training Added to Intradialytic Cycling Lowers Low-Density Lipoprotein Cholesterol and Improves Dialysis Adequacy: A Randomized Controlled Trial. *BMC Nephrol.* **2020**, *21*, 352. [CrossRef]
40. Bogataj, Š.; Pajek, M.; Mesarič, K.K.; Kren, A.; Pajek, J. Twelve Weeks of Combined Physical and Cognitive Intradialytic Training Preserves Alertness and Improves Gait Speed: A Randomized Controlled Trial. *Aging Clin. Exp. Res.* **2023**, *35*, 2119–2126. [CrossRef]

Disclaimer/Publisher's Note: The statements, opinions and data contained in all publications are solely those of the individual author(s) and contributor(s) and not of MDPI and/or the editor(s). MDPI and/or the editor(s) disclaim responsibility for any injury to people or property resulting from any ideas, methods, instructions or products referred to in the content.

MDPI
St. Alban-Anlage 66
4052 Basel
Switzerland
www.mdpi.com

Journal of Clinical Medicine Editorial Office
E-mail: jcm@mdpi.com
www.mdpi.com/journal/jcm

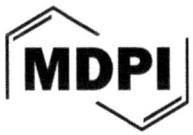

Disclaimer/Publisher's Note: The statements, opinions and data contained in all publications are solely those of the individual author(s) and contributor(s) and not of MDPI and/or the editor(s). MDPI and/or the editor(s) disclaim responsibility for any injury to people or property resulting from any ideas, methods, instructions or products referred to in the content.